ON DISEASES OF THE LIVER.

BY

GEORGE BUDD

GYAN

Published by

Gyan Publishing House
5, Ansari Road
Daryaganj, New Delhi-110002
Phone: 011-47034999, 9811692060
E-mail: books@gyanbooks.com

Distribution Network
gyanbooks.com
India, USA, Canada, UK, Australia, France

ISBN: 978-93-6280-279-8 (HB)

First Published, 1845

2nd Impression 2023

Printed at: Gyan Press, Delhi.

ON DISEASES OF THE LIVER
Author: GEORGE BUDD

ON

DISEASES OF THE LIVER.

By the same Author.

ON THE

ORGANIC DISEASES AND FUNCTIONAL DISORDERS

OF

THE STOMACH.

One Vol. Octavo.

ON

DISEASES OF THE LIVER.

BY

GEORGE BUDD, M. D., F. R. S.,

PROFESSOR OF MEDICINE IN KING'S COLLEGE, LONDON; LATE FELLOW OF CAIUS COLLEGE, CAMBRIDGE.

With Colored Plates and Wood-cuts.

THIRD AMERICAN,

FROM THE THIRD AND REVISED LONDON EDITION.

PHILADELPHIA:
BLANCHARD AND LEA.
1857.

AMERICAN PUBLISHERS' NOTICE.

THE present volume has been reprinted without alteration from the Third English Edition. As but few weeks have elapsed since its appearance in London under the careful revision of the author, it will doubtless be found fully brought to the present state of the subject, and entitled to the continued confidence of the profession, as the standard authority on this class of diseases.

PHILADELPHIA, *October*, 1857.

PREFACE TO THE FIRST EDITION.

THE materials of which the present volume is composed accumulated gradually during eight years in which I had been engaged in hospital practice. For the first three of those years, I was the visiting Physician to the Seamen's Hospital, Dreadnought, where my attention was especially called to diseases of the liver, which are there very frequent among men who have been much in India, and other hot climates.

The chapter on abscess of the liver formed the substance of the Gulstonian Lectures, which I had the honor to deliver at the College of Physicians, in 1842, and which were printed in the *Medical Gazette*.

In pursuing my investigations, I have had great help from my friend and former colleague, Mr. Busk, the accomplished surgeon of the Dreadnought, who was not only ever ready to give me his most valuable aid when we were acting together, but who has ever since continued to call my attention to all cases of special interest occurring in his practice. All who are versed in the recent progress of anatomy may form some judgment of the great value of Mr. Busk's assistance, in a scientific point of view, but only those who have the happiness to enjoy his friendship can appreciate the singular disinterestedness with which it was given.

I am also much indebted to my friend, Mr. Bowman, for microscopic specimens illustrating the structure of the liver, and for some interesting cases which he has placed at my disposal, as well as for the readiness with which he has on several occasions aided me by his intimate knowledge of structure.

To Dr. Inman, of Liverpool, and to Dr. James Russel, of Birmingham, my former pupils, I am likewise indebted for some valuable cases which they have been kind enough to send me.

This account of the opportunities I have had of studying the diseases of the liver, and of the great assistance I have derived from others, will, I fear, lead the reader to expect more information in the following pages than he will find. To prevent disappointment, it is right, therefore, that I should add, that while I was in office at the Dreadnought, many opportunities were turned to little profit, from the ignorance which then prevailed as to the real structure of the secreting element of the liver; and that, since, many have been quite lost from my time and attention having been absorbed in the business of teaching. It is hoped, however, that, with all its imperfections, of which no one can be more sensible than myself, the work will contribute to render the diagnosis of diseases of the liver more certain, and their treatment, therefore, more rational and satisfactory.

DOVER STREET, *June*, 1845.

In publishing the Second Edition of this work, I am desirous of expressing my obligations to Dr. L. S. Beale, for the readiness with which, on numerous occasions, he has made for me chemical analyses requiring much labor and skill.

March, 1852.

CONTENTS.

INTRODUCTION.

CHAPTER I.

ON CONGESTION OF THE LIVER.

CHAPTER II.

ON THE INFLAMMATORY DISEASES OF THE LIVER.

CHAPTER III.

ON DISEASES WHICH RESULT FROM FAULTY NUTRITION OF THE LIVER, OR FAULTY SECRETION.

CHAPTER IV.

ON DISEASES WHICH RESULT FROM SOME GROWTH FOREIGN TO THE NATURAL STRUCTURE.

CHAPTER V.

APPENDIX.

EXPLANATION OF THE PLATES.

PLATE I.—Gall-stones.

The drawings for these plates, with one exception, were taken from preparations in the museum of King's College, to which reference is made.

Fig. 1—Represents small, irregular gall-stones, composed of inspissated and altered bile, cemented by mucus. From a dry preparation (No. 263), which exhibits 279 gall-stones, all of this kind, in the bladder in which they were found. The bladder is enlarged, but its coats seem not to have been thickened.

Fig. 2—Represents a section of a large calculus, composed almost entirely of cholesterine. It existed alone in the gall-bladder, and weighed three drachms. (Prep. 264.)

Fig. 3—Sections of two gall-stones from the same bladder, composed chiefly of cholesterine, stained by the coloring matters of bile. There were three other gall-stones, precisely of the same kind, in the bladder. (Prep. 280.)

Fig. 4—Three calculi from the same bladder, two of them sawn through to show their structure. The bladder contained a great number of calculi (some have been lost, and thirty-two are still left in the preparation) of the same kind; all of them having a crust of pure cholesterine, and all those of which a section has been made having a hollow in the centre. (Prep. 284.)

PLATE II.—Gall-stones.

Fig. 1—Sections of two gall-stones of peculiar structure, from the gall-bladder of a woman who died in King's College Hospital, of cancer of the liver, at the age of 51. The bladder was somewhat contracted at its middle, so as to form two pouches in which the stones were contained, and its coats were much thickened. (Prep. 279.)

FIG. 2—Gall-bladder and cystic duct containing calculi. The calculi have all a crust of pure cholesterine. (Prep. 269.)

FIG. 3—Gall-bladder filled with calculi, which have all a crust of pure cholesterine. From a man, 64 years of age, who died in King's College Hospital, of softening of the brain. No disease of the liver was suspected. (Prep. 261.)

PLATE III.

FIG. 1—Represents small abscesses which formed in the liver in consequence of injury done to an hydatid cyst. See p. 109.

FIG. 2—Represents one of the encysted tumors of the liver described in page 421.

PLATE IV.

FIG. 1—Represents a portion of liver thickly studded with minute spots of melanotic cancer. From a preparation in King's College Museum. (Prep. 324.)

Plate 1

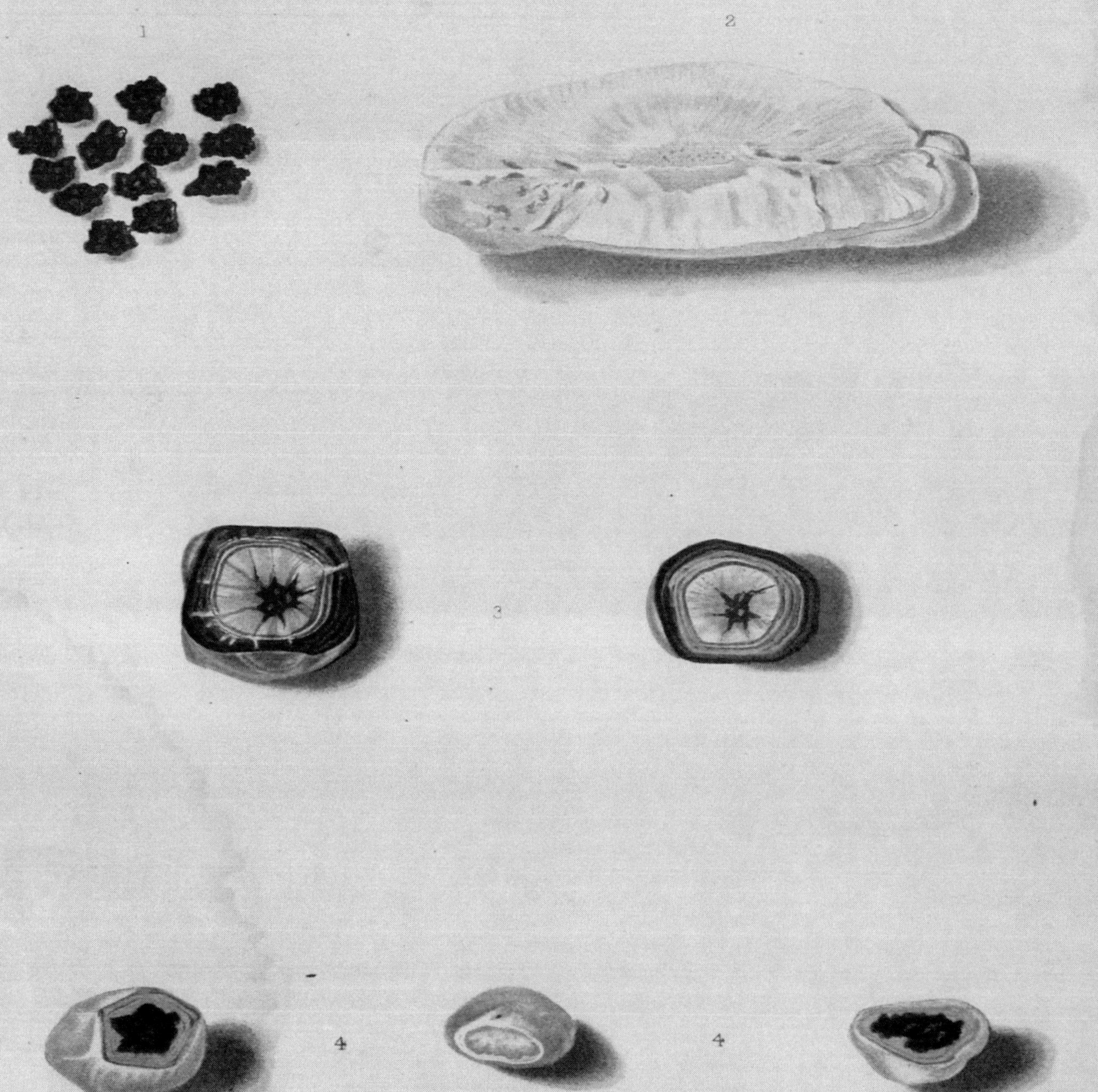

T.Sinclair's lith Phila.

Plate 2

1

2

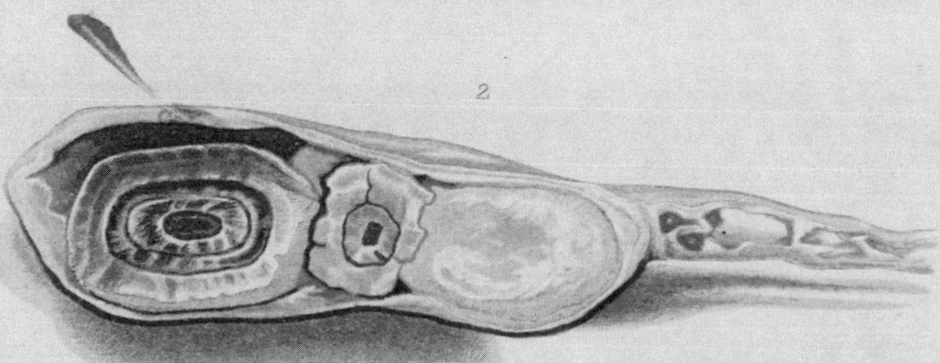

3

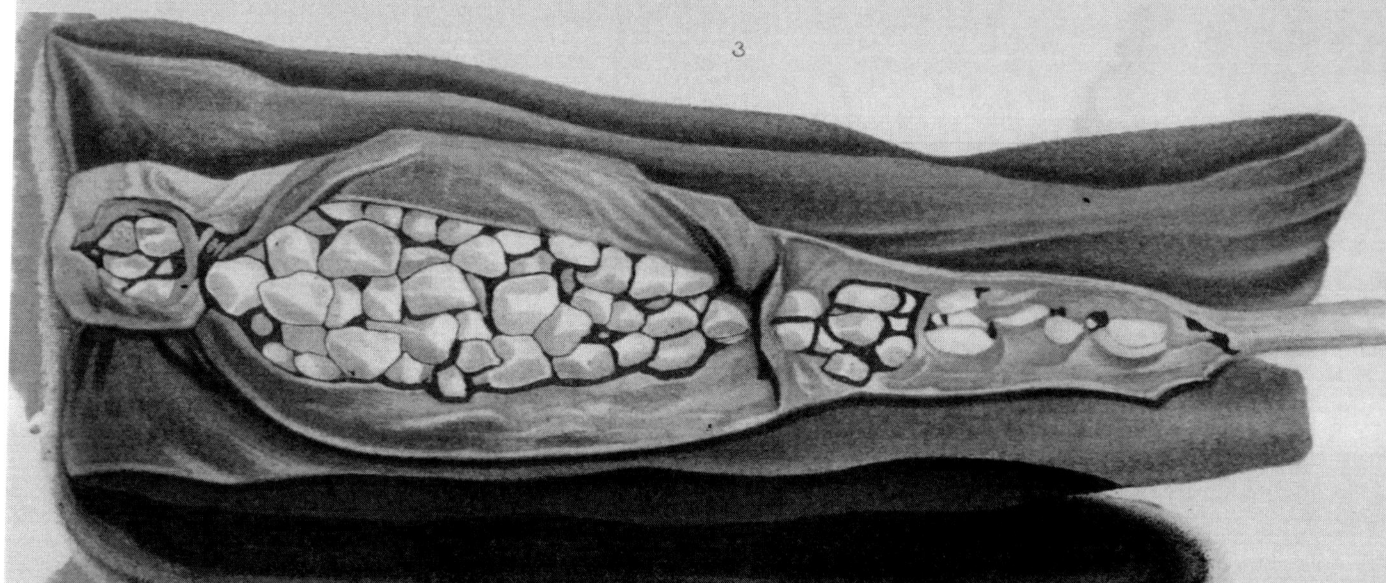

T. Sinclair's lith Phila.

Plate 3

1

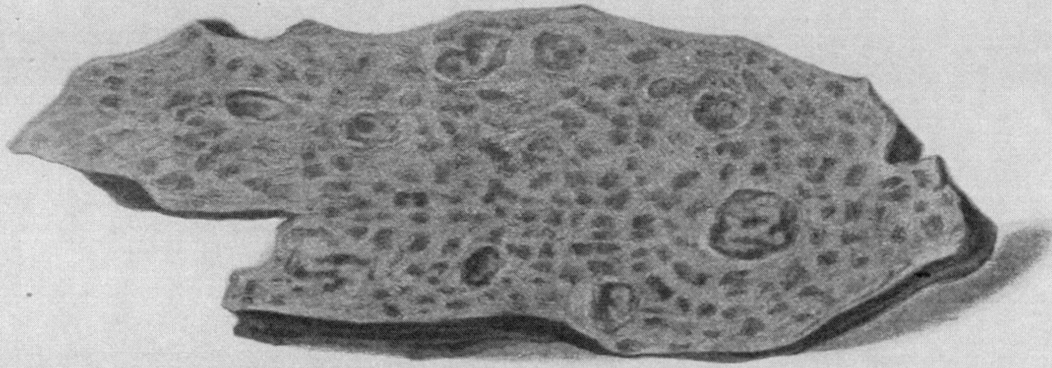

2

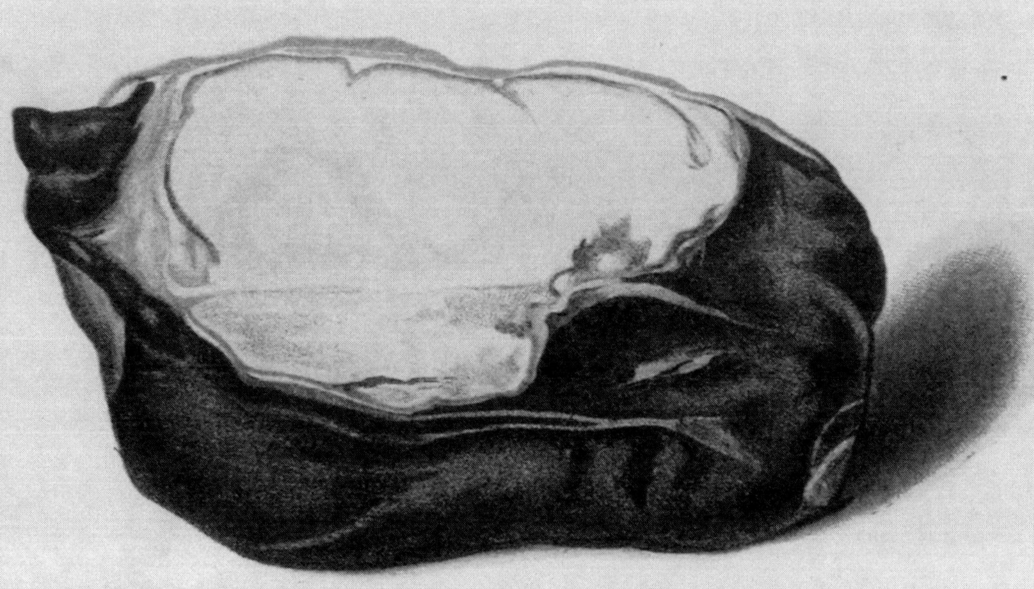

T Sinclair's lith Phila.

Plate 4

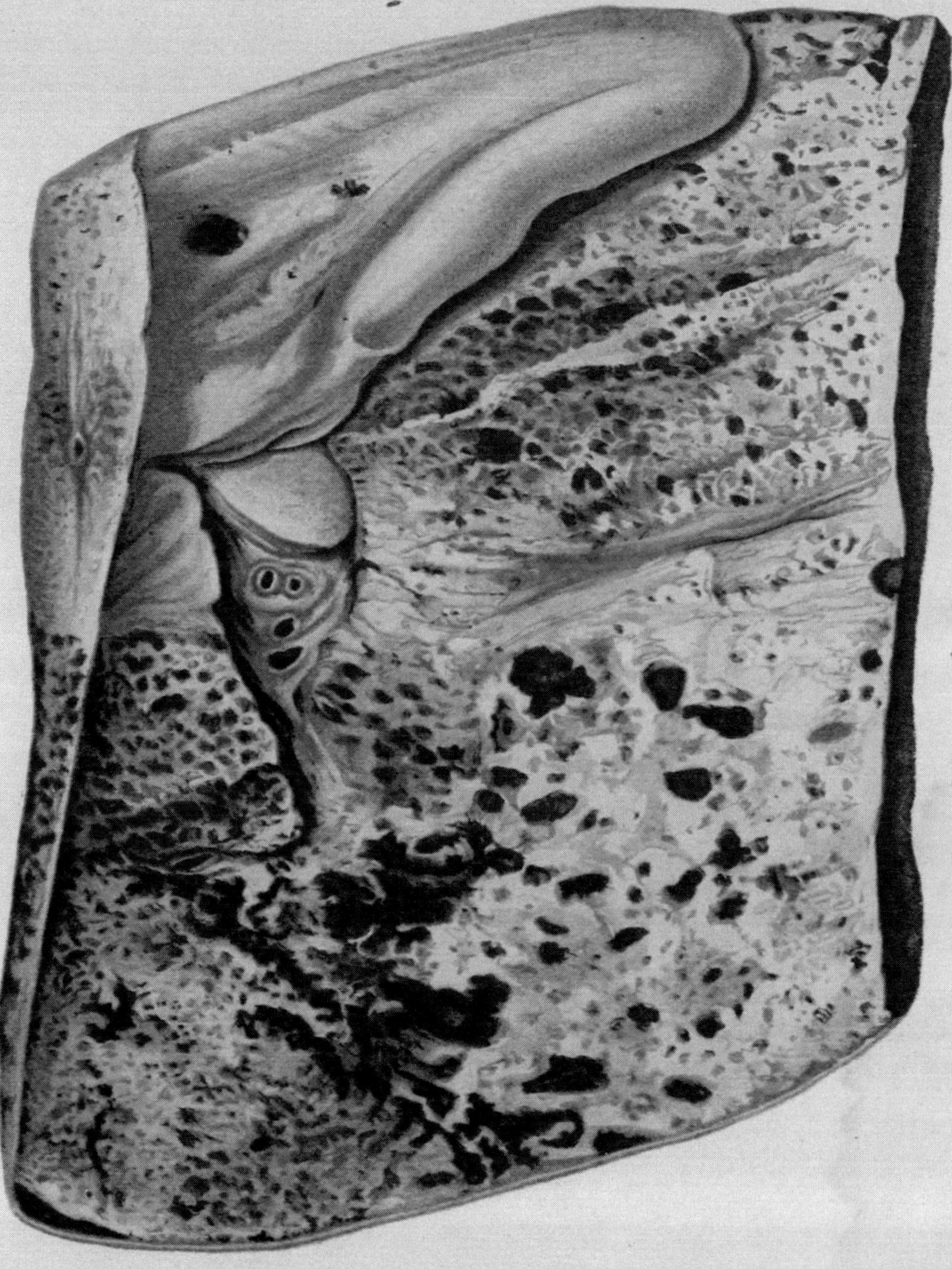

T Sinclairs lith Phila

ON

DISEASES OF THE LIVER.

INTRODUCTION.

Vagueness of our knowledge of Liver Diseases.—Structure of the Liver—Cause of the variations in its form, size, and color.—Physical qualities and composition of the bile.—Source and uses of the bile.—Cholagogue medicines.

In writing a book on Diseases of the Liver, I shall hardly be accused of having undertaken a needless task. There are no other diseases of such frequent occurrence which it is so difficult to discriminate, and for the treatment of which the medical practitioner has so few trustworthy guides. There is, again, no class of diseases at all equal to this in importance on which so few treatises have lately been written.

Diseases of the liver occupied a much larger space in the medical literature of former times than they do in that of our own. Before the functions of the liver had been much investigated, and before its intimate structure was known, physicians saw, in the large size of this organ, in its existence in animals differing widely in organization and habits, and in the obvious relation of its secretion to the process of digestion, sufficient evidence of its great importance in the animal economy, and of the serious evils that must result from derangement of its functions.

This evidence has been confirmed and extended by the more explicit results of modern inquiry. Guided by the comparatively recent discovery, that a gland may be regarded as being essentially a network of capillaries investing a secretory duct, anatomists have found a liver, in the form of cæcal tubes opening into the intestinal canal, in almost the lowest animals, and have thus furnished in its favor the surest testimony that can be given to the importance of any organ—namely, its all but universal presence in the animal kingdom.

The circumstance, then, that so few treatises on diseases of the liver have lately appeared, must be owing, not to their being considered less important, but to the unsatisfactory state of our knowledge respecting them. The precision lately given to our knowledge of many other diseases by the employment of new methods of investigation, has created a demand for more exact information on diseases of the liver than any one has possessed.

The unsatisfactory state of our knowledge of these diseases will scarcely be wondered at, if we reflect that many circumstances have conspired to render the study of them peculiarly difficult.

One of the most influential of these circumstances is, that, owing to the color and the close texture of the liver, it is difficult, with the imperfect means of research hitherto employed, to recognize and distinguish in the dead body the various effects of disease, unless it has gone on to disorganization or complete change of structure.

In an organ whose texture is spongy, as the lung, disease produces such striking changes, that we can at once distinguish their different forms, and thus learn to connect them with the symptoms observed during life; but in organs naturally solid, and also nearly of the color of blood, as the liver and the kidney, these changes, and especially the traces of the various kinds of congestion and inflammation, are far less obvious, and to detect and discriminate them requires a knowledge of intimate structure which has only lately been obtained, and, even with that knowledge, a very close and attentive inspection.

In the case of the kidney, the impediment which these conditions offer to the morbid anatomist is well illustrated by the fact, that a disease so common and so fatal as granular degeneration of this organ, and signalized during life by such marked symptoms as general dropsy and albuminous urine, has been left to immortalize, by its discovery, the name of a living physician; and that even now, notwithstanding the interest it has excited for seventeen years, and the attention given to it by the best anatomists of this and other countries, the real nature of the morbid change in which it essentially consists is a matter of doubt.[1]

Another circumstance unfavorable to the study of diseases of the liver is, that we can obtain but little direct evidence of its physical condition during life.

When the *lungs* are the seat of disease, we may discover, by the sense of hearing, whether any portion of them near the surface contain the natural quantity of air, or whether this, in whole or in part, be displaced by some denser matter; whether the surface of the pleura be roughened by fibrine, or its sac distended by fluid; whether the bronchial tubes be free, or more or less choked by secretions.

If the *heart* be the organ affected, we may not only trace its outline, and estimate the strength of its ventricles, but, by the same sense of hearing, we may penetrate its interior, and ascertain the condition of its valves. The whole physical structure of the organ is, as it were, laid open to us.

We have it in our power, indeed, to explore the liver by *touch*, and by *percussion*, but we cannot, by these means of investigation, penetrate its surface, and discover changes in its consistence and texture. They only enable us, in some cases, to trace its outline, to discover any striking inequalities of its surface, and to form a tolerable estimate of its bulk. This, indeed, is valuable information, and more than we can learn of the kidneys by similar means. But in investigating the diseases of the latter organs, we have the more than equivalent advantage that, day by day, we can measure the quantity, and ascertain the composition of the urine secreted; that is, we can tell precisely the manner in which their functions are performed.

The secretions of the liver, on the contrary, cannot be collected and analyzed during the life of the patient; indeed, until lately, they could scarcely be analyzed at all, as the most celebrated chemists were not even agreed as to what are the normal constituents of bile.

Thus, to detect and distinguish the diseases of the liver, practitioners had little more than the signs of functional disturbance—

[1] Since this was written, much has been done to elucidate the morbid changes in Bright's disease of the kidney; especially by Dr. George Johnson, whose admirable papers on this subject have been published in the *Medico-Chirurgical Transactions*.

signs, in all cases, of doubtful import, and here, if we except that of jaundice, more than commonly obscure and equivocal. We cannot, then, feel surprised that our knowledge of these diseases should be more imperfect, our diagnosis of them less sure, and our treatment, consequently, more tentative and empirical, than of the diseases of any other organ of equal importance.

Very recently, two of the impediments to the study of diseases of the liver have been in some degree removed. By the researches of chemists, we have obtained more precise knowledge of the composition and uses of bile; and by the labors of Kiernan and Bowman in this country, and of Müller and Henle in Germany, we have been taught the intimate structure of the organ; so that now, by the naked eye or the microscope, we can distinguish the various changes of its texture produced by disease.

It is impossible to explain or to understand the morbid appearances of the liver, without referring to its intimate structure, and as some points relating to this have been only lately made out, I shall commence with a short account of it.

Perhaps the best way to get an idea of the structure of the liver, is to examine under the microscope—

1st. A thin slice of liver in which the portal and hepatic veins are thoroughly injected.

2d. A small particle taken from the lobular substance of a fresh liver, in which the bloodvessels are empty, as in an animal killed by bleeding.

From the first specimen, we may learn the distribution of the minute portal and hepatic veins, and the intermediate capillaries. The annexed wood-cut (Fig. 1) has been made from a portion of the liver of a frog, which I selected from numerous specimens of injected liver made by Mr. Bowman. It represents, on a magnified scale, a small branch of the hepatic vein, two or three small branches of the portal vein, and the intermediate capillaries. It appears that the capillaries have nearly the same relation to the branches of the portal vein as they have to those of the hepatic vein. It is difficult, from this specimen, to tell which branch is portal, which hepatic; the smaller branches of both being, as it were, hairy with capillaries, springing directly from them on every side, and forming a close and continuous network.

If we imagine views similar to that in the wood-cut, made by

Fig. 1.

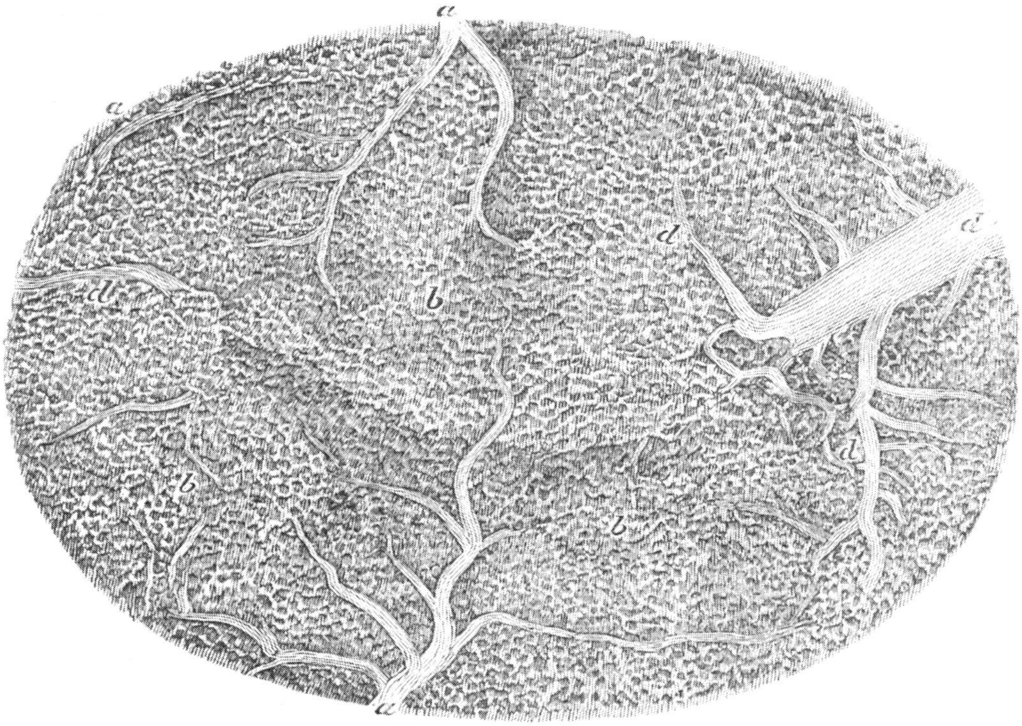

a a, twigs of the portal vein ; *d*, twig of the hepatic vein ; *b*, intermediate capillaries.

slicing the liver in various directions through the branch of the hepatic vein, or through one of the branches of the portal vein, there represented, we shall perceive that the entire organ, abstracting the canals in which the trunk and branches of those veins run, is occupied by a close network of capillary bloodvessels, continuous in every direction throughout its substance. The capillary vessels of this network are immediately concerned in secretion. The vessels of larger size serve merely to convey the blood to them, or carry it from them.

These capillaries are of comparatively large size, being always one-third wider than the diameter of the blood-globule, and sometimes nearly twice as wide, and their coats, which have no areolar tissue about them, appear very thin and delicate.[1]

But although the capillaries form a continuous network throughout the substance of the liver, no part of the portal blood traverses the entire network. The whole mass of capillaries is divided by the minute branches and twigs of the portal vein into small, tole-

[1] See an admirable article on Mucous Membrane, by Mr. Bowman, in Todd's *Cyclopædia of Anatomy and Physiology*, in which several points in the minute structure of the liver, noticed in this chapter, were first published.

rably defined masses; and is likewise partitioned in a similar way by the minute branches and twigs of the hepatic vein, which are intermediate to, or, as it were, dovetailed with, the branches and twigs of the portal vein. In effect of this, the blood conveyed through any branch of the portal vein to a small mass of capillaries, having performed its part in secretion, and been drained of the principles of bile, passes out of the liver through an intermediate or adjacent branch of the hepatic vein; so that the entire mass of capillaries is duly supplied with fresh portal, or biliary, blood.

In tracing even large branches of the portal and hepatic veins, it is seen that they generally run transversely, or that the directions of the two orders of vessels cross each other.

In consequence of this arrangement of the minute vessels, if we cut into a liver in which, as is usual after death, the branches and twigs of the hepatic vein and the capillaries immediately terminating in them are full of blood, while the branches and twigs of the portal vein and the capillaries immediately springing from them are empty, the cut surface will be mapped out into small, tolerably equal, and somewhat pentagonal spaces, having the outline, formed by the portal twigs, pale, and the centre, into which a twig of the hepatic vein enters, red. The small masses, of which these pentagonal spaces are sections, have been termed *lobules* of the liver. They have been described by Malpighi, Kiernan, Müller, and others, as isolated from each other, and each invested by a layer of areolar, or, as it used to be named, *cellular*, tissue. In the pig, in which the lobules of the liver were first noticed, and, according to Müller, in the polar bear, they are thus invested, but in man, as is clearly shown by the injected preparations of Mr. Bowman, and in most other animals, they are not distinct, isolated bodies, but merely small masses defined more or less distinctly by the ultimate twigs of the portal vein and the injected or uninjected capillaries immediately contiguous to them. The ultimate twigs of the vein are, as it were, hairy with capillaries, springing directly from them on every side, and forming a close and continuous network. The lobules appear distinct isolated bodies only when seen by too low a power clearly to distinguish the capillaries.

The real nature of the lobules, and the manner in which they are formed, will perhaps be better understood by reference to the annexed wood-cut (Fig. 2), for which I am indebted to the kindness of Mr. Bowman. It represents on a magnified scale six lobules of the liver, and was made from a drawing under the microscope of

Fig. 2.

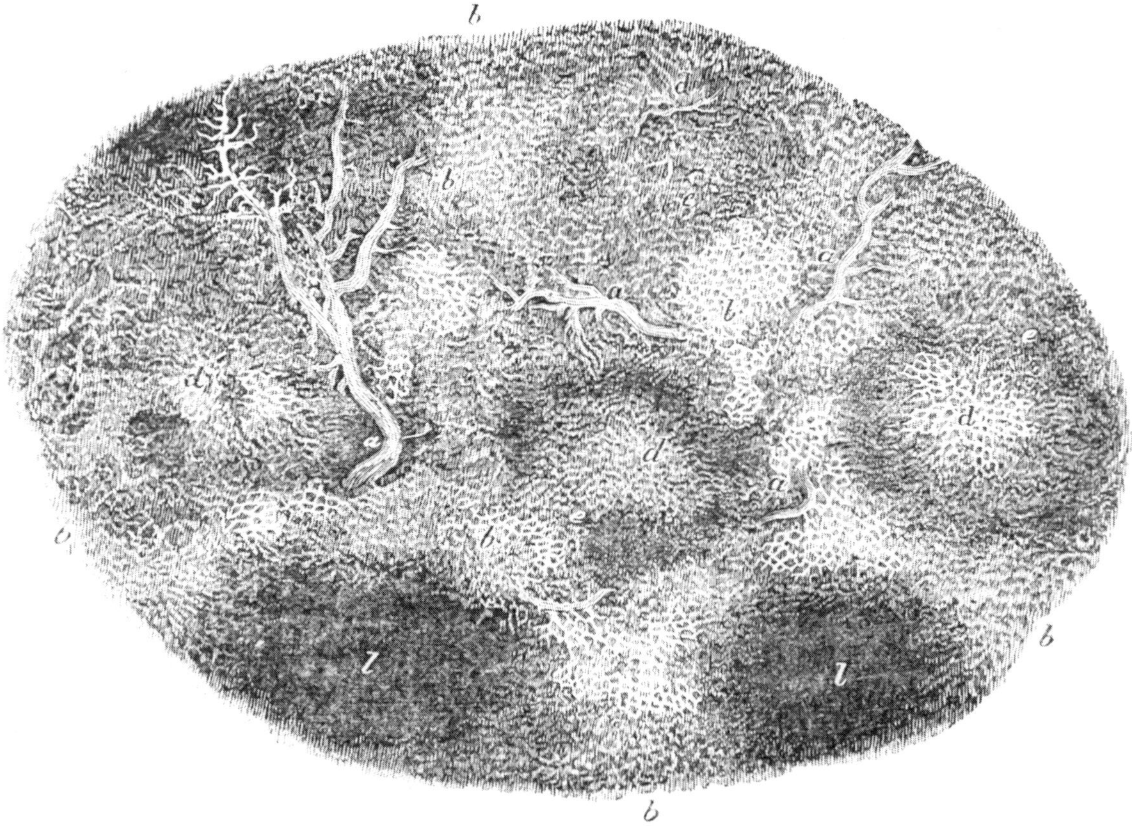

the section of the liver of a cat, partially injected through the portal vein, and also through the hepatic vein; *a a a*, represent minute twigs of the portal vein injected; *b b b*, capillaries, likewise injected, immediately springing from them, and serving with them to mark the outline of the lobules; *d d d*, capillaries in the centres of the lobules, injected through the hepatic vein; *e e*, places at which the size injected into the portal vein has met that injected into the hepatic vein, so that all the intermediate capillaries are colored and conspicuous; *l l*, centres of lobules into which the injection has not passed through the hepatic vein.

It has been stated that the capillaries have nearly the same relation to the small branches and twigs of the hepatic vein as they have to those of the portal vein. This statement requires some qualification. The branches of the portal vein are each accompanied to their smallest twigs by a branch of the hepatic artery, and by a branch of the hepatic duct. Frequently, with a branch of the vein there are two branches of the artery and two branches of the duct. These vessels, which are very much smaller than the corresponding portal vein, run up (as seen in Fig. 3[1]) on one side of it, and of course on that side the capillaries do not spring so immediately from the venous trunk; in other words, the lobules are not in such immediate contact with the vein as on other sides. The capillaries terminate in twigs which go to the vein through the space which the presence of the artery and duct necessarily interposes between the lobules and the vein.

With the artery and duct in the portal canals there is also some areolar tissue, which surrounds these vessels, and is continued in a

Fig. 3.

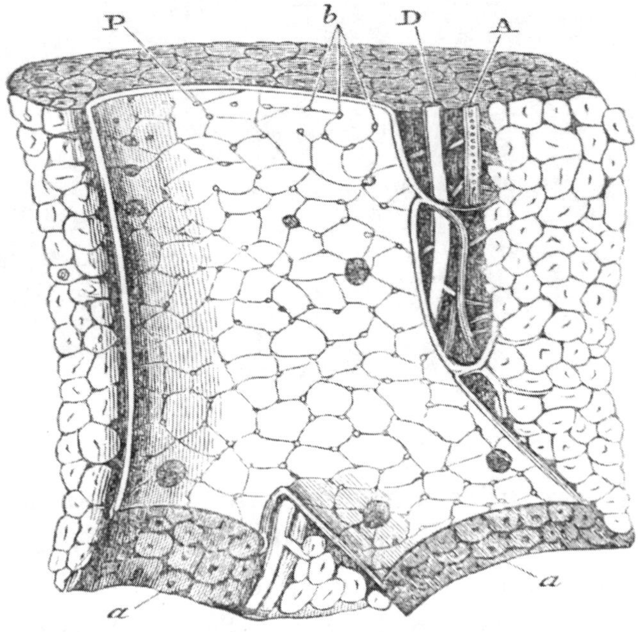

Longitudinal section of a small portal vein and canal. P, the portal vein; A D, the accompanying artery and duct; *a a*, portions of the canal from which the vein has been removed; *b*, orifices of ultimate twigs of the vein springing immediately from it.

thin layer round the branches of the portal vein itself. This layer separates by a small space the lobules from the branches of the vein, and makes the coats of the latter appear thicker than those of the hepatic veins, and their outline more distinct; and also allows them to collapse when empty.

[1] This diagram and the two following are copied from the admirable paper on the Liver in the *Transactions of the Royal Society* for 1833, by Mr. Kiernan, to whom we are in great part indebted for the exact knowledge we now have of the distribution of bloodvessels in the liver, and of many other points of its structure.

The hepatic veins are not accompanied by any other vessels, and are not surrounded by areolar tissue. They are, in consequence, everywhere in immediate contact with lobules, and do not collapse when cut across. In the small branches, the coats are thin and transparent, and capillaries, or the ultimate twigs formed from the capillaries, enter them directly on every side. In the larger branches, the coats are thicker and opaque, and the ultimate twigs unite to form larger twigs before they enter the vein. This is shown in Fig. 4, copied on a smaller scale from a diagram by Mr. Kiernan. The trunks and large branches of the hepatic vein, like the iliacs and the inferior vena cava, contain longitudinal (muscular) fibres.

Fig. 4.

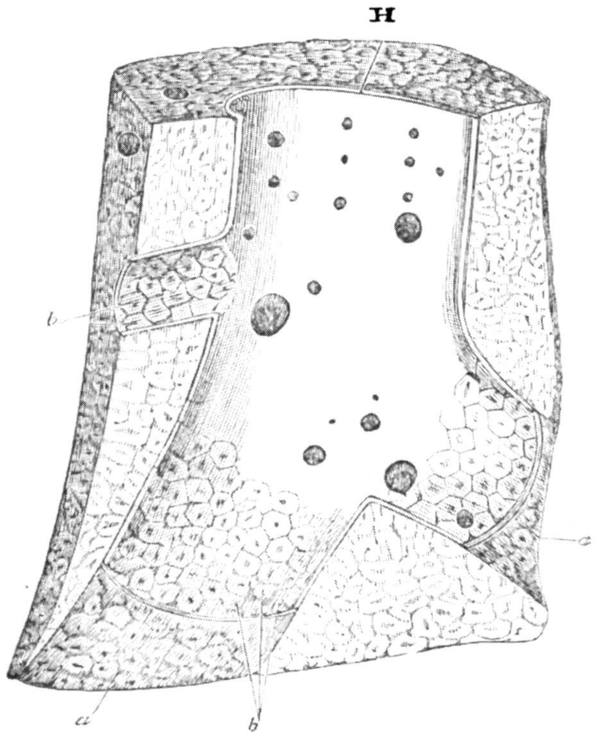

H, longitudinal section of an hepatic vein; *a a*, portions of the canal, from which the vein has been removed; *b b*, orifices of ultimate twigs of the vein, formed by the capillaries of single lobules.

To complete our view of the bloodvessels of the liver, we must now consider the hepatic artery.

We have already seen that a branch of the artery accompanies each branch of the portal vein and hepatic duct. It has been shown by Mr. Kiernan, that the hepatic artery is distributed to, and nourishes, the coats of the gall-bladder and gall-ducts, the ligaments of the liver, its capsule, and the coats of the portal and hepatic veins; and that the blood conveyed to all these parts by the artery passes into veins which terminate in branches of the portal vein, and thus traverses the capillary plexus of the lobules, like blood returned from the other abdominal viscera.[1] These veins, which originate in the liver, and feed the portal vein with the blood brought by the hepatic artery, constitute what Mr. Kiernan has called the *hepatic* origin of the portal vein. No arteries enter the lobules of the liver.

The blood brought by the hepatic artery is distributed chiefly to the ducts. Mr. Kiernan remarked that "when the arteries are well injected, the larger ducts, from the extreme vascularity of their coats, may be mistaken for injected arteries, whilst in the coats of the vein, no vessels will be detected without the aid of the magnifying glass." The blood of the hepatic artery not only nourishes the coats of the excretory portion of the ducts, but furnishes the materials of their proper secretion.

Fig. 5.

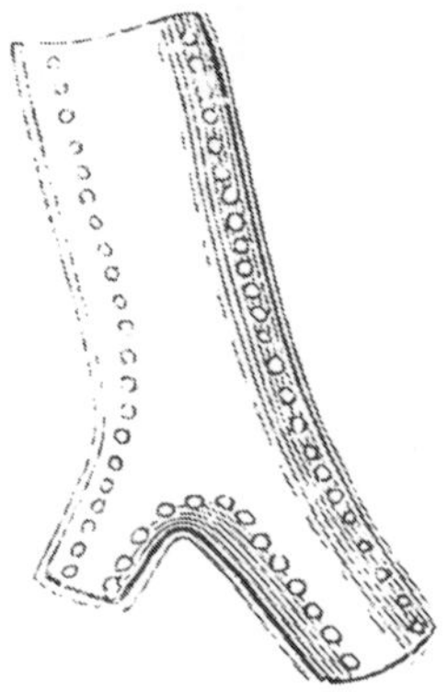

Diagram representing the arrangement of the follicles in a small gall-duct.

The ducts, as we have seen, accompany the portal veins, and their ramifications, like those of the veins, can be traced to the lobules of the liver. The finest *interlobular* branches of the ducts are very small, being, according to Dr. Beale, only $\frac{1}{3000}$ of an inch in diameter, and consist of a simple tubular membrane lined by a delicate epithelium. The large ducts have a complex structure, leading to the inference that they must have some important function besides serving as channels for the bile. Their coats are thick, and their inner surface presents a great number of small cavities or follicles, which, except in the largest ducts, where they are distributed irregularly, are arranged in two lines on opposite sides of the canal. The large ducts are, besides, connected by numerous tortuous branches—the *vasa aberrantia*—which have likewise follicles in their walls, and which anastomose so as to form a network not immediately connected with the lobular structure.[2]

[1] It appears from specimens injected by Mr. Bowman, that some of the arterial capillaries of the capsule return their blood, not into a branch of the portal vein, but immediately into the adjacent capillary plexus of that vein.

[2] For further particulars regarding the structure and arrangement of the ducts, and other points in the minute anatomy of the liver, the reader is referred to an

Having obtained a conception of the distribution of vessels in the liver, we may next consider the other elements of its structure.

This is, perhaps, best done by examining under the microscope a small particle taken from the lobular substance of a fresh liver, empty of blood and uninjected.

In such a specimen there is seen under the microscope a mass of nucleated cells, with here and there a fibre from one of the torn vessels. When the animal died fasting no other objects are visible, but when it was killed while digestion was going on, and in a state of health, the cells are surrounded by fine granular matter, having an active molecular (Brownian) movement.[1]

Fig. 6.

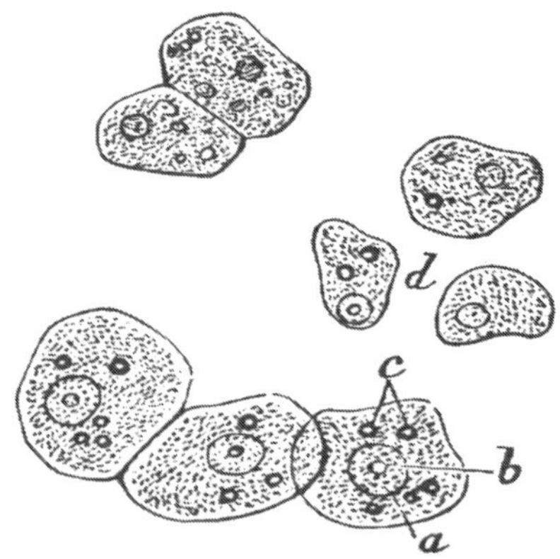

Nucleated cells of the liver. *a*, the nucleus; *b*, the nucleolus; *c*, fat-globules; *d*, cells of small size, detached.

The cells are flattened, irregular in form, but somewhat spheroidal, and have each a nucleus, which again contains a central pellucid spot, the nucleolus. They are of various sizes. The largest are usually about the one-thousandth of an inch in diameter; others are very much smaller, as if not yet fully developed. In some livers the cells, generally, are smaller than in others.

The cells contain oil-globules and amorphous granular matter. Their color and transparency depend on the color and quantity of the matter they contain, which vary very much in different cases, partly according to the nature of the food and the time, with reference to the digestive process, when death occurred. They are usually of a light brown, and almost transparent, but in some subjects we find them yellowish and opaque.

If, while looking at this mass of nucleated cells, we imagine the delicate and now invisible capillaries to be filled with blood or colored size, and thus rendered conspicuous, we shall perceive that the whole liver, excluding the canals in which the portal and hepatic veins run, is a solid plexus of capillary bloodvessels, the meshes of which are filled with nucleated cells.

elaborate paper by Dr. Beale, published in the *Phil. Transactions* for 1856, and entitled "On the Minute Arrangement of the Biliary Ducts, and on some other points in the Anatomy of the Liver of Vertebrate Animals."

[1] Bernard, Leçons de Physiologie Experimentale, p. 162, 1855.

These spheroidal cells are not, however, the only nucleated cells found in the liver.

Fig. 7.

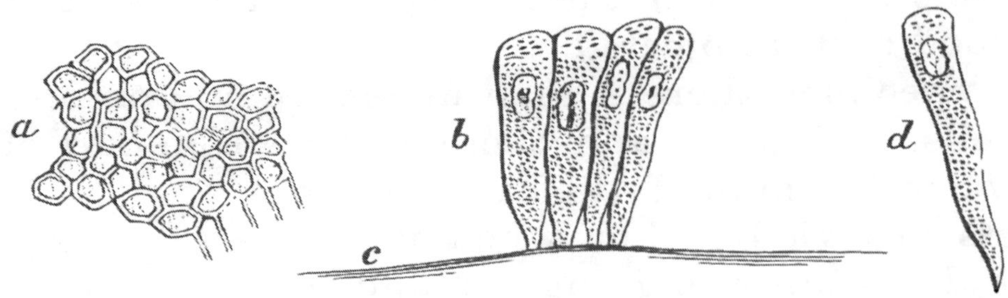

Nucleated cells of the gall-bladder, as seen under a high power. *a*, pavement formed by the union and apposition of the cells; *b*, side view of four cells; *c*, the basement membrane; *d*, a detached cell.

The mucous membrane of the gall-bladder and gall-ducts, like the excreting ducts of other glands, in fact, like all mucous membranes, is composed, as Mr. Bowman has shown, of an extremely thin, transparent membrane, without pores or visible structure, whose external or secreting surface is coated with nucleated cells. These cells, by their apposition and union, form a kind of pavement on the transparent membrane, which, serving as their basis of support, has for this reason been named by Mr. Bowman the *basement*-membrane. The bloodvessels, lymphatics, and nerves ramify on the opposite, deep, or inner surface of the basement membrane.[1]

But although mucous membranes are alike in structure, being all composed of a basement membrane, *paved*, if we may so express it, with nucleated cells, yet the cells differ much in form and appearance in different situations.

In the convoluted, or secreting tubules of the human kidney, the cells, like those of the lobules of the liver, are spheroidal. In the gall-bladder and large gall-ducts, as on the villi of the small intestine, the cells have the form of prisms.

If the gall-bladder be slightly bruised, a portion of the bile taken from it exhibits under the microscope hundreds of these prismatic cells, and the opaque mucus sometimes found in an inflamed gall-duct is almost made up of similar cells. In the smaller ducts the cells are shorter and smaller, and in the finest interlobular branches

[1] For ample details on this point I may refer the reader to the article Mucous Membrane, in *Todd's Cyclopædia*.

they are flattened and very small, forming a delicate tessellated epithelium, and presenting a striking contrast to the much larger cells in the lobular substance.[1]

The researches of Purkinje, Henle, Bowman, and Goodsir, leave no doubt that the nucleated cells are the immediate agents of secretion.

It is not in the liver only that the cells perform this office, for it seems established as a general law, that all true secretion, whether in animals or in plants, is effected by the agency of cells; that, "however complex the structure of the secreting organ, these nucleated cells are its really operative part." In each secreting organ, the secreting cells have a peculiar power to form, or to withdraw from the blood, the secretion proper to the part.

In such of the glands of animals as have excreting ducts, the nucleated cells withdraw from the blood the peculiar principles of the secretions, which they elaborate more or less, and then, in one way or another, whether by bursting, or dissolving, or by some unknown mode, discharge through the excreting ducts.[2] The cells in the lobular substance of the liver sometimes undergo very striking changes from the exercise of this secreting function.

On examining these cells of the liver under the microscope, it is seen that most of them inclose small spheroidal globules, which are recognized by their dark outline, or high refractive power, to be globules of oil or fat.

In ordinary livers these oil or fat globules are small, and few in number; but in the fatty condition of the liver so often found in persons dead of phthisis, and in that induced by keeping animals exclusively on fatty substances, they are so large and numerous as to distend the cells to double their natural size, and consequently to cause a great increase in the volume of the liver.[3] The cells at

[1] See the paper by Dr. Beale, before referred to.

[2] It appears that cells are not only the immediate agents of secretion, but that they are concerned in all active vital operations. It has been proved by the researches of Schwann and others, that all tissues possessing distinctly vital endowments originate, directly or indirectly, in the transformation of cells; and it has been further stated by Dr. Carpenter, "that *all the most active vital operations* in the animal, as in the vegetable organism, *are performed by tissues which retain their original cellular constitution with little or no change.*" See a paper by Dr. Carpenter, On the Mutual Relations of the Vital and Physical Forces, in the *Phil. Trans.* for 1850, part ii.

[3] See Lancet, January, 1842.

the circumference of the lobule usually contain a larger amount of oil than the cells near its centre.

Fig. 8.

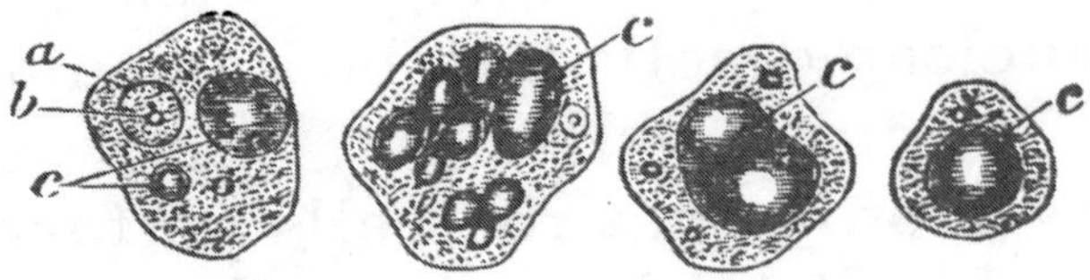

Nucleated cells, from a liver in a state of fatty degeneration. *a*, nucleus ; *b*, nucleolus ; *c c c c*, fatty globules. (*Bowman.*)

From the high refracting power of oil-globules, ocular proof is thus afforded that fatty matters taken into the system in too great quantity pass from the blood into the nucleated cells in the lobules of the liver. There can be no doubt that after undergoing more or less change, they pass in some way or other from these cells into the excreting ducts.

Again, the cells, instead of having their usual light brown tint, are sometimes deeply stained by the biliary pigment. In cells taken from the roundish yellow masses in cirrhosis, or from any portion of a liver that has a well marked yellow or green tint, yellow or green particles can be seen, having, under the microscope, exactly the same appearance as the precipitated coloring matter of the bile. The usual light brown color of the cells is most probably due to the biliary pigment. Mr. Goodsir has given a long list of animals in which he observed in the cells of the liver, or of cæcal tubes supplying the place of a liver, matter of an amber tint, or of various shades of brown, according to the animal examined, but in each having nearly the color of the bile. It is, therefore, most probable that the coloring matter of the bile is formed or withdrawn from the blood by the cells in the lobular substance, and that in some way or other it passes from these into the excreting ducts.

It has long been a subject of discussion, how the bile, supposed to be secreted in the lobules, passes into the ducts—in other words, how the ducts terminate on reaching the lobules? Mr. Kiernan inferred that the duct is continued for some distance into the lobule, forming there a plexus which interlaces with the plexus of capillary bloodvessels, and, in the paper which has been so often referred to, has given a figure representing this arrangement. But he meant the figure to be a diagram only; and confesses that he failed to obtain such a view of the ducts as is there represented. He was led to believe that the ducts terminate in this way, partly by the appearances presented by specimens in which the ducts had been well injected, and partly from observing that the ducts discovered by Ferrein in the left lateral ligament (which Mr. Kiernan regards as a *rudimental* liver where the elements of the organ are unravelled), divide, subdivide, and at length terminate in plexuses of minute ducts, having bloodvessels ramifying on their outer surface.

Dr. Handfield Jones and other observers have believed that the ducts terminate in blind extremities on reaching the lobule, instead of forming a plexus within it, and that the chief agents in the secretion of bile are the cells lining these ducts, and not the cells in the lobular substance.

The latest researches on this point are those of Dr. Beale, and they have convinced him that the inference of Mr. Kiernan is correct. By pouring a continuous stream of water into the portal vein, he not only succeeded in emptying the liver of blood, but a portion of the water returned by the ducts, and almost entirely emptied them of bile. In a liver thus prepared, after allowing the water to drain off, he injected, in succession, the hepatic duct and the portal vein by differently colored fluids, and thus obtained specimens in which some of the lobules were to a certain extent injected from the duct as well as from the vein. In these specimens, he says, in some situations, the cell-containing network in the lobules is seen to have a limitary membrane distinct from the walls of the capillary bloodvessels, but in the greater part of the lobule, where the two membranes come into close contact, they are incorporated, so that really the majority of the cells in the lobules, except where they are in contact with each other, are only separated from the blood in the vessels by one thin layer of delicate, structureless membrane. From these and other observations, Dr. Beale is led to the inference that the lobule is originally composed of two distinct interlacing networks—one containing the secreting cells, the other the blood—as Kiernan supposed; but that the walls of these two sets of tubes gradually become incorporated, except in those situations where the capillary network is less dense, or where the meshes of the cell-containing network are more widely separated from each other, in which situations the tubes containing the liver-cells have permanently a limitary membrane distinct from the wall of the capillary bloodvessels.

If the duct be continuous with the network within the lobule the tube widens, and its function must change, when it begins to form the lobular network, for the duct where it reaches the lobule is much narrower than the cell-containing network within the lobule, and contains cells several times smaller and of a different kind.

We have already alluded to the areolar tissue of the liver. This tissue, which serves to protect the essential elements of the organ is, in man, spread in a dense layer over its surface, forming the proper capsule of the liver, and is continued into its interior in the portal canals. It is in greatest quantity on that side of the portal vein on which the duct and artery run, but a thin layer of it completely invests the branches—at least all the considerable branches—of the vein. It gradually diminishes in amount as the vessels get smaller, and cannot be traced into the capillary network.

To make up the rest of the organ there remain the lymphatic vessels and the nerves.

The liver is very richly furnished with lymphatic vessels, some of which are of large size.

The superficial lymphatics ramify in the proper capsule of the liver. Mr. Kiernan states that after injecting these vessels in the human liver, the peritoneal coat may be removed without injuring them; or the peritoneal coat may be first removed, and the absorbents afterwards injected.

They are spread over the whole surface of the liver, forming a close network. Those on the convex surface unite to form branches, some of which pass through the diaphragm to lymphatic glands in the posterior or anterior mediastinum; while others (chiefly those of the left lobe) run to the glands about the cardiac orifice of the stomach and the adjacent portion of the vena cava. The lymphatics on the concave surface of the liver also take different courses: those on the right lobe run chiefly to glands between the vena cava and aorta, just above the origin of the inferior mesenteric artery; those on the left lobe, to the glands situated along the lesser curve of the stomach.

The deep-seated lymphatics of the liver ramify in the portal canals, beyond which they have not been traced. No vessels of this kind accompany the hepatic veins. They seem to be very closely connected with the ducts. If the ducts be injected, bile and the matter of injection are frequently forced into the lymphatics. About the gall-bladder, too, the lymphatic vessels are very numerous and large.

The lymphatics of the gall-bladder pass to glands adjacent to the duodenum and pancreas; those from the interior of the liver run some of them to these glands, others to glands situated on the lesser curve of the stomach, near the cardiac orifice.[1]

The nerves (derived from the hepatic plexus) enter the liver at the transverse fissure, and run in the areolar tissue in the portal canals. According to Dr. Handfield Jones, nervous threads, which have the usual character of organic nerves, consisting almost wholly of "gelatinous" fibres, are spread in great number over the branches of the portal vein and of the hepatic artery. The larger threads, most of which are parallel to the vessels, continually divide and unite with other threads, so as to form a plexus with elongated meshes. The gall-ducts and the branches of the hepatic vein are also supplied, but very much more sparingly, with nerves of the same kind.

The liver also receives some nervous filaments, which come directly from the phrenic nerve, and are distributed to the coats of the hepatic veins. It is conjectured by M. Bernard that these filaments from the phrenic nerve govern the contraction of the longitudinal fibres which the coats of the hepatic veins contain.

No nervous filaments have been traced into the lobules of the liver.[2]

A knowledge of the structure of the liver enables us to explain the variations so often met with in its size, form, and texture, as well as the various shades of color of which it is susceptible, and which have so taxed the descriptive powers of morbid anatomists.

The mass of the liver is, as we have seen, made up of a plexus of capillary bloodvessels, the meshes of which are filled with nucleated cells containing the peculiar principles of the biliary secretion.

[1] Beautiful plates, showing the course of the lymphatics of the liver, may be seen in Mascagni's work on the lymphatic vessels. "Vasorum Lymphaticorum Historia et Iconographia," 1787.

[2] Medical Gazette, July 14, 1848.

The *size* of the liver will, of course, vary in some measure with the degree of congestion; that is, with the quantity of blood in the capillary bloodvessels; but it depends much more on the number and volume of the cells. If, as in fatty degeneration of the liver, the cells are distended with oil-globules, the lobules are large and unusually distinct, the edges of the liver are rounded, and the liver is much increased in size, and thickened. If, on the contrary, the cells be few and small, the lobules will be small, and the lobular structure distinguished with difficulty, unless different portions of the lobules be differently colored by partial injection of the capillaries; and the whole liver will be small and thin, or, as it were, flattened.

The size of the liver may also be increased by the interstitial deposits of the various products of inflammation; by dilatation of the ducts; and by the growth of cancerous or other tumors. But independently of conditions affecting its structure, the liver may be much altered in form by external pressure. By tight lacing, for instance, the length of the liver from above downwards is often much increased, and its lower portion flattened. The portion of liver above an aneurismal tumor may also be very much flattened, without any marked change of structure. Flatulent distension of the large intestine, even, if long continued, may much alter its outward form.[1]

The *firmness* of the liver varies, not only with the firmness of the capillary vessels, the quantity of blood they contain, and the proportion of fibrin in the blood, but also in some measure with the state of the cells. A large quantity of oil in the cells tends to render the liver unusually soft.

The liver is, however, liable to be much changed in texture by other conditions. It is sometimes extremely soft and frangible, in consequence of chemical changes that there is reason to believe may take place after death; and, in spirit-drinkers, it is often rendered hard, and tough, and granular, by the contraction and induration

[1] A short time ago, I met with a remarkable instance of this in a man who died, after having been paraplegic many months, in consequence of disease of the dorsal vertebræ. The large intestine, which had been greatly distended with gas from the commencement of the paraplegia, was found of very large size, and lodged in a deep groove which it had formed in the liver. A cast of the liver was taken, which is now in the museum of King's College.

of coagulable lymph, deposited, in consequence of inflammation, in the areolar tissue in the portal canals.

The *color* of the liver depends on the quantity of blood in the capillary vessels, and on the quantity of oil, and of biliary coloring matter, in the cells.

The tint due to the blood varies from pale to a deep venous red, according to the empty or congested state of the capillaries; that due to the cells from a light fawn to a deep olive, according to the quantity of oil-globules and of biliary coloring matter they contain. The actual tint of the liver is the combined effect of the tints due to the vessels and the cells, respectively.

In persons who have died of hemorrhage from the stomach or intestines, or of chronic dysentery, or in great general anæmia, as in the advanced stage of granular kidney, the liver is always found very anæmic, and its color depends almost entirely on the state of the cells. In portions of liver of an orange or green tint, the coloring matter on which this tint depends may always be seen in the cells.

It very commonly happens that the capillaries are only partially injected after death, and that the liver, in consequence, presents two colors—a yellowish color, and a red; the former belonging to the uninjected portion, the latter to the injected portion, of each lobule. This gave rise to the notion, which, until the researches of Mr. Kiernan, was held by all anatomists, that there are two substances in the liver—a yellow substance, and a red; which were supposed to constitute, respectively, the medullary and the cortical part of each lobule.

It was Mr. Kiernan who first showed conclusively that the mottled appearance so frequently observed in the liver is owing to part only of its bloodvessels being full of blood; and that in the great majority of cases in which it exists, the hepatic veins and the capillaries that terminate in them are the full vessels; the portal veins and the capillaries that spring from them, the empty ones.

When the twigs of the hepatic vein and the capillaries that terminate in them are filled with blood, while the portal twigs and the capillaries that immediately spring from them are empty, the central portions of the lobules, where the vessels are full, form isolated red spots, while the margins of the lobules, where the vessels are empty, have a color which varies from yellowish white to greenish, according to the quantity of oil-globules and of coloring matter which the cells contain.

This appearance is represented in Fig. 9.

Fig. 9.

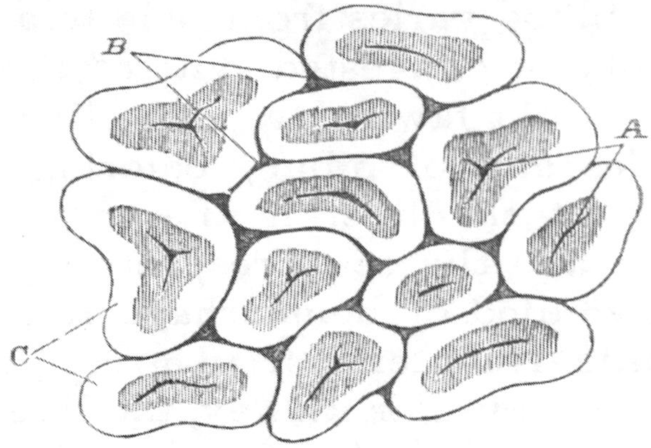

Rounded lobules on the surface of the liver. A, centre of the lobules, red from congestion of the hepatic twigs and adjacent capillaries; C, margins of the lobules, pale, from the capillaries being there empty; B, spaces between the lobules, occupied by twigs of the portal vein. (Diagram after *Kiernan*.)

When more of the vessels forming the capillary network are filled, the appearances are somewhat different. As the injection extends backwards from the hepatic to the portal twigs, it passes, as before remarked, from lobule to lobule at those points where adjacent lobules are connected by their capillaries; and when the injection has nearly, but not quite, reached those twigs of the portal vein that go to define the lobules, all the capillaries of the lobules will be full, except those immediately surrounding the portal twigs. A section of the liver will still present a mottled appearance, but now the pale portions will be in spots, where the uninjected twigs of the portal vein are divided, and the red portion will form a band continuous throughout the liver. (Fig. 10.)

When the entire capillary network is filled, the whole liver is red, but, as was observed by Mr. Kiernan, the central portions of the lobules are still usually of a deeper red than the marginal portions.

It appears, then, that after death the blood in the liver tends to collect especially in the central portions of the lobules. An opinion has been expressed by Mr. Bowman, that this circumstance is owing to the capillaries in the marginal portions of the lobules being subject to greater pressure, in consequence of the cells being there often more distended with oil and larger.

Fig. 10.

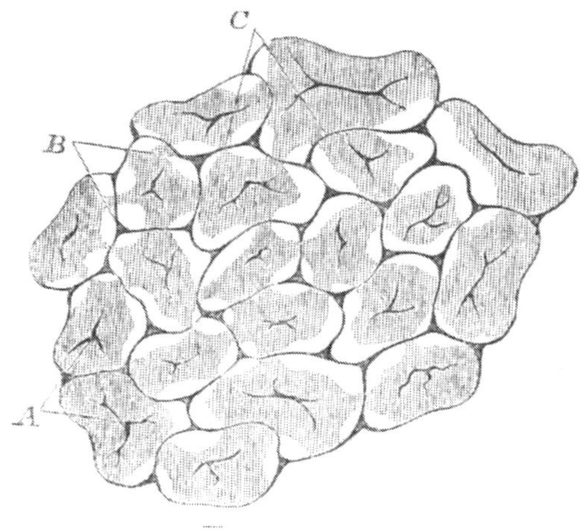

Lobules on the surface of the liver. A, centres of the lobules, red from congestion of the hepatic twigs and adjacent capillaries; C, places where capillaries uniting contiguous lobules are congested; B, pale spots, where the capillaries springing from the portal twigs are uninjected. (Diagram after *Kiernan*.)

Many circumstances, to be noticed in the following pages, leave little doubt that this opinion is true.

When, for example, the liver is in a state of fatty degeneration, and the cells in the lobules are everywhere gorged with oil, and also in what has been termed the scrofulous enlargement of the liver, where the lobules are enlarged by the infiltration of some morbid deposit, the capillaries of the lobules are usually empty throughout, and the entire substance of the liver is, in consequence, unusually pale.

Again, when, from the retention of biliary matter, the cells in the marginal portions have a yellow tinge, it often happens that while the centres of the lobules are deeply injected, and are consequently of a deep red, the marginal portions, or parts of them, are quite empty of blood, and have the yellow color that is due to the cells only. A section of the liver presents, in consequence, that striking contrast of colors which suggested the term "nutmeg" liver.

It occasionally happens, however, that the portal veins, and the capillaries immediately springing from them, are found alone injected. The margins of the lobules, and the interlobular spaces, are then red, forming a continuous red band, while the centres of the lobules appear as isolated pale spots. (Fig. 11.)

From the pale, uninjected portion being in isolated spots, this condition looks very like that represented in Fig. 10. It was remarked, however, by Mr. Kiernan, that the injected substance

Fig. 11.

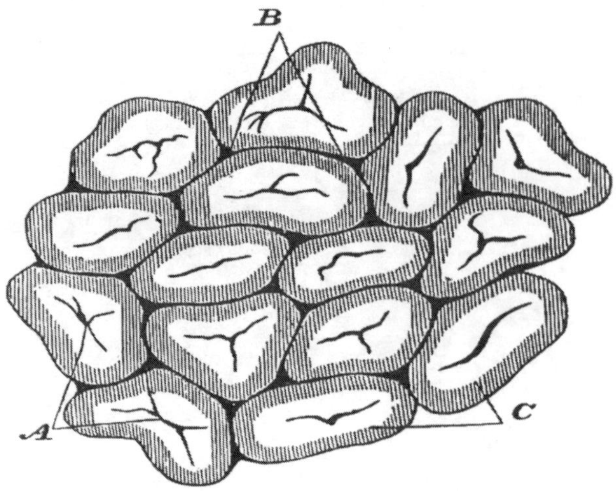

Lobules on the surface of the liver. A, twigs of the hepatic vein in the centres of the lobules, surrounded by uninjected capillaries; C, margins of the lobules, red from the capillaries there being congested; B, spaces between the lobules, occupied by injected twigs of the portal vein. (Diagram after *Kiernan.*)

never has the deep red color that it has when the central portions of the lobules are the part injected.

All that is known of this form of partial injection of the capillaries is contained in the few observations of Mr. Kiernan, who states that it is very rare, and that he has met with it in children only.

Having examined the structure of the liver, we may next consider the composition and uses of the Bile.

We have seen that the gall-ducts—the channels of the bile—if they do not form terminal plexuses within the lobules, can at least be traced to them; and it is therefore a fair inference that the constituents of the bile are derived, at least in part, from the nucleated cells in the lobular substance. In its passage through the ducts the matter furnished by the lobules becomes mixed with that secreted by the ducts themselves, which, if we may judge from the large quantity of blood the ducts derive from the hepatic artery and the numerous involutions of their mucous membrane, must be considerable in amount. Secretion is always going on, both in the lobules and in the ducts, and the compound fluid derived from these two sources probably passes continuously along the ducts as far as the junction of the hepatic duct with the cystic.

When the stomach and duodenum are empty, part only of the bile flows along the common duct into the duodenum; the remainder passes down the cystic duct into the gall-bladder.

During digestion, on the contrary, the gall-bladder contracts, and part of the bile accumulated in it, together with all which is brought by the hepatic duct, is poured into the duodenum.[1]

In the gall-bladder, the bile loses, by absorption, some of its more watery parts, and is further modified by the addition of the proper secretion of that cavity. After death, if it be not soon removed from the body, it becomes still further altered. Its more liquid part continues to pass out, giving a greenish stain to the tissues in contact with the gall-bladder, while the serum of the blood and the gaseous and liquid contents of the intestines and the juices of the liver itself pass in the opposite direction through the intervening tissues into the gall-bladder, and become mixed with the bile.

The bile in the gall-bladder is of a greenish-yellow color, which varies much in depth, according to the composition of the bile itself and its degree of concentration. If much diluted or thinly spread over a white surface, its color is yellowish, but if concentrated and seen in mass, it is of a dark green or olive, sometimes approaching to black. It has been described as having a peculiar sickly odor, somewhat like that of melted fat, but the odor of healthy human bile, when fresh and not mixed with intestinal gases, is scarcely perceptible. Bile has a nauseous bitter taste, which leaves behind it a smack of sweetness. It is more or less viscid, has an unctuous feel, and in many of its physical properties has much in common with soap. It combines readily with water in any proportion, mixes freely with oil or fat, and foams, when stirred, like soapy water; and is, indeed, like soap, in common use for cleaning articles of dress, and especially for taking out grease. It will be seen, hereafter, that these properties are probably closely related to one of the physiological uses of bile. When evaporated, it leaves inspissated mucus, and a variable proportion of a yellowish-green matter, which is very bitter, and which dissolves almost completely in water and in alcohol. Bile is heavier than water but its density varies much according to its composition and degree of concentration. That from the gall-bladder of the ox has usually a specific gravity between 1.026 and 1.030. Cystic bile has been generally supposed to have an alkaline reaction, but M. Bouisson and Dr. Kemp, who have lately made observations on this point,

[1] Bouisson—De la bile et de ses variétés physiologiques, et de ses alterations morbides. Paris, 1843.

state that when fresh and perfectly healthy, it is neutral—a statement confirmed by the still more recent as well as more extensive observations of Gorup-Besanez.

Under the microscope, bile, if diluted, gives a yellow stain to the glass, but often presents no definite objects. If, on the contrary, it be dark colored and concentrated, it shows amorphous particles of yellowish-green matter, which is usually collected into small roundish masses, and is the matter obtained by evaporating the bile.[1] In addition to this, a few prismatic cells from the mucous membrane of the gall-bladder may be seen, and now and then some oil-globules or small plates of cholesterine. The oil-globules are, probably, usually derived from the lobules of the liver. The plates of cholesterine are generally, if not always, formed in the gall-bladder. They may be there formed, by precipitation, from the bile, which usually contains a certain quantity of this substance in solution; or they may be derived from the coats of the gall-bladder itself. When the coats of the gall-bladder are, as it is termed, ossified, or when the mucous coat is much thickened or otherwise altered in structure, the bile in the gall-bladder generally contains visible cholesterine.

The bile in the hepatic ducts is less viscid, and much less bitter, than that in the gall-bladder, and is usually of a bright yellow, even when that in the gall-bladder is dark-green or olive-colored. Under the microscope, it gives a light yellow tinge to the glass, and presents some prismatic cells, but seldom any other object. In the numerous specimens of bile taken from the hepatic ducts that I have examined, I have never seen plates of cholesterine. The darker color and bitterer taste of cystic bile are, no doubt, mainly owing to its greater concentration. In persons who have fasted some time before death, the bile in the gall-bladder is usually very viscid and dark-colored.

There are probably more important differences between cystic and hepatic bile than those which result from different degrees of concentration, but little is known on this point.[2] It is very difficult to collect bile from the hepatic ducts in quantity enough for a

[1] See Bouisson, op. cit., p. 16.

[2] Dr. Kemp has lately communicated to the Royal Society some researches which show that the mucus of the bile and the mucous membrane of the gall-bladder exert a highly catalytic action on the constituents of the bile, and that the analysis of bile left in contact with this mucus must consequently lead to varying and unsatisfactory results. See Proceedings of the Royal Society for May, 1856.

complete analysis, and consequently chemists, in their study of this fluid, have confined themselves almost exclusively to bile taken from the gall-bladder. Most chemists, indeed, have been content with bile from the gall-bladder of the ox, which can be obtained in a healthy state, and in sufficient quantity for analysis, more readily than human bile.

Cystic bile contains *water*, the proportion of which, of course, varies very much according to the time the bile has remained in the gall-bladder, or rather according to its degree of concentration. In the often-quoted analysis of bile from the gall-bladder of the ox, by Berzelius, the water amounts to 904.4 parts in 1000. The quantity of water may be readily ascertained by evaporation.

Bile also contains *mucus*, derived from the gall-bladder and gall-ducts, the relative quantity of which, like that of the water, varies very much in different specimens. In the ox-bile analyzed by Berzelius, it amounted to 3 parts in 1000. Lehmann states that the relative quantity of mucus in any specimen of bile varies very much with the manner in which the bile is withdrawn from the bladder; that if it be pressed from the bladder with force, a large quantity of epithelium is detached from the lining membrane of the bladder, which counts in the analysis as mucus; and that when he used every precaution to avoid this source of error, he found in ox-bile only 1.34 parts in a thousand, and in human bile 1.58 parts in a thousand.[1] The quantity may be determined by adding to bile a sufficient quantity of alcohol, which precipitates the mucus in flakes, while it dissolves the proper biliary matter. The mucus may also be precipitated by acetic acid. It is chiefly to this ingredient that bile owes its viscidity. When the mucus is in large quantity, the bile can be drawn out into threads.

Bile likewise contains a considerable proportion of *soda*, and certain organic constituents, to which last it owes its color and its bitterness. The organic constituents are very readily decomposed, and enter into new combinations with the substances employed to separate them. In consequence of this, different chemists, by employing different methods of analysis, have obtained very different results, but all agree that these organic ingredients are allied to fat in composition, and contain a large proportion of carbon. Late researches have shown that they also contain a certain quantity of sulphur.

[1] Lehmann, Physiological Chemistry, translated by Dr. Day, vol. ii. p. 68.

The principles to which bile owes its color may be separated from those to which it owes its bitterness. The coloring matters are entirely removed by filtering bile through animal charcoal, and are also thrown down from solution by precipitates of barytes and other earthy salts.

In addition to these constituents, bile contains chloride of sodium, and in smaller proportions phosphate of soda and the earthy phosphates.

Chemists have also obtained from bile a small quantity of cholesterine, and of other forms of fat, for the most part saponified. In certain states of disease, cholesterine exists in large quantity in the bile of the gall-bladder, forming the chief part of most gall-stones; but in healthy bile it is in very small quantity, and in solution. It is not seen under the microscope.

The following is the composition of bile from the gall-bladder of the ox, according to the analysis by Berzelius already referred to:—

Water	90.44
Biliary matter, with fat	8.00
Mucus of the gall-bladder	0.30
Osmazome, chloride of sodium, and lactate of soda	0.74
Soda	0.41
Phosphate of soda, phosphate of lime, and traces of a substance insoluble in alcohol	0.11
	100.00

There has been, of late years, an active controversy respecting the state and relations of the organic constituents of bile. The subject has engaged the attention of many distinguished chemists, and their labors have led to several successive changes of opinion, which it is both interesting and instructive to consider.

Berzelius, in his later researches, separated from his biliary matter a green and a yellow coloring matter, and small quantities of fat and fatty acids, and obtained a matter which he termed *biline*, and which he considered the chief and the peculiar constituent of bile. Biline, which is composed of carbon, hydrogen, nitrogen, sulphur, and oxygen, is a soft substance, of a light yellow color, without smell, and having a bitter, and at the same time a sweetish, taste.[1] It is soluble in water and in alcohol, insoluble in ether,

[1] Berzelius conjectured that the sweet taste might be due to glycerine, engendered by saponification of the fat contained in the bile.

and, when obtained by evaporation from alcohol, reddens litmus-paper. It is readily metamorphosed by various agents, and especially by heat and acids.

Most chemists have inferred that the organic constituents of bile are combined in some way with the soda.

M. Demarçay, in an elaborate paper published in 1838,[1] advanced the opinion that bile is not a very complex secretion, as it was then generally supposed to be, but that its essential principles consist of a single resinous acid, which is combined with the soda, forming a substance analogous to soap. He termed this resinous acid *choleic acid*, and consequently considered bile, abstracting the mucus and coloring matters, to be little more than *choleate of soda*.

This view of the composition of bile brought us back to the doctrine which, before the elaborate researches of Thenard and others, was generally held, that the bile is an animal soap whose base is soda: a doctrine which seemed sanctioned by the physical qualities of bile already noticed—by its solubility in water, its consistence, its ready frothing, the readiness with which it takes up spots of grease or fat, and by the fact, then known, that it contains a fatty matter and an alkali.

The subsequent researches of Dr. Kemp, Liebig, and others, tended to confirm the conclusions of Demarçay; but the organic substance which is united with the soda, from being readily decomposed, was found to vary somewhat in its properties, according to the process by which it was obtained.

In ox-bile, this compound of the organic principles of the bile with soda (that is to say, *bile* freed from water, mucus, coloring matter, and fat) consists, according to the analysis of Dr. Kemp,[2] of the following ingredients:—

Carbon	59.90
Hydrogen	8.90
Nitrogen	3.40
Oxygen	17.63
Sulphur	3.10
Soda	6.53
Chloride of sodium	0.54
	100.00

[1] Annales de Chimie et de Physique, tom. lxvii. p. 177.

[2] Chemical Gazette, vol. iv. p. 472.

The opinion that the organic constituents of bile are combined with the soda, was to some extent further confirmed by Dr. Platner, of Heidelberg, who succeeded in causing fresh ox-bile, which had been dried by evaporation in a water-bath, and freed from mucus, and from the greater parts of its salts, by repeated solution in alcohol, to crystallize. He says: "For this purpose nothing further is necessary than to add ether repeatedly to as strong an alcoholic solution of the bile as possible, and then to set it aside in a cool place. The principal and most important constituent of the bile then crystallizes; but from one-sixth to one-fourth of the bile used does not crystallize, but remains as a yellowish-brown syrupy liquid. I have not been able to separate this in any manner from the crystals; consequently, I can say nothing more concerning its nature. It is, however, evidently a different substance from the principal constituent of the bile, perhaps even a product of its decomposition."[1]

Crystals thus obtained have been analyzed by F. Verdel, under the direction of Liebig. After separation of the chloride of sodium, with which they are contaminated, he found that they were composed of[2]—

Carbon	59.87
Hydrogen	8.91
Nitrogen	4.22
Oxygen	16.18
Sulphur	3.83
Soda	6.99
	100.00

It will be seen that the result of this analysis does not differ much from that of the analysis of the dried and purified bile, by Dr. Kemp, which is given above.

Many attempts have been made to elucidate the composition of bile by studying the products of its decomposition.

It was found by Mulder that when ox-bile undergoes decomposition spontaneously, or by the prolonged action of hydrochloric acid, it is resolved (with the exception of the fats, coloring matters,

[1] Chemical Gazette, vol. iii. p. 186. Muller's Archiv. 1844. Heft v. See also Chem. Gaz., vol. ii. p. 515. Muller's Archiv. 1844. Heft ii.

[2] Chemical Gazette, vol. iv. p. 486.

and salts) almost entirely into three products—*taurine*, ammonia, and a substance which forms various acids, differing from each other merely in containing different proportions of the elements of water. All these acids pass into a well-characterized acid, *choloidic acid* (Demarçay), and, as the ultimate product of decomposition, into *dyslysine*.[1]

Taurine, which contains nitrogen and all the sulphur of the bile, is a neutral body, and forms beautiful transparent six and four sided prisms, with oblique terminal faces. It is readily dissolved in water, but is insoluble in alcohol. The composition of taurine, which is expressed by the formula $C_4H_7NS_2O_6$ is as follows:—

Carbon	19.28
Hydrogen	5.73
Nitrogen	11.25
Sulphur	25.70
Oxygen	38.04
	100.00

Choloidic acid, which contains no nitrogen or sulphur, is a white substance, easily reduced to powder, insoluble in water, and very sparingly soluble in ether, but readily soluble in alcohol. It combines with alkalies, forming salts, which are soluble in water and in alcohol, but insoluble in ether; and which have a purely bitter taste. It consists (dried at 212° F.) of—

Carbon	72.18
Hydrogen	9.77
Oxygen	18.05
	100.00

and is expressed by the formula $C_{48}H_{39}O_9$.

Dyslysine is a tasteless, resinous substance, insoluble in water and in cold alcohol, sparingly soluble in boiling alcohol, but soluble in ether. Its composition is expressed by the formula $C_{48}H_{36}O_6$.

Some researches on ox-bile, recently made by Dr. Strecker,[2] in

[1] Chemical Gazette, vol. v. p. 317.

[2] See Chemical Gazette, vol. vi. p. 49; or, Comptes Rendus, Décembre 13, 1847. Chem. Gazette, vol. vi. p. 149; or, Comptes Rendus, xxvi. p. 38. Chem. Gazette, vol. vii. p. 49; or, Ann. der Chem. und Pharm., lxvi. p. 1.

the laboratory of Liebig, have given us more insight into its constitution. They have shown that the biliary matter which is combined with the soda (the choleic acid of Demarçay), may be resolved into two acids; both containing hydrogen, and one of them containing sulphur.

The acid that is free from sulphur ($C_{52}H_{43}NO_{12}$) may be further resolved into glycine, the sugar of gelatine ($C_4H_5NO_4$), and an acid, which contains no nitrogen, to which Dr. Strecker has given the name *cholalic acid.* This acid, which is the *cholic acid* of Demarçay ($C_{48}H_{40}O_{10}$), when boiled with strong hydrochloric acid, or when exposed to a high temperature, is converted, by the loss of part of its water, into choloidic acid, and ultimately, by a still further loss of water, into dyslysine.

The sulphuretted acid of ox-bile ($C_{52}H_{45}NO_{14}S_2$) may, in like manner, be resolved into cholalic acid and taurine. It has, therefore, a similar constitution to its fellow acid, with taurine in the place of glycine. When acted on by strong acids it yields taurine, choloidic acid, and dyslysine.

If we use the simpler term, *cholic acid,* to express the cholalic acid of Strecker, the two acids above mentioned, of which glycine and taurine are respectively the adjuncts, may therefore be termed *glyco-cholic* and *tauro-cholic* acid.

Tauro-cholic acid contains six per cent. of sulphur. Now, as the dried and purified bile of the ox contains only three per cent. of sulphur, it follows that, in ox-bile, glyco-cholic and tauro-cholic acids exist in nearly equal proportions.

Dr. Strecker has further shown that tauro-cholic acid, and its compound with soda, dissolve cholesterine very readily; while glyco-cholic acid has very little solvent action upon it. He has thus rendered it probable that tauro-cholic acid is the chief solvent of the cholesterine of the bile.

An admirable test for cholic acid, whether it exist alone or in combination with glycine and taurine, or in the form of its derivative, choloidic acid—which may, therefore, be considered a test for bile—was discovered a few years ago by Pettenkofer, in the change of color produced in it by addition of sugar and sulphuric acid. The following are directions for applying the test:—

Dissolve the alcoholic extract of the fluid to be tested for biliary matter in a little water; then mix with it a drop of a solution of any kind of sugar (in the proportion of one part of sugar to four parts of water); and afterwards add to the mixture pure sulphuric acid, free from sulphurous, in drops. If biliary matter be present, the fluid now becomes turbid, but on the gradual addition of sulphuric acid it clears again. For the first few moments its color is yellowish, but it soon becomes red, and passes through purple to a deep violet.

In using the test, care must be taken not to employ too much sugar, which is rendered brown or black by sulphuric acid; and also properly to regulate the temperature of the fluid, which should nearly reach, but not much exceed, 120° F. Sufficient heat may generally be produced by the addition of the sulphuric acid.

The bile of the ox, when perfectly fresh, seems to be very constant in composition. In the numerous specimens, analyzed by different chemists, at different times and in different countries, the chief constituents have been in very nearly the same relative proportions. The same is probably true of other animals. Dr. Strecker could find no difference between the bile of a dog fed upon flesh, and that of a dog which had been kept on a vegetable diet.

It was long ago stated by Dr. Kemp (*Cambridge Phil. Trans.*, vol. viii. p. 1), that human bile differs in some respects from that of the ox. After the discovery of sulphur in bile, it was found that this ingredient exists in very different proportions in the bile of different animals. Dr. Bensch found that while dried ox-bile, free from mucus and coloring matter and fat, contained, after deduction of the ash which it leaves on calcination, from 3.5 to 4 per cent. of sulphur:[1]—

	Sulphur.
The bile of the calf contained	5.62 per cent.
" sheep "	6.46 "
" goat "	5.55 "
" bear "	6.38 "
" wolf "	5.03 "
" fox "	5.56 "
" chicken "	5.57 "
" dog "	6.21 "
" serpent "	7.20 "

Dr. Strecker has analyzed the bile of various kinds of fish, and of many of our domestic animals, and his investigations show that

[1] Chemical Gazette, vol. vi. p. 50; or, Comptes Rendus, Déc. 13, 1847.

the bile of most animals contains essentially the same organic constituents, but that, in different animals, the organic substance containing sulphur, and that which contains no sulphur, are in different proportions.

The most striking deviations were found in the bile of the pig, which contains an extremely small quantity of sulphur, and in the bile of marine fish, where the soda of ox-bile is replaced in great part by potash. It is certainly, as stated in the account of Dr. Strecker's investigations, published in the *Chemical Gazette*, vol. vii. p. 430, "a remarkable circumstance that the bile of marine fish living in sea-water, which is so abundant in soda, principally contains potash; whilst in the bile of the ox, the food of which abounds to such an extent in potash, the ash consists of a large quantity of soda, with mere traces of potash."

Few complete analyses have been made of human bile, which it is more difficult to obtain fresh, and in sufficient quantity, and when wanted, than the bile of many of the lower animals. Human bile resembles ox-bile in its physical qualities, and on decomposition yields the same products—taurine, ammonia, and choloidic acid. There is every reason, therefore, to infer that it is formed of the same constituents, though most probably in somewhat different relative proportions.

Little has been yet said respecting the coloring matters of bile. These, however, are very important, at least with reference to medical practice, because, when they are not duly eliminated by the liver, they tinge the complexion, and impart a darker color to the urine, and thus give early intimation that the secretion of the liver is defective, or that the course of the bile into the intestine is impeded. Of defective action of the kidney, we have no such obvious ocular proof, and it often happens, in consequence, that the various ill effects of it are not traced to their source.

The coloring matters of bile have different tints, of green, yellow, and brown, in different animals. The bile of herbivorous animals is usually green; the fresh bile of carnivorous animals generally varies from a yellow to a yellowish-brown. In animals, however, whose hepatic bile is yellow or brown, the concentrated bile found in the gall-bladder, after long fasting, has always more or less of a green tint. In the bile of the ox, which has been most frequently chosen for analysis, there have been distinguished a green pigment and a yellow pigment; and it has been shown, by

Berzelius, that the green pigment, of which the yellow pigment is probably a modification, is identical with chlorophyl—the green coloring matter of plants. This matter is very readily modified by chemical influences, and its exact composition has not been determined; but it contains a large proportion of carbon and hydrogen, and from seven to nine per cent. of nitrogen. The brown bile-pigment of other animals seems to be also a modification of the same substance. When exposed to the air, it absorbs oxygen, and becomes of a dark green.[1] Nitric acid, also, by its oxidizing influence, renders it of a dark green, which soon, however, passes into various shades of red. A similar change of color is produced, by similar influences, in the leaves of plants. The various shades of yellow, brown, and pink, which the leaves present in autumn, are all owing to the action of oxygen on their coloring matter, when, at the appointed time for their decay, they can no longer resist the chemical influence of the air.

Dr. Bence Jones has given various good reasons for believing that the urine mainly owes its color to the same source; and that the various shades of yellow, brown, and pink, which the sediments of the urine present, like the similar tints of the autumnal leaves, are due to different degrees of oxidation of the peculiar matter to which the green color of plants and of the bile is owing. This hypothesis may serve to account for the influence, frequently to be noticed in the following pages, which organic diseases of the liver have in causing red and pinkish sediments in the urine.

The successive shades of blue, green, and yellow, which are seen in a bruise-mark on the skin, and which are so like the tints of the bile, long ago suggested the hypothesis, that the coloring matters of bile are derived immediately from the red coloring matter of the blood.[2] Late researches tend to confirm this hypothesis, and thus

[1] It has been inferred by Lehmann that the green tint acquired by yellow or brown bile, when long retained in the gall-bladder, likewise depends on the influence of oxygen, which it then abstracts from the circulating blood.—*Physiological Chemistry*, vol. ii. p. 505.

[2] Many considerations render it probable that the coloring matter of bile is derived from that of the blood.

Saunders says: "Green and bitter bile being in common to all animals with red blood, and found only in such, renders it probable that there is some relative connection between this fluid and the coloring matter of the blood, by the red particles contributing more especially to its formation."

A few years ago, Professor Schultz revived this notion, and dressed it up with

render it probable that the peculiar colors of bile, urine, and blood, result from different modifications of the same pigment. The coloring matter of the bile has a strong tendency to combine with bases —with alkalies, metallic oxides, and alkaline earths. With the alkaline earths it forms insoluble compounds, of which the nuclei of gall-stones mainly consist.

The bile, in man, has been supposed to be ultimately derived from two sources. It is clear enough that, in most circumstances, a large proportion of the proper principles of bile is derived from the waste of the body, and is a product of the metamorphosis of the tissues and of materials stored away in the system. In the hybernating animal during its winter sleep, in the fœtus, and probably in the carnivora, these materials are its only source. And under certain conditions, the same must be the case in man also. In protracted abstinence, for example, bile continues to be formed, and sometimes in considerable quantity. Here, the living tissues gradually waste away, and their materials are discharged in the excretions. The three principal outlets at which they make their appearance, are the liver, the lungs, and the kidney. Nitrogen predominates in the compounds which escape through the last-named organ, while the two former separate principally carbon and hydrogen. But while the liver and the lungs have thus much in common, there is this important difference between them: that in the lungs the carbon and hydrogen pass off *burnt*—that is, fully combined with oxygen, as carbonic acid and water—while in the liver they escape only partially combined with oxygen, and still combustible. From which it would appear, that the larger the amount of these elements discharged by the lungs as carbonic acid and water, the less, *cæteris paribus*, must remain *unburnt*, to form the constituents of bile. So that here we already meet with a fundamental and important relation between the secretion of bile

much fanciful speculation. He is of opinion that in the liver the blood sheds the coloring matter of the effete blood corpuscles, and thus becomes revivified.

Bouisson, again, says: " Burdach fait observer, que lorsqu'il se forme du sang rouge dans l'œuf de poule, le jaune fixé au feuillet muqueux acquiert une coloration verdâtre, en sorte qu'il reste démontré qu'il a coincidence entre la sanguification et la séparation d'une matière verte."

Quite recently the same opinion has been advocated on various grounds by Polli, an Italian physiological chemist, by Lehmann, and by G. Besanez, who considers a strong confirmation of it to be the presence (which he has ascertained on several occasions) of a notable quantity of iron in bile.

and the great function of respiration. I shall not, however, dilate upon this topic at present, as we shall again have to consider it in endeavoring to follow the bile to its final destination.

To return from this digression. It appears, then, sufficiently clear, that the proper principles of bile are in part derived, like those of the urine, from the waste of the tissues. There can be little doubt that the nitrogen of the bile is always derived from the metamorphosis of the nitrogenous tissues; but it has been supposed that in man, and in all animals which live on a mixed diet, those articles of food which are devoid of nitrogen also contribute directly to the elements of bile. Liebig, indeed, imagines that, as regards the horse and the ox, he has fully established this by means of quantitative analysis—showing that the bile these animals secrete in a day contains more carbon than all the albumen, fibrin, and casein of their food (the *protein-elements* of modern chemists) put together; more carbon, therefore, than can be derived from the waste of the tissues which these elements go to repair; and that, consequently, the remainder, at least, must needs be furnished immediately by the food, and by those constituents of it which contain no nitrogen. If this be so, there is every reason to presume that these same principles, which form a large and staple ingredient in the food of man, play in him, also, the same part.

But the calculations of Liebig are open to very serious, if not fatal, objections. The calculations are founded on the supposition that a horse or an ox secretes daily thirty-seven pounds of bile, as concentrated as that usually found in the gall-bladder. This would yield about forty ounces of carbon; whereas the animal consumes in the form of vegetable albumen, fibrin, and casein, only about four ounces and a half of nitrogen, which, reckoning from the known composition of these substances, would give not quite sixteen ounces of carbon. The carbon of the bile is, therefore, greater in amount than all the carbon in the protein elements of the food, in the proportion of 40 to 16. Such is the argument. Its weight all depends on the truth of the assumption, that thirty-seven pounds of bile, as concentrated as that usually found in the gall-bladder, are secreted daily—an assumption which, without much stronger evidence of its truth than we have at present, surely ought not to be made the basis of important doctrines, which confessedly rest solely on relations of *quantity*. Considering the size of the gall-bladder of the ox, thirty-seven pounds seem an enormous quantity of bile to be secreted in a day, and if the daily secretion should turn out to be only a quarter the amount—and few physiologists, we imagine, would rate it nearly so high even as this—the argument falls to the ground.[1]

It is clear that before we can draw any safe conclusions on this point, or trace the bile to its ultimate destination, by means of quantitative analysis, we must have some estimate of the quantity of bile daily secreted under ordinary circumstances. This must necessarily be one of the starting points in any such inquiry. Many attempts have been made to estimate the quantity of bile daily secreted by a man in a state of health; but, as might have been expected, the conclusions come to are wide apart, and little confidence can be placed in the greater number of them. Some physiologists, believing the bile to be chiefly excrementitious, and looking to the small size of the gall-bladder and the small quantity of bile ordinarily discharged from the bowels, have estimated it at a very few ounces; while others, regarding the large size of the liver, and believing that most of the bile secreted is again absorbed from the bowel to serve ulterior uses in the body, have rated it, with Burdach and Haller, at from seventeen to twenty-four ounces.

It is plain that the amount of the proper principles of bile secreted in a day must, like that of urinary ingredients, vary widely in different persons, and in the same person under different circumstances. The amount may be modified by the degree of waste in the body; by the activity of respiration; by the quantity of matter thrown off by the kidneys and the skin; and, directly or indirectly, by the quantity and quality of the food.

In some circumstances, a quantity of bile, as large as the estimate of Burdach or Haller, may certainly be secreted for a considerable time together. A very interesting case showing this, was read to the Medico-Chirurgical Society in the spring of 1844, by Mr. W. R. Barlow, of Writtle, Essex.

[1] The hypothesis that a horse or an ox secretes thirty-seven pounds of bile in a day has no other foundation than a calculation by Schultz, that, in an ox, it would take as much bile as this to neutralize the acid of the chyme. It is strange that Liebig should have adopted the estimate so unhesitatingly on the authority of Burdach, who not only states this to be the ground of it, but also draws the inference, that if the estimate be correct, and the ox secrete daily ten pounds of saliva, the quantity Schultz supposed to be secreted by the horse, the quantity of the two fluids secreted in a day would together equal the whole mass of the blood! (See *Burdach's Physiologie*, t. vii. p. 439.)

A strong healthy man, a thatcher, fifty-four years of age, injured himself by lifting a heavy ladder, on the 28th of August, 1843. When seen by Mr. Barlow, the same day, he complained of so much pain in the region of the liver that a rupture of that organ was apprehended. He was very faint, in a cold sweat, and the pulse could scarcely be felt. Some brandy and water was given him, and he recovered sufficiently to be taken to his own house, which was about three miles distant. Five grains of calomel and a grain of opium were given him at night, and an ounce of castor oil the following morning, which operated and produced several natural evacuations.

On the 29th he was bled, and continued the calomel and opium, with a dose of saline mixture, every five hours.

On the 30th it was observed that the evacuations from the bowels were white and without bile, while the urine was dark, as in jaundice. Five grains of blue pill were ordered every six hours.

As the pain in the region of the liver continued, the bleeding was repeated at different times, and a blister was applied over the right hypochondrium. The same medicine was continued till the 15th of September, when a swelling of the size of a walnut was observed over the region of the liver. This gradually increased, and on the 9th of October was so large, and caused so much pain from distension, that it was thought proper to tap it. Seven quarts of fluid were drawn off, which from its color and taste appeared to be pure bile. The pain was instantly relieved, and the swelling entirely subsided.

The fluid collected again, and it was necessary to repeat the tapping on the 21st of the same month, when six quarts and a half of fluid were drawn off. This fluid was analyzed by Dr. Pereira, Dr. G. O. Rees, and Mr. Taylor, and found to be composed in great part of bile. Dr. Rees guessed the proportion of bile in the fluid to be at least eight parts in ten.

On the 31st of October he was tapped again, and seven quarts were drawn off. On the 9th of November the operation was repeated for the fourth time, when six quarts were withdrawn. On the 18th of November he was taken to St. Bartholomew's Hospital, and tapped again, when nine pints of fluid escaped. On the 26th of November he was tapped for the last time, when only three pints escaped. The cyst was not emptied as in the former operations, and he suffered extreme pain from the tapping, which he had not previously done. On the following day, bile appeared in his stools, and the urine was lighter colored. On the 3d of December, the motions were of proper color, containing plenty of bile. The swelling gradually subsided, and towards the end of the month he became quite convalescent. In the beginning of February he was able to walk eight or ten miles; and, when an account of his case was presented to the Society, appeared to be in good health.[1]

It appears here that in twelve days, from the 9th of October to the 21st, thirteen pints of fluid accumulated in the sac. If, as Dr. Rees believed, four-fifths of this consisted of bile, nearly ten pints and a half of bile must have been discharged—not very far short

[1] The Medico-Chirurgical Transactions, vol. xxvii. p. 378.

of a pint a day. The quantity of fluid discharged at the two subsequent tappings was still larger in proportion to the time, but of this fluid no analysis seems to have been made.

In a note appended to the account of this case in the Society's *Transactions*, Dr. Cursham gives references to other cases of a similar kind. One of these, by Mr. Fryer, of Stamford, in the fourth volume of the *Medico-Chirurgical Transactions*, accords in almost every particular with the case just related, except that the subject of it was a boy thirteen years of age, and that the quantity of fluid discharged at the successive tappings was still larger in proportion to the intervals between them. The fluid was not analyzed, but had, it is stated, the appearance of *pure bile*. In this case, as in the former, mercury was given.

We should not, of course, be warranted in assuming from these cases that the same amount of bile is secreted under ordinary circumstances; or, at any rate, in drawing from such an estimate any important physiological inference not warranted by other reasons.

The secretion of bile is continuous, but varies in amount according to the state of digestion. Bidder and Schmidt, in an extensive series of experiments on cats, found that in these animals it attained its maximum from ten to twelve hours after a full meal; and that in continued starvation it gradually and continuously diminishes.[1]

It has long been a question whether the peculiar principles of the bile are formed in the liver, or whether they exist ready-made in the blood, as the result of the waste of the tissues in other parts of the body, and are merely strained off from the blood in the liver. There is now little doubt that the peculiar biliary acids are formed in the liver, through the agency of the secreting cells, for the most distinguished chemists have failed to detect them in the portal blood, and even in the blood of persons affected with jaundice.[2]

[1] See Lehmann, vol. ii. p. 87.

[2] Lehmann states, that he has constantly failed to detect the peculiar biliary acids, even in large quantities of the portal blood of horses, and supposes that chemists who have imagined they have detected these acids in the blood, have been led into error by the circumstance that olein and oleic acid give a reaction on Pettenkofer's test very like that of bile. He states that the reaction of oleic acid differs from that of the bile only in this, that it takes place more slowly, and requires the entrance of atmospheric air. It has also been ascertained, that oil of turpentine, oil of cumin, and some other volatile oils, give a similar reaction on Pettenkofer's test. The rich brown color that must result from the action of the sulphuric acid on the sugar, when cane-sugar is employed in the test, is also likely to mislead.

Again, the peculiar coloring matters of bile cannot, according to Lehmann and other chemists, be detected in the portal blood, and must, therefore, at least for the most part, be formed in the liver itself. It has been clearly shown that the coloring matters of bile are most probably derived from those of the blood, and we are, therefore, led to the inference that the transformation is effected, at least for the most part, in the liver. It will be seen in the following pages that very extensive structural changes in the liver—in the fatty liver, the gin-drinker's liver, the scrofulous liver—may exist without jaundice; and that in those cases in which jaundice results from permanent closure of the common duct, the jaundice sometimes lessens after the lapse of many months, and when the secreting cells of the liver are almost entirely destroyed.

In secreting bile, the liver serves unquestionably very important purposes. The large size of the liver, and its existence in all animals, down almost to the lowest in the animal scale, leave no doubt on this point: but it has long been a question among physiologists—What these purposes are?

At one time it was supposed that the chief purpose of the liver, like that of the kidneys, is to purify the blood, by separating from it noxious and effete principles that result from the waste of the tissues. There can be no doubt that the liver effects a purpose of this kind. Much of the sulphur of the bile, and much of the coloring matters of the bile, are discharged from the intestine, and must be regarded as a real excretion, the result of waste of the organic constituents of the blood or tissues: and the liver must further tend to maintain the purity of the blood, by ridding it of other matters foreign to its composition. It will be remembered that all the blood sent to the stomach and intestines has to pass through this organ before it can again mix with the venous blood from other parts of the body. Now the blood that has come from the stomach and intestines must necessarily be charged with many impurities besides those derived from the mere decay of the tissues. Along the extensive mucous tract with which everything we eat or drink is brought in contact, absorption is constantly going on, and various matters must therefore enter the portal vessels, not fit by their nature to form blood or to serve any other purpose in the body. Many of these substances are intercepted, at least in part, in their transit through the liver, and, according to their kind, are either fixed there, or are gradually cast out of the system with the bile. This, indeed, has been fully proved with respect to many of the metallic salts. In animals poisoned by arsenic, antimony, the soluble salts of lead, and corrosive sublimate, these substances have been found in greater quantity in the liver than in other organs, even when death occurred a considerable time after they were swallowed; and copper, derived probably from cooking utensils and food, has often been found in human bile and gall-stones. The retention of noxious matters in the liver, and their elimination through it, are doubtless the cause of many biliary disorders.

It was long ago conjectured that the liver is a blood-making organ—that, in some way or other, it is instrumental in the generation or restoration of the blood-corpuscles—but no distinct evidence that such is the case was adduced. Modern physiologists and chemists, especially Bernard and Lehmann, have investigated the changes which the blood undergoes in its passage through the liver, by making a chemical and microscopic examination of the blood as it enters the liver by the portal vein, and as it issues from it by the hepatic vein, and their investigations have led to very remarkable results. One of the results of microscopic observation is, that in blood drawn from the hepatic vein the colorless corpuscles are very much more numerous than in blood drawn from the portal vein, leading to the inference that the colorless corpuscles, which appear to be the first stage in the formation of the red corpuscles, are generated in great quantity in the blood in its passage through the liver. Again, the red corpuscles differ in their appearance, and in their chemical and vital properties, in the two kinds of blood. The red corpuscles, in blood drawn from the hepatic vein, have not the same color as those in blood drawn from the portal vein; their capsules, according to Lehmann, do not disappear so readily on the addition of water; and they are not so apt to arrange themselves in rolls. The red corpuscles of the hepatic blood have a sharp outline, and do not exhibit the spotted appearance and irregular forms that have been remarked in the portal blood. These observations show that the visible organic constituents of the blood are much modified in their passage through the liver, and they probably justify the opinion that the chief office of the organ is the generation, or, as it has been termed, the *rejuvenescence* of the blood-corpuscles.

The blood in its passage through the liver undergoes other changes made known to us by chemical analysis. It has been lately discovered by M. Bernard that sugar is habitually formed in considerable quantity in the liver, and that there are, if we may so speak, two secretions going on in the liver—the secretion of bile, which escapes by the gall-ducts, and the secretion of sugar, which is absorbed into the blood. The sugar formed in the liver is the sugar of diabetes, which closely resembles the low sugar of grapes—it turns brown when boiled with liquor potassæ, reduces the salts of copper in Trommer's and Barreswil's tests, rapidly undergoes fermentation on the addition of yeast, and in the polarizing apparatus turns the luminous ray to the right. M. Bernard has investigated with singular ability the conditions which increase or diminish the formation of sugar, and his discovery is one of the most remarkable and most promising achievements of modern science.

The following are the principal points established in this inquiry:—

1. That, in a state of health, sugar exists in the liver of man, and of other classes of animals, carnivorous as well as herbivorous, down to the lowest in the animal scale, but exists in no other organ, except during fœtal life. In the fresh liver of the ox, the quantity of sugar amounts to 1.79 parts in 100. In the livers of two men who had died by the guillotine, it amounted respectively to 1.79 and 2.142 parts in 100.

2. That sugar exists in the liver in animals kept many days without food, and in dogs and other animals long fed entirely on flesh, in whom no sugar is formed in the stomach during the process of digestion—showing that the sugar which exists in the liver is not introduced from without, but is formed in the body, and that independently of the nature of the food.

3. That sugar exists in the blood which has passed through the liver in carnivorous animals and in animals kept some days without food, when there is no sugar in the blood which enters the liver by the portal vein or by the hepatic artery: and that in other circumstances, when sugar exists in the blood entering the liver, there is much more sugar in the blood leaving the liver—showing that the sugar is formed in the liver itself.

Other observations show that the sugar so formed is secreted by the cells of the lobular substance, that it may be formed in the liver in certain amount even after death, and that it is carried out of the liver, not only in the current of blood, but also by the lymphatics. It has not been discovered in the bile, even in animals in whom a biliary fistula has been established, and therefore either does not pass off by the gall ducts, or is absorbed or rapidly transformed in them.

The quantity of sugar secreted varies according to the stage of digestion. Whatever be the nature of the food, the secretion of sugar increases as soon after a meal as intestinal absorption begins,[1] and attains its *maximum* in about four or five hours; it then gradually diminishes until the next meal. In a dog fed on flesh, the proportion of sugar in the blood of the hepatic vein varies from 1 per cent., which is about its amount in the fasting state, to 1½ or 2 per cent., when the formation of sugar has reached its height. We have already seen that the secretion of bile has similar variations in amount, dependent on the digestive process; but it appears from Bernard's researches that the oscillations in the secretion of sugar are not synchronous with the oscillations in the secretion of bile, the greatest secretion of sugar, in dogs, taking place in about four or five hours after a meal, while, according to extensive researches by Bidder and Schmidt, the greatest secretion of bile takes place in these animals from 13½ to 15½ hours after the last meal.[2] The phenomena of disease show that the two secretions are not commensurate. An abundant secretion of bile is not attended with saccharine urine, and an excessive secretion of sugar in diabetes is not, as far as we can judge, necessarily attended by an excessive secretion of bile.

The sugar passing out of the liver by the veins and lymphatics at once enters the general current of blood, and is rapidly transformed. In a healthy animal, the quantity that enters the blood in the intervals of digestion is all transformed in the lung, so that not a trace of it can be found in the arterial blood. During digestion, when its quantity increases, some of the sugar may escape transformation in the lung, and be sent in the arterial blood to every part of the body; but it is not then found in the urine or other

[1] Starchy or saccharine articles of food increase the quantity of sugar in the system, because the sugar absorbed from the intestinal canal is then added to that which is formed in the liver. According to the observations of Bernard, cane-sugar absorbed from the intestinal canal is transformed into diabetic or liver-sugar in passing through the liver.

[2] See Bernard, Leçons, 1854–5, p. 93; Lehmann, Physiological Chemistry, vol. iii. p. 506.

secretions, and must therefore be transformed in the blood. It is only when the secretion is so increased as to constitute disease that the sugar passes off in the urine, and the *diabetic* state is produced. What precise transformation the sugar undergoes in the blood is still uncertain. From some experiments made to determine this point, Bernard concludes that its transformation is not effected by the immediate influence of oxygen—that the sugar is not *burnt* in the lung, and exhaled as carbonic acid—and that it must undergo transformation by the lactic, or some other fermentative process.

The most remarkable results which Bernard has arrived at are those which relate to the influence of the nervous system in controlling and modifying the secretion of sugar.

The principal of these results are the following:—

1. That division of the pneumogastric nerves in the neck arrests the formation of sugar. If this operation be performed on a dog, and the animal be killed three days after, not a trace of sugar can be found in the blood of the hepatic vein or in the substance of the liver itself.

2. A second result, which, on its first announcement, was very startling, is, that in all animals in which he could perform the experiment (dogs, rabbits, guinea pigs), lacerating the floor of the fourth ventricle between the auditory nerves and the par vagum increases the formation of sugar to such a degree that a large quantity of sugar passes off in the urine, and the creature is rendered diabetic. The diabetic state continues some days, until the injury is repaired, after which sugar can no longer be found in the urine. Bernard states that the experiment which led to this singular result was suggested by his having noticed, in making experiments with another purpose, that pricking the pons Varolii at the origin of the fifth nerve caused an abundant secretion of tears and saliva. He further found that irritation of the floor of the fourth ventricle increases the secretion of sugar in the liver when the par vagum has been divided in the neck—showing that the nervous influence exciting the secretion is transmitted to the liver, not down the pneumogastric nerves, but down the spinal marrow. This last conclusion was confirmed by another result, that division of the spinal marrow below the brachial enlargement puts a stop in all cases to the production of sugar.

Bernard hence infers that the nervous influence that ordinarily excites the secretion of sugar is a *reflex* influence—that it passes up the pneumogastric nerves to the nervous centre (medulla oblongata or brain), and thence down the spinal marrow, and along the spinal nerves and the branches of the great sympathetic communicating with them, to the liver.

This inference has been confirmed by the observation that when the pneumogastric nerves are divided in the neck, an operation which usually arrests the secretion of sugar, the secretion may be excited again by galvanizing the upper or central ends of the divided nerves.

The fact that division of the pneumogastric nerves in the neck ordinarily arrests the formation of sugar, shows that an influence is ordinarily transmitted along them to the liver, and Bernard infers that this influence has its origin in the lungs, and that it is excited by the impression made by the air on the nervous filaments in the lung. He states that although the formation of sugar is stopped when the pneumogastric nerves are divided in the neck, it goes on just as usual when the nerve is divided lower down between the lung and the liver.

The readiness with which the presence of sugar can be detected has enabled him to determine the influence of other conditions in increasing or lessening the formation of sugar, and to ascertain that its formation, like the secretion of the salivary and other glands, is increased during the apoplectic state, and that it is arrested by long-continued abstinence from food, by severe pain, and by fever. This last circumstance explains the fact, that sugar cannot generally be found in the livers of persons who die of disease.

The formation of sugar coincidently with the rapid development of the colorless corpuscles of the blood in the liver has suggested to Bernard the theory that, in animals as in plants, the presence of sugar is requisite for the most rapid development of cells; and that whatever other purposes in the animal economy the sugar may serve, its chief use is in the formation of the blood-corpuscles.

It is a curious fact, in connection with these researches, that diabetes may exist when much of the lobular substance of the liver has been destroyed by cirrhosis, and when, in consequence of this disease, the secretion of bile is defective and the passage of blood through the liver much impeded. In the winter of 1840, a man who had long been addicted to spirit-drinking was admitted, under my care, in King's College Hospital, with great ascites and all th other symptoms of the gin-drinker's liver; but, in conjunction with these symptoms he had saccharine diabetes. At the time of his admission to the hospital he was passing daily from ten to twelve pints of urine, of sp. gr. 1040--1045, and containing a large quantity of sugar, the existence of which was ascertained by fermentation. The diabetes continued, without causing any diminution in the quantity of liquid in the peritoneal sac; and on his death, which happened about a month after he entered the hospital, the liver was found to be very large, and to have in a striking degree the "hob-nail" surface that results from cirrhosis.

Many other differences than those yet mentioned have been found between the blood as it enters the liver and as it issues from it.

The blood which enters the liver contains much more fat, especially more oily fat, than the blood which issues from it. According to Lehmann, the solid residue of blood from the portal vein contains, on an average, 3.225 per cent. of fat, while that of blood from the hepatic vein contains only 1.885 per cent.[1]

Another very remarkable difference relates to the fibrin, which almost entirely disappears from the blood in its passage through the liver. In the experiments of Lehmann and Bernard, the fibrin in the portal blood was often in just as large amount, and as contractile, as in the blood of the general venous current, while in the hepatic blood drawn at the same time scarcely a trace of fibrin could be found. Lehmann conjectures that the fibrin which disappears in the liver may help to form the glycine and taurine—the nitrogenous and sulphurous adjuncts of the cholic acid—in the bile.

Again, the blood as it issues from the liver contains much less albumen, less water, and a smaller amount of salts than the blood which enters the liver.

The full extent of the changes which the blood undergoes in the liver has probably not even yet been made out, and our comprehension of the purport and meaning of the changes is very vague, but enough has been discovered to show that the liver modifies and elaborates in a wonderful way the materials of the blood.

Coincident with the chemical changes in the blood is an elevation of its temperature. Bernard found that, in the dog, the tempera-

[1] Physiological Chemistry. Translated by Dr. Day, vol. ii. p. 88.

ture of the blood in the hepatic vein is nearly $\frac{3}{4}°$ F. higher than in the portal vein, and more than a degree higher than in the aorta, and he concludes that the liver, among its other uses, is one of the chief sources of animal heat.[1]

But the uses of the liver are not confined to the changes which it immediately produces in the portal blood. The fact that the bile is poured into the intestinal canal, so near its upper end, is sufficient to show that it is not a merely excrementitious fluid, but that, when it has arrived in the intestine, it has important offices to serve. These offices are related to the function of digestion, on the one hand, and (according to Liebig) to that of respiration, on the other.

It was formerly supposed that the one great use of the bile is to complete the process of digestion, and for this end it was considered quite as essential as the gastric juice itself. That the bile has, indeed, an important relation to digestion is evident from the fact that man and other animals that feed at intervals by large meals have a gall-bladder which allows bile to accumulate when the stomach and duodenum are empty, so as to be poured into the digestive canal in greater quantity when they are full. But there can be no doubt that the part which bile plays in digestion has been much overrated. The recent investigations of chemists have much simplified our views of this process. Since the important discovery that complex nitrogenous principles (albumen, fibrin, casein) identical with those of the blood and tissues of animals exist in plants, and that in the food of herbivorous animals they exist in sufficient quantity to supply the waste of the body, we have been led to the inference that these principles are not *formed*, as was formerly supposed, during the process of digestion, but that they are compounded only by plants, and that they exist ready-made in the food. With respect, then, to these nitrogenous elements of the food, all that appears necessary to digestion, as far as mere chemical changes are concerned, is to effect their solution. Now experiments of a conclusive kind have shown that the gastric and intestinal juices can accomplish this object. Of the non-nitrogenous substances we take as food—the sugar, starch, fat, and oil—sugar is already soluble enough, and starch is altered by the saliva and the pancreatic juice, and thus rendered soluble in the fluids found

[1] Bernard, Leçons, &c., p. 198.

in the stomach and intestines, from which, like the dissolved albuminous matters, it is absorbed into the bloodvessels to be carried to the liver. Fatty matters are not digested in the stomach, and must require, therefore, after they pass into the intestine, some preparation in order to become easily absorbed; for membranes absorb with great difficulty those fluids which do not penetrate them by imbibition, or which, in more familiar phrase, *do not wet them.* But it has been shown by M. Bernard that fatty matters undergo the needful modification by mixing with the pancreatic juice, which acidifies them, and rapidly makes with them a persisting emulsion, and thus enables them to be absorbed both by the veins and by the chyle-vessels of the small intestine.

It appears, then, that all the staminal principles of the food may be digested, or rendered fit for absorption, without the aid of the bile—a fact, indeed, sufficiently established, as regards man, by the observed effects of permanent closure of the common gall-duct. In a future chapter, cases will be related in which the common gall-duct was completely and permanently closed by a gall-stone, so that no bile could flow into the intestine; yet, in spite of the complete absence of bile in the intestine, and of the deep and permanent jaundice which results from this condition, the body was tolerably well nourished for more than twelve months, clearly showing that all the staminal principles of the food must have been digested and absorbed. A case still more remarkable will be related, in which a poor woman lived more than eight months in a state of deep jaundice from obstruction of the common gall-duct, and not only kept up her nutrition during this time well enough to be able to attend to the common duties of life, but, five months after the occurrence of the jaundice, gave birth to an infant, which she continued to suckle up to her death.

Such cases are quite as convincing as the results of direct experiments, and show conclusively that all the staminal principles of the food may be digested and absorbed without the aid of the bile. But it does not follow from this that the bile is of no use in digestion; for the very cases in question show that permanent closure of the common gall-duct destroys life in the end, and generally in little more than twelve months, by causing a gradual impairment of nutrition. Some experiments made by M. Bernard have led him to the conclusion that the gastric juice, when mixed with the pancreatic juice and the bile, has a more solvent action on albuminous substances than the gastric juice alone; and there are many reasons for believing that if the fatty matters which pass out of the stomach can be made into an emulsion and be so fitted for absorption by the pancreatic juice, their absorption is in most cases much promoted by the bile.

Another effect commonly attributed to bile is that of neutralizing the acid that passes from the stomach into the intestines, after having performed its part in digestion. As healthy bile is itself neutral, or but very slightly alkaline, it can only neutralize the acids of the chyme by becoming decomposed. In that case the soda of the bile would unite with the muriatic and lactic acids of the chyme, and bile-acids would be set free. There would be as much free acid in the bowel as before, but this acid, instead of being a sour liquid, like muriatic acid, would be an acid sparingly soluble in water, and probably much less irritating to the bowel. There can be little doubt that a substitution of this kind does take place; for it has been shown by Lehmann, Von Bibra, and others, that choloidic acid, and even dyslysine, are formed from the bile in its passage through the intestine; but the substitution can only take place to a certain extent. The quantity of soda in the bile is too small, even if it were all employed for this purpose, to neutralize the acid of the chyme.[1] The chyme is most probably neutralized, at least in chief part, by the pancreatic juice, and by the secretions of the intestinal canal. The bile may contribute to it also indirectly, by stimulating the coats of the canal, and rendering their secretion more active. If the soda of the bile unite with the acid of the chyme, the characters of the bile as a soap must be destroyed, and, consequently, the bile cannot at the same time perform this office and promote the absorption of fatty matters in the way usually supposed.

Bile has been supposed to prevent by its bitter principle the development of gas in the intestines, and the occurrence of putrefactive changes in the nitrogenous constituents of the food during their passage through the intestines. From the readiness with which bile undergoes decomposition, such an office might seem improbable; but it has been ascertained that bile, out of the body, arrests alcoholic fermentation, and prevents for some time the putrefaction

[1] It was the supposition that the office of the bile is to neutralize the acid of the chyme, that led to the extravagant estimate by Schultz before referred to, viz., that an ox secretes daily 37 lbs. of bile.

of flesh; and it is an observed fact that in jaundice the bowels often become flatulent, and the stools unusually fetid, while, in cases of stricture of the pylorus, when the bowels are confined for days together and bile continues to flow into them, flatulent distension of the intestines seldom occurs.

Collaterally, the bile forwards in various ways the great business going on in the alimentary canal. One of the most obvious of its uses is, to promote the due discharge of the contents of the bowel. If such a phrase may be used—bile is the natural purgative. If poured into the intestine in too large quantity it causes diarrhœa, and if its secretion be deficient, constipation generally follows. Eberle further observed that, in animals, which he made the subject of experiment, and especially in such as had fasted for some time before death, the mucus of the intestine was much more abundant, as far as bile had reached, than below this point.

We have next to consider the final destination of the bile itself. It seems clear that, in man, under ordinary circumstances, the bile which is voided by the bowel can be but a small proportion of the whole amount secreted. For the quantity thus voided is very trifling, and consists chiefly of modified bile-pigment, with cholesterine and taurine. The greater part of the resinous matter of the bile and the soluble salts must therefore be reabsorbed. Liebig states, that in the carnivora the whole of the bile is reabsorbed. The excrements of these animals contain neither bile nor soda; for water extracts from them no trace of any substance resembling bile, and yet bile is very soluble in water, and mixes with it in every proportion. It has been lately advanced by Liebig, on the authority of quantitative analysis, that the portion of the bile reabsorbed is eventually discharged through the lungs, as carbonic acid and water; thus supplying fuel for respiration and supporting animal heat. On account of the novelty and importance of this doctrine, and the high reputation of its author, it is right that the calculations on which the doctrine is based should be closely examined.

Liebig adopts the estimates of Haller and Burdach, that a man in health secretes daily from 17 to 24 ounces of bile; and he assumes that this bile contains 90 per cent. of water, which gives from 816 to 1152 grains of dried bile.[1]

[1] See Liebig's "Organic Chemistry, in its Application to Physiology and Pathology," pp. 64, 65.

Now Berzelius found in 1000 parts of fresh human feces, only 9 parts of a substance similar to bile. Reckoning from this proportion, the daily feces of a man, which do not, on an average, weigh more than 5½ ounces, contain only 24 grains of dried bile at most.

So that, according to this computation, the whole quantity of bile secreted exceeds the quantity that can be detected in the matters discharged from the alimentary canal in at least the proportion of 816 to 24, or 34 to 1.

The chief part of the bile is therefore reabsorbed, and as (Liebig argues) no traces of it are found in the other excretions, the carbon and hydrogen it contains must evidently be discharged through the lungs in union with oxygen, as carbonic acid and water. Whatever intermediate purposes it may serve, this must be the ultimate fate of these, its chief elements.

The estimate of the amount of bile daily secreted—namely, from 17 to 24 ounces, as concentrated as bile usually found in the gall-bladder—is higher than most physiologists would admit. But the proportion it gives of bile secreted to that found in the excrement is so large that even a considerable error in this direction would not vitiate the conclusion, although it would, of course, give too high an estimate of the amount of fuel for respiration furnished from this source. Even at this estimate, the carbon furnished by the bile would be but a small proportion of that given out in respiration. It has been computed that in a grown-up person, taking moderate exercise, $13\frac{9}{10}$ oz. of carbon escape daily through the skin and lungs as carbonic acid. Now 816 grains of dried bile, which does not contain more than 69 per cent. of carbon, gives only 563 grains of carbon, or about $1\frac{1}{5}$ oz.[1] These considerations tend to show that it can hardly be one of the chief purposes of the bile to support respiration, although it seems established by the reasoning of Liebig, that the bile that is reabsorbed, after having served other uses, is applied to this purpose, for which, indeed, it seems singularly fitted by its solubility and the large amount of carbon and hydrogen it contains.

[1] Liebig has made a calculation of this kind with reference to the ox, and concludes that in that animal the bile daily secreted contains 40 ounces of carbon, but he starts with the extravagant estimate of 37 lbs. (as concentrated as that in the gall-bladder) for the amount of bile daily secreted.

Before these researches of Liebig, the opinion was generally held that the bile is mainly excrementitious, and voided by the intestine; and it was supposed to be the chief office of the liver to rid the system of all matters, rich in hydrogen and carbon, that result from the waste of the tissues and are not discharged by the lungs in union with oxygen. The lung and the liver were thus considered to be directly and strictly vicarious in their office, and in support of this view it was alleged that, throughout the animal scale, whenever the lungs are large and active, the liver is small, and *vice versâ*. Thus it was remarked that in all cold-blooded animals—creatures in which respiration is very feeble—the liver is very large and excessively developed when compared with the lungs. But it is a very formidable objection to this theory of vicarious action, that in serpents, whose respiration is extremely feeble, the excrement does not contain a particle of bile. Great stress is laid on the case of the mollusca, animals whose liver is generally immense in proportion to their other viscera. But even if their bile be excreted, that would not disprove Liebig's theory of the use of bile in man and the higher animals, since this professes to rest on entirely independent evidence. The same may be said with regard to the instances of animals in which the bile is poured into the rectum, and is, therefore, probably voided by the intestine.

But, although the old doctrine of vicarious action can no longer be maintained, it is plain enough, especially since the discoveries of Bernard, that there is a direct and fundamental relation between the function of the liver and that of the lung. Fortunately, the activity and effects of the respiratory process are largely under our control. In the vast power we have of modifying these by appropriate regulations, having reference to the great conditions of air, exercise, temperature, and food, we have means much more effectual than any other, in dealing with biliary disorders.

Of these disorders, on the other hand, the neglect of such regulations is by far the most fruitful source.

Thus, for example, may be explained many of the bilious disorders of hot climates. If, in such climates, the food be not regulated in accordance with the smaller needs of the economy as to animal heat, an excess of bile is formed, and disorder of the stomach and intestines—bilious vomiting, and diarrhœa—is the consequence.

Hence, also, the general repugnance to rich meats, and the greater tendency which these and spirituous liquors unquestionably have to produce diseases of the liver, in hot seasons and in tropical climates.

In the same way may be explained the greater frequency of bilious disorders in middle life, when men begin to take less exercise, and their respiration becomes less active, while, on the other hand, the tendency to indulgence at table but too often increases.

We may also often see inverse evidence of these relations in the effect of pure air and active exercise, in relieving various disorders that result from repletion, and from the retention of principles which, if not burnt in respiration, should pass off by the liver as bile. Every sportsman must have remarked the effect of a single day's hunting in clearing the complexion. It has, no doubt, much the same effect on the liver as on the skin.

The secretion of the bile is influenced not only by the general conditions just mentioned, but also by the state of the liver itself, and especially by the number and activity of the cells in its lobular substance.

Not unfrequently, in bodies examined in our hospitals, considerable portions of the liver are found atrophied, from adhesive inflammation in or about branches of the portal vein. In consequence of the obstruction of those vessels, the portions of liver to which they carried blood, waste, and if such portions be near the surface, the capsule is drawn in, and the surface appears puckered, or fissured, according to the size and direction of the obstructed veins. Again, hydatid and other tumors may cause atrophy of portions of the liver, by the pressure they exert on its substance, or on the vessels which supply it.

But in effect of acute disease, without any permanent obstruction of vessels, the vitality of the cells may be permanently damaged, and their power of reproduction perhaps impaired.

In persons who die of yellow fever, the liver presents various morbid appearances, which have been minutely described by Louis, that depend not on the products of inflammation, or on the state of the vessels, but on the condition of the cells. The damage done to the liver in this way may last for years. It is probable that the bilious disorders of many men on their return to this country from India and other hot climates, are in great measure owing to permanent injury done to the secreting element of the liver.

In most persons, perhaps, a portion of the liver may waste or become less active, without sensible derangement of health. They have more liver, as they have more lung, than is absolutely necessary. In others, on the contrary, the liver, from natural conformation, seems only just capable of effecting its purpose in favorable circumstances. They are born with a tendency to bilious derangements. This innate defect of power in the liver has its counterpart in the deficient respiratory power in persons with vesicular emphysema of the lungs, and like this latter defect, and most other peculiarities of physical structure, is no doubt frequently inherited. Persons who inherit this feebleness of the liver, if we may so term it, or in whom, in consequence of disease, a portion of the liver has atrophied, or the secreting element of the liver has been damaged, may suffer little inconvenience as long as they are placed in favorable circumstances and observe those rules which such a condition requires; but whenever from any cause—as a hot climate, gross living, indolent habits, constipation—a more abundant secretion of bile is requisite to purify the blood, the liver is inadequate to its office, and they become bilious and sallow. In the management of such cases, we have two objects to fulfil—first, to enjoin those conditions and rules of life that render a plentiful secretion of bile less needful; and secondly, to endeavor to render the liver itself more active.

The chief conditions to diminish the quantity of matter which the liver is called on to excrete, are, a light diet, with water for drink; active exercise; early rising; and a cool or temperate climate.

Various medicines seem to fulfil to a certain extent the second object, that of rendering the liver more active, and increasing in this way the secretion of bile. Mercury, iodine, the salts of soda, muriate of ammonia, and taraxacum, when given in proper doses, have undoubtedly an action of this kind. The first and the last of these medicines, especially, have long been in this country the chief resources of the physician in the treatment of chronic hepatic disorders. The marked temporary benefit often resulting from mercury given for this effect has, from the difficulty of distinguishing the various diseases of the liver, and the consequent indiscriminate use of the drug, led to great evils. This medicine was at one time, by English practitioners, given almost indiscriminately, and long persevered in, for disorders of digestion, many of which did not depend on fault of the liver at all, but on local disease of the stomach or intestines, or on faulty assimilation, the result of debility, which the prolonged use of the mercury but too often increased. Of late, these evils have much abated; but still, before the real nature of the disease is ascertained, mercury is often tried in cancer, and other incurable organic diseases of the liver, in which this and other powerful and lowering remedies can only do harm.

Pepper, ginger, and other hot spices, are also supposed, and perhaps justly, to render the liver more active and increase the secretion of bile. The great relish with which they are eaten by our countrymen in the East and West Indies gives considerable sanction to this opinion.

Most purgatives, especially rhubarb and senna, have perhaps an effect of the same kind, and may fitly be styled, in the language of our fathers, *cholagogues*. Many persons have succeeded in warding off bilious attacks to which they had been long subject, by taking habitually before dinner a few grains of rhubarb. A rhubarb pill will often relieve a slight bilious disorder, even before it has purged.

We may suppose these medicines to excite the secretion of the liver, either by virtue of the impression they make on the stomach and duodenum, or by their becoming absorbed in the stomach and intestines, and subsequently excreted by the liver. Spices probably act chiefly in the former way, and excite the secretion and flow of bile, as they do that of saliva, by the impression they make on the mucous membrane adjacent. Mercury, iodine, and other medicines, probably excite the secretion of the liver chiefly, if not solely, by becoming absorbed into the blood, and passing out of the system with the bile.

We have, indeed, little positive evidence in favor of this theory, by regarding the liver merely, because not many analyses of any kind have been made of human bile, and very few attempts have been made to discover different medicines in it.

Autenrieth and Zeller[1] state that they found mercury in the bile of animals treated by mercurial frictions; and copper, derived probably from cooking utensils and food, has often been detected in human bile and gall-stones. Bouisson[2] states, that the coloring principles of madder and some other substances pass off in the

[1] Bouisson, p. 14, who takes this fact from Reil's Archiv. fur die Physiologie, vol. viii. p. 252; 1807, 1808.

[2] Bouisson, p. 303.

bile; a fact which, if established, would lead us to expect that some principles of rhubarb, senna, and taraxacum might pass off in it likewise. Iodide of potassium and prussiate of potash have been injected into the blood of animals, and been subsequently detected in the bile.[1]

Most medicines that act as diuretics are no doubt excreted by the kidneys. Nitre, iodide of potassium, asparagus, and most other medicines of diuretic action, for which we have chemical tests, or which we can detect by our senses, have been found in the urine. The active principle of squills, our chief expectorant, probably passes off by the lungs, for all the onion tribe, of which squills is one, taint the breath. It would seem, indeed, not only that most medicines that increase the secretion of a gland pass out of the system through it, but conversely, that nearly everything foreign to its own secretion, that drains off through a gland or mucous membrane, excites its secreting function.[2]

Medicines that pass off in this way through a gland, not only increase its activity, but may also alter the qualities of the secretion, and act directly on the surfaces over which the secretion passes; and when the secretion is unhealthy, or these surfaces are diseased, these latter effects of the medicines may be far more important than the first.

We have examples of this in the efficacy of alkalies in preventing the deposit of lithic gravel in the urine; and in that of the balsams and of various vegetable astringents, in certain diseases of the bladder and urethra. As might have been expected, our knowledge of the effects of different medicines on the qualities of the bile, and on the mucous membrane of the gall-bladder and gall-ducts, is very scanty. We cannot ascertain during life the composition of the bile, and of course cannot tell in what way, or in what degree, our medicines change it. But there are, unquestionably, medicines which do change it. Experience long ago led physicians to infer that if some medicines, as mercury, owe their chief virtue, in hepatic disorders, to their increasing the quantity of the bile, there are others, whose chief merit consists in their altering its quality. Alkalies, especially soda, ether, and turpen-

[1] Bernard, Leçons, 1854–5, p. 301.

[2] On the same principle, undoubtedly, various abnormal matters that find their way into the portal blood, cause sudden and copious fluxes of bile.

tine, have been supposed to render the bile thinner, and have, on this account, been at various times recommended as remedies for gall-stones. Hitherto, it has been impossible to fix the value of medicines of this class. They are given empirically, generally with a vague notion only of what is amiss; and according to the chances of individual experience, or the fashion of the day, are rated at one time much above their worth, and at another time, in effect probably of this very over-estimate, are altogether discarded.

Medicines which alter the urine, or act on the bladder or urethra, have more permanent favor, because, from being always able to collect and analyze the urine, we have better opportunities of fixing their value.

CHAPTER I.

CONGESTION OF THE LIVER.

Congestion of the liver from impediment to the flow of blood through the lungs or heart—Effects of this—Congestion from other causes—Hemorrhage.

ONE of the simplest morbid conditions of the liver is *Congestion*—that is, an undue accumulation of blood in the capillary vessels.

Congestion of the liver, as of other organs that have an active function, may arise from various causes, and be, if we may so speak, of different kinds. The simplest kind, and which may therefore be fitly considered first, is that which results from some mechanical impediment to the return of blood through the veins to the heart.

Examples of congestion arising from this cause are most frequently met with in persons with organic disease of the valves on the left side of the heart. In such persons it often happens that when the circulation becomes much impeded the liver grows larger, so that its edge can be felt two or three inches below the false ribs. If the circulation be relieved by bleeding, or by diuretics, or by rest, the liver returns to its former size. This enlargement, from what may be termed *passive* congestion, often takes place, and again subsides, very rapidly, according to the varying conditions of the general circulation.

Without any unnatural impediment to the passage of the blood through the chest, a transient congestion of the liver of this kind is produced in man by running, or other violent bodily exertion. Under the influence of such exertion the circulation is very much quickened, more blood is brought to the liver than can pass readily through its dense plexus of capillary vessels, and the liver becomes gorged with blood. This happens especially after meals, when the vessels of the portal system are charged with the products of digestion, and when more blood is detained in the liver by the activity of its secreting function. The gorged state of the vessels of the liver impedes the passage of blood through the splenic vein, and thus leads to temporary engorgement of the spleen. It has been conjectured that this rapid and transient engorgement of the liver is the cause of the stitch in the side which fast running so commonly causes. In horses, dogs, and other animals, made for fast running, there is, as Bernard has pointed out,[1] a special provision to meet this emergency. Some vessels of considerable size pass directly from the trunk of the portal vein to the vena cava, so that some of the blood of the portal vein can enter the general current of the vena cava without traversing the capillary plexus of the liver.

Enlargement of the liver from passive congestion is, in general, unattended with pain, and the only complaint made by the patient is of a sense of weight or fulness in the right hypochondrium. The turgid state of the capillary vessels in the lobular substance of the liver, and the slowness of the current through them, must, however, tend to lessen the functional activity of the liver, and it impedes the elimination of bile, so that it often happens that after a few days the symptoms above mentioned are succeeded by a sallowness of the complexion, which, in some cases, passes into decided jaundice—the jaundice, like the enlargement, soon disappearing when the general circulation is relieved.

In all organs, a state of congestion produces analogous effects. The unnatural fulness of the capillary vessels, and the slowness of the current through them, lessens the activity of the nutritive processes, and causes the organ to do less of its proper work, and do it more slowly. If the brain be congested, the sensations are blunted, volition is less vigorous, and the mental power is diminished; if the lungs be congested, the exhalation of carbonic acid is lessened; if the kidney be congested, the urine is more scanty; if a muscle be kept congested, it soon tires, and only slowly recovers its fatigue.

It is, then, in accordance with a general law, that when the liver is kept in a state of passive congestion, the secretion of bile is diminished. The jaundice in such cases does not, however, seem

[1] Leçons de Physiologie, 1854–5, p. 164.

to depend on diminished activity of the secreting cells, but rather on impediment to the passage of bile from the lobules and through the small gall-ducts, caused by the pressure exerted upon the ducts by a gorged state of the bloodvessels. When the liver is examined after death, it frequently contains not only an unusual quantity of blood, but also, as was remarked by Mr. Kiernan, an accumulation of biliary matter in the lobular substance.

This *biliary congestion*, as Mr. Kiernan termed it, like the gorged state of the bloodvessels, of course tends to increase the size of the organ.

Enlargement of the liver must take place in some measure in all cases where the vessels are turgid, but the degree of enlargement will depend on the time the congestion has lasted, and on the previous condition of the organ. The longer the vessels are kept distended, and the more yielding the surrounding tissues, the greater, of course, will be the enlargement. In young persons, and in persons in whom the liver is healthy and its capsule thin, it will necessarily enlarge much more for a given force of distension, than in persons in opposite circumstances. When, in consequence of an interstitial deposit of lymph, the liver has become unnaturally firm and tough, an impediment to the free passage of the blood from it towards the heart, unless it be long continued, will produce but little increase of its size; but will cause the same, or even greater, pressure on the other elements of its texture, and be as apt, therefore, or even more apt, to cause secondary biliary congestion.

The changes in the appearance and texture of the liver produced by congestion are such as these considerations would lead us to expect. The liver, from the turgid state of its bloodvessels, is more or less enlarged, somewhat more friable than it otherwise would be, and of a deep red color: the central portions of the lobules having, however, a deeper hue than the marginal portions. Occasionally, the liver is at the same time in a state of biliary congestion, and, in consequence, if any portions of the lobules be uninjected, they have a deeper yellowish or greenish hue than is natural to them. If the biliary congestion be long kept up, the function of the cells in the congested lobules is arrested, or rendered less active, and the cells seem to become impaired in their vitality and powers of reproduction: the liver is thus permanently injured in its secreting element. Now and then, in persons who die of valvular disease of the heart of long standing, the liver is found much diminished in size and weight, without presenting any marks of inflammation or other striking change; and this may occur in persons who have led temperate lives—where, consequently, the atrophy can only be explained by the influence which the long-continued congestion has had in impairing the functional activity and nutrition of the cells. The wasted condition of the muscles of the legs that so constantly results from serious valvular disease of the heart affords another and familiar example of atrophy thus produced.

Andral, and many other writers, have remarked that congestion of the liver from impeded circulation through the chest, when long continued, often leads to organic disease; and they have thus accounted for the frequent association of organic disease of the liver with organic disease of the heart. The changes in the liver really attributable to disease of the heart consist, at first, in distension of the capillary bloodvessels, and in accumulation of biliary matter in the lobules, resulting from impediment to its escape through the small gall-ducts. If this impediment be kept up, the biliary matter, as long as there are cells enough to separate it from the blood, goes on accumulating faster than it can escape; but whenever the cells are long prevented from discharging their contents, they seem to lose their fertility, and consequently diminish in number. In another chapter cases will be related where from the passage of bile through the common gall-duct having been long stopped, the liver had entirely lost its lobular appearance, and contained no nucleated cells in the lobules—so that when a portion of it was examined under the microscope nothing was seen but free oil-globules and irregular particles of greenish or yellow biliary matter.

Many writers have stated that disease of the heart produces *cirrhosis* of the liver; meaning by that term the hardened and granular state of the liver so frequently found in drunkards, which is caused by the interstitial deposit of fibrin from adhesive inflammation, and which often, like congestion of the liver, leads to accumulation of biliary matter in the lobules, by impeding its escape through the small gall-ducts. But disease of the heart does not of itself lead to this form of disease, or, indeed, to *inflammation* of any kind. Among the many persons who die in our hospitals of diseased heart consequent on rheumatic fever, the liver is seldom found tough and granular from the presence of foreign fibrous tissue, except in such of them as have drunk spirits to excess. But although disease of the heart does not directly lead to inflammation of the liver, it yet, by causing more or less stagnation of the blood in the capillaries of the liver, gives greater effect to spirituous liquors, or to any other deleterious agent that is absorbed from the intestinal canal, and thus mixed with the portal blood. This point will be again noticed in a subsequent chapter on Adhesive Inflammation of the Liver.

Congestion of the liver, from mechanical impediment to the onward current of the blood, is generally brought under our notice, not as a disease of itself, but as a consequence and a complication of valvular disease of the heart, or of some other condition that prevents the free passage of the blood through the chest. But although a secondary disorder, its results are very important. If it continue long, it leads to bilious contamination of the blood, often already impure by defective action of the lungs and the kidneys; and in other ways much aggravates the condition of the patient.

The congestion of the liver may be relieved directly by general or local bleeding, or by medicines, such as sulphate of magnesia and bitartrate of potash, which cause a copious drain from the portal system of veins; and, indirectly, by medicines, such as small doses of blue pill, which increase the secretion of bile. In cases of dropsy from disease of the heart, when the liver is gorged and the complexion sallow, small doses of blue pill, in conjunction with diuretics or purgatives, are often productive of extraordinary benefit.

Under such circumstances, it is almost needless to remark, it is very important that the patient should take very sparingly of fermented drinks, and abstain from rich dishes, and, indeed, from all articles of food likely to add to the congestion of the liver.

Hitherto we have considered only that kind of congestion which results from mechanical hindrance to the backward current of the venous blood. But congestion—that is, undue accumulation of blood in the vessels—may result from totally different conditions.

The large vessels serve merely as channels to convey to the different tissues of the body the blood from which the materials of their nutrition are drawn. The process of nutrition is dependent on a mutual affinity between the blood and the tissues, by virtue of which each part withdraws from the blood, through the thin walls of the capillary vessels, those materials which its proper nutrition requires: and the equable distribution of the blood through the body depends not merely on its more obvious conditions—on the propulsive power of the heart, on the suction power of respiration, and on there being a free passage for it through the arteries and the veins—but also on this mutual action, or affinity, between the blood and the tissues, which is being constantly exerted in every part of the body as long as its nutrition continues. Modifications of this affinity, leading to congestion, or undue fulness of the vessels, may result from changes either in the tissues or in the blood. Thus, if a part be injured in any way—if the skin be cut, or a bone be broken—provided the vitality of the tissues be not destroyed, there is immediately set up a process of inflammation, or of repair, and one of the first results of this process is an increased flow of blood to the part, and a turgid state of its vessels. So, again, if any part be the seat of a cancer, or of any other morbid growth, there is, at once, by virtue of this increased and faulty nutrition of the tissues, an increased flow of blood to the part, and, after a time, the vessels of that part are found to have grown larger. So, indeed, it is generally: wherever an important vital process is going on, there is an increased flow of blood to the part, and a congestion, if it may be so termed, or an accumulation of blood in the vessels, by which the vital action is maintained. And there can be no doubt that this increased flow of blood, and this turgescence of the vessels, is secondary to the vital action, and the result of it; and that it is caused by the modification of the affinity between the blood and the tissues which the action in question produces.

Congestion of the liver originating in changes in its tissues need not detain us here. It is a mere concomitant of the process of inflammation, or of the growth of a cancer, or of some other structural change, and belongs, therefore, to those conditions—conditions which will be considered in subsequent chapters. But, as already observed, congestion may result, not only from a change in the tissues which the blood nourishes, but also from a change in the blood itself. All abnormal changes in the relation of the blood to any organ affect the circulation through that organ. Foreign matters in the blood, which are eliminated by a gland, necessarily affect in some way or other the circulation through it—sometimes causing a more active nutrition of the gland, and thus increasing its functional activity—sometimes causing more or less stagnation, and consequently accumulation, of blood in the capillary vessels, and thus arresting or diminishing its function. If the natural elements, even, of any secretion, be in undue quantity in the blood, they may lead to a state of congestion of the secreting organ. All this is strikingly illustrated by the kidney. Diuretic medicines, when given in proper doses, like the natural constituents of the urinary secretion, cause, for a time, more active nutrition of the kidney, and increase the quantity of urine. Other foreign matters, and, indeed, these same diuretic medicines in too large doses, and even the natural elements of the secretion when in undue quantity, clog the kidney, by leading to more or less stagnation of blood in the capillary vessels; and the congestion so produced has the same effect as congestion caused by mechanical hindrance to the return of the venous blood, and leads to hemorrhage from the kidney. The liver, from its situation and office, is peculiarly exposed to congestion from such causes. All the matters absorbed by the bloodvessels in the intestinal canal have to pass through it. Its lobular substance is the first filter, if we may so term it, through which the impure liquid must strain. All the alcoholic drinks, all the noxious ingredients that may chance to be present in our food, and such hurtful products of faulty digestion as are readily soluble, are immediately—before they have been diffused throughout the whole mass of the blood, and before they have been submitted to the influence of oxygen—carried to the liver, and more or less influence the circulation through it. Without any excesses in diet the liver, in accordance with the general law just stated, contains much more blood after meals, when the products of digestion are conveyed to it and its secreting functions are actively performed. Amid the continual excesses at table of persons in the middle and upper classes of society an immense variety of noxious matters find their way into the portal blood that should never be present in it; and the mischief which this is calculated to produce is enhanced by indolent or sedentary habits. The consequence often is, that the liver becomes habitually gorged. The same, or even worse effects, result in the lower classes of our larger towns, from their inordinate consumption of gin and porter.

Different persons are, of course, affected in different degrees by excesses of this kind. Persons of large frame, with active respiration, engaged in active pursuits, and who, from natural conformation, have a vigorous liver, can indulge almost with impunity in habits that would be fatal to others.

The congestion of the liver we are now considering has the same effects as the congestion produced by impediment to the return of venous blood to the heart. It causes enlargement of the liver, a sense of fulness and of weight in the right hypochondrium, and, after a time, by diminishing the secreting activity of the liver, and by impeding the passage of bile through the small gall-ducts, causes also a bilious tinge of the complexion, which, in some cases, passes into decided jaundice. These disorders are, of course, often accompanied by disorders of other organs, and by such derangement of the general health as the faulty habits of life mentioned above are apt to engender. If the congestion be long kept up, it seems permanently to impair, like the simpler kind of congestion we have before considered, the vitality and the power of reproduction of the secreting cells: and thus permanently lessens the power of the organ, and in some degree changes its structure.

In congestion of the liver so produced, great benefit results from saline purgatives, especially the sulphate of magnesia or of soda, in conjunction with senna; from occasional small doses of blue pill; from active exercise, and exposure to the fresh air—especially horse exercise, which combines exercise of the most exhilarating kind, with free exposure to the air—and from a restricted diet. Under the influence of such measures, the congested state of the liver speedily subsides; the bile is secreted more abundantly, and flows more freely; the sallowness of complexion disappears; and if the congestion have not lasted long enough to cause permanent damage to the liver, the health, as far as this organ is concerned, is restored.

The articles of food which tend most to clog the liver—from which, therefore, persons with congestion of the liver should most carefully abstain—are rich dishes and fermented liquors; which, like the organic principles of bile, contain a large proportion of hydrogen and carbon.

Congestion of the liver from unhealthy states of the blood now and then occurs in other circumstances. Thus, in the hot state of ague, in some instances, great congestion of the liver, as of the spleen, comes on rapidly, and again rapidly subsides when the fit of ague is past.

Congestion so produced, like the forms of congestion already considered, causes more or less enlargement of the liver, but is of too short duration to give a tinge of yellow to the skin.

We have most efficient means of preventing this kind of congestion in quinine and the other antidotes to the marsh poison.

Congestion of the liver occasionally results from other morbid states of the blood, the nature of which is unknown, and which have not been traced to their source. In a person dead of purpura hæmorrhagica, I have found the liver and the spleen very large, and of the dark color of a Morello cherry, from the great quantity of blood they contained. From the researches of M. Andral, it would seem that a great diminution in the proportion of the fibrin in the blood is an occasional cause of such congestions.

There is reason to believe that, independently of any primary change in the blood or in the tissues of the liver, the current of blood through the liver may also be modified and a state of congestion be induced by causes of disturbance which have their origin in the nervous system;[1] but, at present, our knowledge on this subject is very vague.

Nothing has yet been said of hemorrhage of the liver as a result of congestion. Hemorrhage is a common result of congestion in many other organs, but in the liver it is extremely rare. Now and then, however, it does occur; more especially, according to the observations of Rokitansky, in children, when the liver is much congested from suffocative catarrh, or some other condition that impedes the passage of the blood through the chest. The hemorrhage may take place in the substance of the liver or at its surface, or in both situations at once. When it takes place in the substance of the liver it may cause but little pain, and do but little other mischief. After a time, the blood, like blood effused elsewhere, is absorbed, and no sign of the accident remains; or the only sign of it that remains is a scar, the origin of which can seldom be traced. The hemorrhage thus escapes detection. When hemorrhage takes place at the surface of the liver, the blood may collect under the

[1] It has been shown by Bernard that irritation of the floor of the fourth ventricle, while it increases the production of sugar in the liver, causes increased vascularity of it; that the apoplectic state increases the various secretions, and therefore the vascular fulness of the secreting organs; and that division of the sympathetic nerve in the neck in rabbits immediately causes persisting vascular congestion of the corresponding side of the head.

capsule, and form a palpable tumor; or may even rupture the investing membranes, and thus become effused into the peritoneal sac. It then, of necessity, causes much pain and tenderness, which are more or less widely diffused, according to the nature of the injury. The pain and tenderness are, however, seldom of long continuance. The effused blood does not inflame the serous membrane, and, in consequence, the pain and tenderness disappear entirely, or much abate, in the course of a few days.

Hemorrhage of the liver may result from other conditions. A few years ago, through the kindness of Mr. Busk, I had an opportunity of examining the liver of a man who died of apoplexy, from softening of the brain, in the last stage of granular disease of the kidney, and in whom profuse hemorrhage of the liver occurred six weeks before death, in consequence, as it seemed, of some excess in eating and drinking. The symptoms resulting from this hemorrhage were intense and continuous pain and tenderness in the epigastric region, and in the left side of the belly. The pain abated much at the end of two days, and soon ceased to excite complaint: but some degree of tenderness remained almost up to the time of death. Two days after the accession of these symptoms a deeply-seated, firm, tender tumor was detected in the epigastric region. At some subsequent examinations this tumor was felt, but it seemed to have diminished in size.

The liver was of natural size, although the left lobe was larger in proportion than usual, and descended in front of the stomach, so that it could be felt in the epigastrium during life. It had no unusual adhesions to the surrounding parts. The surface was of natural color and appearance, except in two places; one on the inferior surface of the left lobe, and the other on the anterior part of the convex surface of the right lobe. In these two places, the proper capsule of the gland was separated from its substance by very firm coagula, which in some parts presented the appearance of the fibrinous laminæ met with in aneurismal sacs, while other portions of the coagula were more recent.

The clot on the convex surface of the right lobe occupied a space about four inches in diameter, and was about half an inch thick in the middle. The clot under the left lobe was not quite so large, but was thicker, and the capsule of the liver by which it was covered had been ruptured towards the anterior edge of the liver, during life; and, in consequence of this rent, blood had been effused in considerable quantity in the peritoneal sac. This effused blood formed moulded coagula of various sizes, and of various degrees of firmness and decoloration, as if they were of various dates. A large mass of this kind, remarkably firm, was situated between the liver and the stomach, which was very small, and completely hidden by the liver and coagula.

The substance of the liver and the gall-bladder appeared to be sound.

In such a case as that just related it seems impossible to recognize hemorrhage of the liver during the life of the patient. The symptoms, indeed, correspond exactly to the nature of the injury; but there were no circumstances that rendered such an injury probable. When, however—as from disease of the heart, or in a fit of ague—the liver is known to be greatly congested, and when there is no reason to presume that it is the seat of any other organic disease, such a train of symptoms as that mentioned above might, perhaps, lead to the suspicion, or even justify the opinion, that hemorrhage had occurred; but, as already observed, such an event, under any circumstances, is very rare.

CHAPTER II.

INFLAMMATORY DISEASES OF THE LIVER.

SECT. I.—*General Remarks on the Classification of Inflammatory Diseases of the Liver—Suppurative Inflammation and Abscess of the Liver.*

THE inflammatory diseases of the liver are usually divided into *acute* and *chronic;* but this division is essentially faulty in practice, because the terms are applied, not with reference to the kind of inflammation or the rapidity with which it works its effects, but to the severity, merely, of the local symptoms. Now, inflammation of the liver running rapidly into abscess, if deep-seated and of small extent, may give rise to but few and obscure local symptoms, and would consequently be styled *chronic* during the life of the patient; while inflammation involving the surface of the liver, even when causing the slow effusion of coagulable lymph only, will be attended with well-marked local symptoms—with great pain and tenderness—and would be termed *acute.*

We shall never have faithful descriptions of inflammatory diseases, or unerring rules for their treatment, until we arrange them, not according to their mere outward characters or the prominence of particular symptoms, but according to the nature of their causes; for it is a truth that cannot be too strongly enforced, that it is the nature of the *cause* of an inflammatory disease that mainly determines its course and character and the influence of remedies over it.

To take, for example, the inflammatory diseases of the knee-joint:—

If inflammation of the synovial membrane of the knee-joint be excited by a penetrating wound and the consequent admission of air, it causes speedy suppuration, and generally destroys the joint.

If it be occasioned by the presence of pus in the blood, it is attended with very little effusion and swelling; but, as in the former case, it leads to the formation of pus; and that so soon, and with such slight local symptoms, that pathologists have even inferred that the pus, instead of being formed by a process of inflammation in the joint, is actually deposited there, ready made, from the blood.

If the inflammation be excited by the peculiar cause of rheumatism, it is attended with severe pain, and often with much effusion; but the fluid effused is never purulent, and is almost always absorbed after some days, leaving the motions of the joint free and its structure uninjured.

If the inflammation be gouty, it is attended with still more severe pain and with greater effusion; but the fluid effused here differs in quality from the fluid effused in rheumatism, and when its aqueous part is absorbed, particles of lithate of soda are often left on the synovial membrane, and in the areolar tissue about the joint. These, perhaps by mechanical irritation, occasion fresh attacks of inflammation, which lead to fresh deposits of lithate of soda, and, at length, the joint is completely crippled.

If the inflammation be excited by the specific poison of gonorrhœa, it is attended, like gouty inflammation, with abundant effusion, which distends the synovial capsule, and causes great swelling. There is seldom much pain or fever, but the disease is very obstinate—the swelling, in spite of all the remedies we yet know of, often lasting weeks or months.

Thus we may have—to take the last two examples—to treat two cases of inflamed knee. The appearance of the joint is exactly alike in the two cases, and in both there is great swelling from fluid effused into the synovial capsule. We give colchicum in both; in one case the inflammation rapidly subsides under the remedy, and the effused fluid is quickly absorbed; in the other the malady pursues its course as if nothing had been done. And why this difference? The parts affected are the same, and the changes, in outward appearance, exactly alike in the two cases. One might readily be mistaken for the other. The reason is simply this—the morbid changes are, in one case, the effect of the specific principle of gout; in the other, that of the poison of gonorrhœa; and although they are alike in the two cases in those characters that most strike the eye—in the distension of vessels and the effusion of fluid—they differ in more essential particulars.

The instance here adduced is a simple one, but every department of pathology abounds with illustrations of the same truth; thus leading to the conviction that we can never foresee clearly the result of an inflammatory disease, or foretell the effect of our remedies on it, unless we have ascertained its cause, or know at least the particular character of the inflammation. It is, in a great measure, our ignorance of the causes and particular characters of the diseases we have to treat that renders the practice of medicine so uncertain.

At present it would be premature to attempt to arrange the inflammatory diseases of the liver with reference solely to their causes; but, as the nature of the cause mainly determines the character of the inflammation and its mode of termination, some approximation to such an arrangement will be obtained by classing them according to their effects. I propose, therefore, to range the inflammatory diseases of the liver under the following heads:—

1st. *Suppurative* inflammation, or that which leads to suppuration and abscess;

2d. *Gangrenous* inflammation;

3d. *Adhesive* inflammation, or inflammation that causes effusion of coagulable lymph;

4th. Inflammation of the veins of the liver;

5th. Inflammation of the gall-bladder and gall-ducts;

And to consider, as far as our present knowledge permits, the various causes of these different forms of inflammation, and the modification of each form according to the particular cause that excites it. In following out this plan, I shall speak first of the causes of that form of inflammation of the liver which leads to suppuration and abscess.

Suppurative Inflammation and Abscess of the Liver.

With the view of discovering the causes of inflammation of the liver that leads to suppuration and abscess, I have tabulated the chief circumstances of sixty-two cases in which one or more abscesses were found in the liver after death. Seventeen of these cases occurred in my own practice—fifteen at the Seamen's Hospital, in sailors, most of whom had been in the East, and two in King's College Hospital; sixteen are published in the works of

Andral[1] and Louis,[2] and were most of them collected in the hospitals of Paris; and twenty-nine are recorded in the splendid work by Annesley, on the Diseases of India.

In the following remarks frequent reference will be made to these cases.

The most obvious cause of abscess of the liver, and which may therefore be fitly placed first, is—

1st. A blow, or other mechanical injury. But this is by no means a frequent cause. In the sixty-two cases of abscess of the liver to which I have alluded, there is only one—a case recorded by Andral—in which the disease was clearly traced to a blow. In this case (*Clin. Med.*, tom. iv. obs. xxviii.) there were two large abscesses on the convex surface of the right lobe—the usual seat, probably, of abscesses produced in this way.

The rarity of inflammation and abscess from accidental injury shows how effectually the liver, when of its natural size, is shielded by the ribs.[3]

2d. A second and far more frequent cause of abscess of the liver is suppurative inflammation of some vein and the consequent contamination of the blood by pus.

Very soon after morbid anatomy began to be studied, it was noticed that, in persons who die some days after a severe injury or surgical operation, there are often collections of pus in the lungs, the liver, the joints, between the muscles, and in various other parts of the body. These collections of pus form very rapidly—in some cases in three or four days—and often with very slight local symptoms; and, when occurring in the lung, are strictly circumscribed, or immediately surrounded by perfectly healthy pulmonary tissue. These circumstances suggested the notion—at one time generally received and still held by some eminent pathologists—that the pus is not formed by a process of inflammation in the parts in which we find it, but that it is all brought with the blood from the original seat of injury and merely *deposited* in those parts. The abscesses

[1] Clinique Médicale, t. iv.

[2] Mémoires ou Recherches Anatomico-pathologiques sur diverses maladies.

[3] Since the analysis in the text was made, I have been consulted by a gentleman in whom an abscess of the liver resulted from a blow received through a fall in hunting; and notes of another case in which abscesses of the liver seemed to have resulted from a blow have been kindly sent me by my friend, Mr. Erlin Clark. The strange thing is that the event is not of more frequent occurrence.

found in the lungs and liver in such cases have in consequence been very generally spoken of as *deposits* of pus.

An examination of pus through the microscope is sufficient to show that it cannot be deposited in the way supposed. Pus-globules are larger than blood-globules, and therefore could not escape bodily from the vessels without the blood-globules escaping as well. This circumstance is perhaps of itself sufficient proof that the pus of these scattered abscesses is not simply *deposited* from the blood, but that it is formed, as in other cases, by a process of inflammation in the parts in which we find it.

Other and more conclusive evidence on this point has been furnished by the researches of MM. Dance and Cruveilhier. They have shown that although in most of such cases fully formed abscesses immediately surrounded by perfectly healthy pulmonary tissue exist in the lungs after death, yet in other cases in which death happens earlier, instead of abscesses there are small circumscribed, indurated, or hepatized masses. In some instances the abscesses are formed in succession, so that in the same lung there may be found all intermediate stages between commencing induration, or hepatization, of a small circumscribed portion of the pulmonary tissue and a small circumscribed abscess. This circumstance, indeed, did not escape the observation of Morgagni,[1] whose sagacity nearly led him to the discovery of what at present seems to be the true mode of formation of these abscesses.[2]

He inferred that pus carried to the viscera from distant parts is

[1] Speaking of abscesses of the same kind that result from injuries of the head, Morgagni says—

"Fac enim relegas quas tibi novissimè descripsi, Valsalvæ observationes. Nempe tubercula plerumque invenies sive in pulmonibus, sive in ipso etiam jecore non omnia fuisse suppurata, quin plura interdum glandulosi corporis firmitudinem adhuc referentia. Quid? si ægro moriente, necdum ulla essent quæ pus habere inciperent." (Epist. li. art. 23.)

[2] His words are—

"Videtur autem secundum eas observationes, quibuscum, ut puto, Molli nellii conjungi potest observatio, pus in viscera aliunde invectum, non puris forma semper deponi, sed haud raro saltem nonnullas ejus particulas cum sanguine permistas, et prorsus disjunctas, in angustiis quibusdam, fortasse glandularum lymphaticarum, hærere, easque, ut in venereorum bubonum productione fit, obstruendo, aut irritando, eoque humores præterituros retinendo distendere, et multo copiosioris quam quod advectum est, puris generationi, a rigoribus illis, et horroribus significatæ, causam præbere. Qua ratione illud quoque intelligitur, quomodo multo plus puris in visceribus, et caveis corporis sæpe deprehendatur, quam modicum vulnus dare potuisset."

not always deposited as pus, but that often some of its globules become arrested in the narrow channels of the body, and there, by obstruction or irritation, cause congestion, and give occasion to the formation of a much greater quantity of pus than is brought there by the blood.

The mode of formation of these abscesses is well illustrated by an experiment made more than half a century ago by Dr. Saunders, and related by him in his admirable work on the structure and diseases of the liver. He injected ʒij of quicksilver into the crural vein of a dog. No ill effects were observed the first day, but at the end of this the dog became feverish, and after two or three days had cough and difficulty of breathing, which continued until its death. On examination after death, Dr. Saunders found the lungs studded with small indurated masses, which he calls tubercles, and small circumscribed abscesses. In the centre of each was a small globule of mercury.

Here the globules of mercury, like the globules of pus in suppurative phlebitis, became arrested in the capillary vessels of the lungs, and each globule, acting perhaps by mere mechanical irritation, caused circumscribed inflammation and abscess. The inflammation was circumscribed because the irritation that excited it acted only at particular points.

In the dog experimented on by Dr. Saunders the lungs were the only organs in which abscesses were found. The reason of this is obvious. All the mercury conveyed directly to the lungs became arrested in their capillaries. No globules passed through to cause inflammation and abscess of other organs.

In the same way, in some cases of suppurative phlebitis consequent on injury of the head or limbs or on amputation, abscesses are found in the lungs only; and they are usually found in the lungs in greater number than in other internal organs. After the lungs, the liver is the organ in which they are most frequent—a circumstance attributable in some measure to the large quantity of blood that flows to the liver, and to the slowness of the current through its capillary network, but perhaps still more to those vital or other attractions by which matters of particular composition are there detained and excreted.

In the liver the abscesses are often scattered, as in the lungs, but they are usually larger and less regular in their outline—a consequence, it would seem, of the anatomical fact noticed by Mr. Bowman, that the lobules of the liver are not distinct bodies, separated from each other by a layer of areolar tissue, but that their capillaries form a continuous network throughout the entire organ.

For a long time it was strongly objected to the doctrine that the scattered abscesses consequent on injuries and surgical operations are formed in the way here supposed, that in many such cases no inflamed vein can be detected after death. This objection was much weakened by the important observation made by Mr. Arnott, that the effects of suppurative phlebitis bear no relation to the size of the vein or to the extent of the portion inflamed, and that even in cases rapidly fatal the portion of vein inflamed is often very small. Mr. Arnott infers, no doubt rightly, that in many cases we fail to discover the source of the mischief on account of the small size of the vein or the small extent of the portion inflamed.

Another important observation has been made by Cruveilhier, which almost entirely removes the objection I have stated. It is that, after operations or injuries, where a bone has been divided or broken, the portion of vein inflamed, the source of the subsequent mischief, is often within the bone. He maintains that operations and injuries that involve bones are those most frequently followed by scattered abscesses, and that inflammation of the veins in the interior of bones is more apt to cause them than inflammation of the veins of other textures. He accounts for this by the circumstance that the vascular canals of bone cannot collapse like the vessels of other textures, and further supports his opinion by the following experiments:—

The marrow was removed from the thigh-bone of a dog, and mercury put in its place. At the end of five days the dog died, and the mercury was found strewed through the lungs. Each globule was the centre of a small hepatized mass. (*Cruv.*, liv. xi.)

In another dog, a single globule of mercury was placed in the medullary cavity of the femur. A month afterwards it was found in the lungs, divided into many very small globules, each the centre of a small abscess.

The observation of Cruveilhier, that injuries which involve bones are those most frequently followed by scattered abscesses, includes, as a particular instance, the fact, long ago noticed, that injuries of the head are often followed by abscesses of the liver. From the researches of Mr. Arnott in this country, and of MM. Dance and

Cruveilhier in France, no doubt remains that the abscesses in such cases result from suppurative inflammation of a vein, either in the soft parts or between the tables of the skull.

Many false theories of the mode of formation of the abscesses of the liver, consequent on injuries of the head, have been maintained under the erroneous impression that abscesses exist in the liver only. It was, however, long ago remarked by Morgagni that, in these cases, there are often abscesses in the lungs, heart, spleen, and other organs, as well as in the liver. The abscesses in the liver attracted more attention than those in the lungs, on account, perhaps, of their larger size, and of their being more conspicuous from the stronger contrast between the color of pus and the natural color of the organ.

There is a close analogy between the secondary abscesses from phlebitis and secondary masses of cancer.

A cancer of the breast may be the source of cancerous tumors in the lungs and liver, just as an inflamed vein in the arm may be the source of abscesses in the same parts. The abscesses and the secondary cancerous tumors will be scattered in the same manner, and immediately surrounded by healthy pulmonary or hepatic tissue. The lungs and the liver are the organs in which secondary cancerous tumors, as well as the abscesses from phlebitis, are most frequent. The cancerous tumors and the abscesses have in each organ the same form and seat; and, in the lungs, both have a great predilection for the surface.

These points of resemblance can hardly be explained, except on the supposition that the germs of the two diseases—cancer-cells and pus-globules—are disseminated in the same manner through the veins.

It may be considered then established, that the abscesses which form in the liver and other organs, after surgical operations and injuries of the head or limbs, are owing to suppurative inflammation of a vein and the consequent contamination of the blood by pus. The globules of pus, mingled with the blood, are conveyed to the capillary vessels of the lungs, and, it would seem, by becoming mechanically arrested there, excite each circumscribed inflammation and abscess. If any of the globules pass through the capillaries of the lungs to the left side of the heart, they are sent in the arterial current to other organs, and becoming arrested in the capillaries of these organs, excite, as in the lungs, inflammation of limited extent, rapidly passing on to abscess.

These scattered abscesses are most commonly found after operations or injuries, because suppurative inflammation of the inner surface of a vein is most commonly caused by mechanical injury of its coats; but they may obviously result from suppurative phlebitis set up in any other way. I have met with two instances in which scattered abscesses in various organs seemed to result from a collection of pus that had formed, from some cause which I could not discover, between the periosteum and bone of the upper arm; another instance, in which their source was probably a large tuberculous cavity in the lungs.

Perhaps, then, we are justified in concluding in all cases in which we find collections of pus rapidly formed in different parts of the body, that the immediate cause of these scattered inflammations is some irritating substance conveyed there by the blood; and in most of the cases where the abscesses in the lungs are small and circumscribed, that this irritating substance is pus, derived from inflammation of the inner surface of a vein.

In cases in which we cannot find the inflamed vein, the facts, that the abscesses are scattered in the same way, and occupy the very same anatomical seat as in those cases in which the source of the pus is known—that this kind of dissemination and the anatomical seat occupied are also the same as in the case of injected mercury and secondary cancer—are conclusive in showing that the agent arrives by the blood, and almost conclusive, when abscesses are found in the lungs, that this agent is a pus-globule.

The proportion of cases of this kind, in a given number of cases of abscess of the liver, will, of course, vary with the frequency of abscess of the liver from other causes.

In India, where other powerful causes of abscess of the liver are in operation, the proportion will be small. In the cases published by Annesley, there is not one that we can, from his description, place in this category.

In the seventeen cases that have fallen under my own care in the Seamen's Hospital and in King's College Hospital, there is only one that clearly belongs to this head. In that instance abscess of the liver, with abscesses of the lungs and collections of pus in various joints, resulted from phlebitis caused by the operation of bleeding.

In sixteen cases collected by Louis and Andral, in Paris, where abscess of the liver from other causes is less frequent, there are four which may be placed in this category; one, in which the abscesses were consequent on venesection (Louis, *Obs.* 2); another in which they were consequent on childbirth (Louis, *Obs.* 1); a third (Andral, *Obs.* 23) where with abscesses of the liver there were lobular pneumonia of the left lung, gray hepatization of the right, and pus between the vertebral column and pharynx: a fourth (Andral, *Obs.* 26) in which there was gray hepatization of the lower lobe of the left lung, and pus in the mediastinum.

As yet, I have alluded only to inflammation of those veins that return their blood immediately to the vena cava, in which case the pus formed in the inflamed vein is at once conveyed to the capillaries of the lungs. Sometimes it is all arrested there, and abscesses form in the lungs only. More generally, however, some of the pus passes through the capillaries of the lungs to be distributed with the arterial current, and abscesses, though commonly still most numerous in the lungs, are found also in other parts of the body. But when pus is formed in one of the veins that feed the vena portæ, it will be carried directly to the liver, *will generally all be arrested in the close plexus of capillary vessels that goes to make up its lobular substance*, and abscesses will be found in the liver only. The liver, from the closeness of the vascular network in its lobular substance, or from the affinities which are there at work, has a remarkable power to arrest and to fix or eliminate foreign substances conveyed to it by the blood. Cruveilhier found, that if mercury be injected into one of the veins that feed the vena portæ, it will be stopped in its course through the liver, and will cause circumscribed abscesses there, just as it does in the lungs when injected into the crural vein.

He injected mercury into one of the mesenteric veins of a dog. At the end of twenty-four hours the dog died, and the surface of the liver was found sprinkled with small spots of a deep red color, which extended four or five lines into its substance. In the centre of each of these red masses was a small globule of mercury. (*Cruv.*, liv. xi.)

In another instance, having met with a dog having an umbilical omental hernia, he injected mercury into one of the small veins of the omentum. The dog was killed about ten weeks after, and the liver found studded with a countless number of what Cruveilhier calls tubercles, in the centre of each of which was a globule of mercury.

Some of these tubercles had two distinct layers: the outer, albuminous or tuberculous; the inner, puriform.

In these two experiments the different stages of suppurative inflammation are seen. At first, there is a spot of a deep red color; this passes to suppuration and abscess; and the matter of this abscess, acting as a source of irritation, excites around it inflammation of a kind which leads to effusion of albumen or fibrin, and thus forms a cyst for the matter.

The veins that feed the vena portæ are little exposed to accidental injury, but some of their branches are divided in operations on the rectum and for strangulated hernia; and, as might have been anticipated, these operations are sometimes followed by abscess of the liver.

Cruveilhier relates a case where abscesses of the liver were immediately consequent on repeated attempts to return a prolapsed rectum.

The patient, a man of sixty, had been subject to prolapsus many years. The bowel protruded at the first effort to empty it, but was usually returned without difficulty. When he sought assistance on the last occasion, it had been down twenty-four hours, and was replaced only after repeated and violent attempts, which gave him much pain.

The same day the expression of his countenance altered, and his pulse became small and unequal. He soon fell into a state of prostration, with a cold skin, vomiting, hiccough, stupor, but without pain, and died on the fifth day.

A great number of small abscesses, some superficial, others deep-seated, were found in the liver. The hepatic tissue for a short distance round each of them was of a brown slate-color, and softened. (*Cruv.*, liv. xvi.)

Dance mentions a case in which abscesses formed rapidly in the liver after an operation for cancer of the rectum, where cauterization was practised: another, in which they were consequent on a simple operation for fistula; and two others, in which they followed the operation for strangulated hernia, where a portion of irreducible omentum suppurated externally. (*Archives Générales*, t. xix. p. 172.)

Since the publication of the second edition of this work, Dr. J. Jackson, formerly of Calcutta, has sent me notes of three cases, in which abscesses of the liver that proved fatal seemed to have resulted in Europeans in India from operations for the removal of piles.

There can be little doubt that in most of these cases, if not in all, the abscesses in the liver were the consequence of phlebitis caused by the operations.

It is an important circumstance, and one to which I shall again have to refer, that in none of the cases were abscesses noticed in other organs. The pus furnished by the inflamed veins was, it would seem, all stopped in its passage through the liver; and abscesses formed in the liver only.[1]

3d. The consideration of these cases leads us naturally to a third cause—I believe by far the most frequent cause—of abscess of the liver: namely, ulceration of the large intestine, or, more generally, of the intestines, the stomach, the gall-bladder, or gall-ducts—parts which return their blood to the portal vein, to be thence transmitted through the capillaries of the liver.

A connection between abscess of the liver and dysentery has long been noticed, but the two diseases are associated far more frequently than has been generally imagined. Of the twenty-nine cases recorded by Annesley, there are twenty-one, or nearly three-fourths, in which there were ulcers, more or less extensive, in the large intestine; and two other cases in which the large intestine was contracted or strictured, in consequence, no doubt, of dysentery at some former period. It is not unlikely that in some of the remaining cases ulceration of the intestines existed but was not noticed.

Of the fifteen fatal cases which fell under my own observation at the Seamen's Hospital, the state of the intestines was not noticed in two. In eight of the remaining thirteen cases there were ulcers

[1] In some instances the abscesses in the liver may cause inflammation of the hepatic vein, and thence disease of the lung, or some pus may traverse vessels establishing a direct communication between the portal vein and the vena cava. According to Bernard a free communication of this kind exists in the horse and some other animals made for running, and is not entirely wanting in man.—Bernard, *Leçons de Physiologie Experimentale*, 1855, p. 165.

in the larger intestines, and, in one other case, two ulcers in the stomach; so that, in nine of thirteen cases, or in nearly three-fourths, there were ulcers in the large intestine or stomach. In another of these cases, without ulceration of the stomach or intestine, there was ulceration of the common gall-duct.

Of the two cases that have fallen under my care in King's College Hospital, the abscess of the liver was associated with dysentery in both. Yet the condition of the two patients, in other respects, was very different. One of them was a man who had served seven years in the army in India, and who became affected with dysentery in that country; the other, a poor woman who had long lived in London, and whose disease came on in this city.

In the sixteen cases collected by Andral and Louis, who seem not to have suspected any connection between abscess of the liver and ulcerated intestine, ulcers are noticed in the large intestine and in the lower end of the ileum, in two cases;[1] in the lower end of the ileum only, in one case;[2] in the stomach, in four cases;[3] in the gall-bladder, in one case.[4]

In one of the cases in which the stomach was ulcerated, the ulcer communicated with the abscess, which was in the left lobe of the liver. It is fair to conclude, as Andral does, that in this case (Andral, *Obs.* 31) the ulcer was caused by the abscess opening into the stomach. Excluding this case, there are still seven cases out of fifteen, in which there was ulceration of some part of the extensive mucous surface that returns its blood to the portal vein.

The fact will appear still stronger, if we recollect, that in one of these sixteen cases the abscess of the liver was caused by a blow; that in four others it seemed the consequence of phlebitis; and that in none of these five cases were there any ulcers in the stomach, intestines, or gall-bladder. So that in seven out of eleven cases, in which the abscesses were not the consequence of a blow or of general phlebitis, there was ulceration of the stomach, the small or large intestine, or the gall-bladder.

It is impossible to suppose that this is a mere coincidence of diseases having no relation to each other. In another of these eleven cases (Andral, *Obs.* 32) the abscess of the liver was obviously consequent on chronic disease of the stomach, and after death, the

[1] Andral, Obs. 25; Louis, Obs. 3.
[2] Andral, Obs. 24.
[3] Andral, Obs. 27, 30, and 31; Louis, Obs. 4.
[4] Louis, Obs. 5.

lining membrane of the stomach was found in some parts so softened as to resemble liquid mucus. In this last case, and in the three cases in which there was an ulcer in the stomach, the state of the large intestine is not noticed.

Here, again, I may adduce, as a further support to my position, the analogy of cancer. Cancer of the stomach is frequently followed by disseminated cancerous tumors in the liver, and in no other organ. In a subsequent chapter I shall refer to numerous instances of this kind from those storehouses of pathology—the *Clinique Médicale* of Andral, and the *Anatomie Pathologique* of Cruveilhier. It would seem that cancer cells, like pus-globules, usually, if not always, become arrested in the liver, and do not pass through to become the germs of cancerous tumors in other organs.

The association of dysentery with abscess of the liver is noticed by most physicians who have treated of either of those diseases.

Dr. Cheyne, speaking of the dysentery of Ireland, says, that in the majority of his dissections the liver was apparently sound; but that in two cases he found abscesses in its substance. (*Dublin Hospital Reports*, vol. iii.)

In two of the four cases of abscess of the liver, published by Dr. Abercrombie, there were ulcers in the large intestine.[1] It is remarkable that Dr. Abercrombie should have considered the association of the two diseases accidental. He says: "Dysentery is often accompanied by diseases of neighboring organs, especially the liver, in which are found in some cases abscesses, and in the protracted cases chronic induration. These are to be regarded as accidental combinations, though they may considerably modify the symptoms." (*Diseases of the Stomach*, &c., 2d edition, p. 266.)

Annesley, much struck with the frequent association of the two diseases, and impressed with the importance of establishing their true relation, confesses his inability to do so. He supposes that, in some cases, the abscess is consequent on the dysentery; that, in others, the dysentery is the mere consequence of the disease of the liver; while, in a third order of cases, the disease of the liver and that of the larger intestine are coeval, or so nearly coeval, that it is almost impossible to decide which had priority. (*Annesley*, vol. ii. p. 199.) And, indeed, in India, it must be extremely difficult to discover the relation between the two diseases, on account of the

[1] Diseases of Stomach, &c.; 2d edition: cases 93 and 130.

great prevalence of other disorders of the liver that are not easily distinguished from abscess during the life of the patient.

In the cases that fell under my own care in the Seamen's Hospital I experienced the same difficulty, and generally found it impossible to tell, from the history of the case, which had priority—the disease of the liver or the dysentery.

In some cases, however, it was impossible to resist the conclusion, that the abscess of the liver was not only consequent on the dysentery, but caused by it.

On the 12th of March, 1838, four men, Brown, Flett, Crere, and Davies, were brought into the hospital from the same vessel, the *Renown*, in a dreadful state of dysentery. The *Renown* had just come from Calcutta, and had lost many of her crew from dysentery between Calcutta and the Cape. At the Cape, having but five men before the mast remaining, she shipped seven fresh hands, among whom were Brown, Flett, Davies, and Crere, at that time in perfect health. Some of the original crew continued to suffer from dysentery after leaving the Cape, but these new hands had good health until, between the Western Islands and the Channel, when they had got into cold weather, they were attacked, one after another, with dysentery of the most severe kind. Two of these men died soon after their admission to the hospital; the others recovered sufficiently to leave it.

In the two fatal cases, I found the state of the large intestine exactly the same. From the ileo-cæcal valve to the rectum, the mucous membrane was almost entirely destroyed by sloughing. In one of these cases, the liver contained three small abscesses, not encysted, and evidently quite recent; in the other, the liver, as far as I could then judge, was perfectly healthy.

Now, the primary disease in the two cases was obviously the same, produced by the same cause; and as disease of the liver was only found in one of them, we must infer that it was secondary, the consequence of the dysentery. Among many cases of dysentery, there may be only one in which abscesses form in the liver, just as among many cases of amputation or of injury of the head, there may be only one in which abscesses form in the lungs and other organs.

In another case that fell under my care in the Seamen's Hospital, the patient had dysentery at the Isle of France. The violent symptoms subsided after two months, and he continued his work for four years. At the end of that time, while on his passage home from the East, diarrhœa recurred, and he had, for the first time, pain in the right side and shoulder. These symptoms had lasted three months, when he was brought into the hospital. He died soon afterwards.

On examination, I found a superficial abscess on the convex surface of the right lobe of the liver. The mucous membrane of the small intestine was quite healthy to within two inches of the ileo-cæcal valve. Immediately above that valve were three ulcers (the largest about the breadth of half a crown), in most part of which the muscular coat of the intestine was laid bare. In their immediate vicinity were many other ulcers, about the size of smallpox marks, which had not eaten through the mucous membrane. The mucous membrane about these ulcers was not softened or unusually vascular. In the cæcum was a single ulcer, the size of a crown-piece, having the same appearance as the larger ulcers in the small intestine. The mucous membrane in the whole cæcum was much softened; in the rest of the large intestine, it was in all respects healthy. The mesenteric glands in the neighborhood of the cæcum were enlarged, and softened to a pulp, of a pinkish color. There was no ulceration of the stomach or gall-bladder; no enlargement of the patches of Peyer or of the solitary glands of the small intestine.

The sequence of events, in this case, seemed to be dysentery, which had left a few chronic ulcers in the cæcum and lower end of the small intestine; at the end of four years, recurrence of dysenteric symptoms; inflammation and abscess of the liver. The abscess of the liver clearly dated from the recurrence of the dysenteric symptoms, when the patient first felt pain referable to the liver. An abscess so superficial could not have existed without manifest symptoms.[1]

If the liver-disease had been the cause of the dysentery, it would, in all probability, have produced more extensive ulceration. Irritating bile might cause ulcers of the large intestine, and scattered ulcers, but it could hardly affect, so exclusively, such a small portion of the gut.

I might adduce other instances, which I should, perhaps, weary

[1] Compare this case with Obs. 25 of Andral, where suppurative inflammation of the liver occurred in the course of chronic enteritis.

the reader by relating, in which there could be little doubt that the abscesses in the liver were secondary to dysentery.

We are led, then, to the conclusion, admitted by Annesley, that abscess of the liver is in some cases consequent on dysentery, and caused by it.

The question now arises: Is it not so caused in all the cases, or in most of the cases, in which the two diseases are associated?

Annesley thought not, from the circumstance that, in India, the symptoms of liver-disease sometimes appear as soon as those of dysentery; in other cases, even before them.

The circumstance that the symptoms of liver-disease appear as soon, or nearly as soon, as those of the dysentery, does not prove that the former disease is not dependent on the latter. In the case above cited from Cruveilhier, in which abscesses in the liver were caused by the rough handling of a prolapsed rectum, the symptoms commenced almost immediately after the injury, and at the end of five days, when the man died, the matter in the abscesses was fully formed. After an amputation or injury, inflammation of a vein may occur, pass on to suppuration, and contaminate the system, in less than forty-eight hours. Supposing, then, the suppurative inflammation of the liver to be excited in the same way in dysentery, it might be expected that its symptoms would, in some cases, appear almost as soon as those of the primary disease.

But, in India, it sometimes happens that the symptoms of liver-disease precede those of dysentery. This, also, is what might have been expected.

In India, derangements of the liver, consisting in excessive and perhaps vitiated secretion of bile and inflammation of the gall-ducts, are very common; the consequence, it would seem, of the heat of the climate and the free living in which the English in India indulge.

Adhesive inflammation of the liver, terminating in induration and cirrhosis, is also very common there, as in this country, from spirit-drinking. Now, although neither of these disorders may terminate in suppurative inflammation of the liver and abscess, yet they present nearly the same symptoms, and may be readily mistaken for it. If, then, a person with any such derangement of the liver should be taken with dysentery, and have abscess of the liver in consequence, it is very natural that the dysentery should be ascribed to pre-existing suppurative inflammation of the liver.[1]

If the explanation I have offered be rejected, we are almost driven to conclude, as Annesley does, that the dysentery in these last cases is caused by the passage of irritating bile. Now, if this were the case, we should expect to find the most evident marks of disease in the gall-ducts and the upper part of the small intestine—parts with which the irritating secretion comes first in contact; but, instead of this, these parts are almost always perfectly healthy in cases in which abscess of the liver is associated with the most destructive forms of dysentery. The whole of the large intestine may be a complete slough, while the gall-bladder and gall-ducts and the small intestine almost down, or even quite down, to the ileo-cæcal valve, are perfectly healthy, and the bile in the gall-bladder is of its natural consistence and color. Annesley, indeed, makes a distinction between what he calls *simple* dysentery and *hepatic* dysentery; and states that in simple dysentery, or dysentery unconnected with liver-disease, the inflammation of the large intestine generally stops abruptly at the ileo-cæcal valve, while in *hepatic* dysentery the lower part of the small intestine is often inflamed as well as the large intestine. He believes that in the latter cases the small intestines become diseased from the irritating quality of the bile. Annesley is right in stating that in dysentery connected with abscess of the liver, the lower extremity of the ileum is often found diseased as well as the large intestine. It was so in five of the fifteen fatal cases of abscess of the liver I treated at the Seamen's Hospital, but it not unfrequently presents just the same marks of disease in cases of simple dysentery.

I have met with many cases of simple dysentery in which the ulceration of the bowel did not stop short at the ileo-cæcal valve, but extended twelve or eighteen inches up the small intestine. Cruveilhier has given a plate in which this is very faithfully represented; and in three out of eight cases of simple dysentery, in which Annesley has given an account of the dissections (vol. ii. Cases 172, 173, 179), the lower end of the ileum was diseased as well as the large intestine.

The proper reading of these facts seems to be, that the disease

[1] Cases 71, 75, 77, of Annesley, are probably examples of this sequence—chronic disease of the liver, dysentery, abscess of the liver.

of the bowel in dysentery is, in some cases, strictly limited to the large intestine, while in others it creeps a little way up the small intestine; in some cases, it causes abscess of the liver, in others not.

In no case, whether of simple or hepatic dysentery, is the upper part of the small intestine ulcerated. The ulcers of the small intestine, if any exist, are always near the ileo-cæcal valve.

There can be no doubt that a copious flow of irritating bile may cause diarrhœa, and may prevent the ulcers of dysentery from healing; it may, perhaps, cause ulceration of the bowel; but it is very improbable that it causes the early and extensive ulceration and gangrene of the large intestine, which occurs in Asiatic dysentery, and often destroys life in a few days, while the small intestine, almost in its entire length, remains perfectly healthy.

The more probable explanation is that which I have before given; namely, that in these cases the patient had some derangement of the functions of the liver, which was followed by dysentery, and then by abscess; and, consequently, that in all the cases, or most of the cases, in which abscess of the liver and dysentery are associated, the former disease is the consequence of the latter.

If irritating bile cause ulceration of the intestine, it may be the remote cause of abscess of the liver, through the disorder it first occasions in the intestine.

Admitting dysentery, or ulceration of the bowel, to be a source of abscess of the liver, it is obvious that the liver does not become involved by spreading of the inflammation, but through injury to the nervous filaments of the sympathetic, or, which is much more likely, by some contamination of the portal blood.

The portal blood may be contaminated either by *pus*, formed by suppurative inflammation of one of the small intestinal veins; or by matter of other kind resulting from softening of the tissues; or by the fetid gaseous and liquid contents of the large intestine in dysentery, which must be absorbed and conveyed immediately to the liver. It seems probable that contamination of the first kind usually gives rise to small scattered abscesses; of the last, to diffuse inflammation, and a larger, perhaps single, collection of pus. If the morbid matter be such that it does not mix readily with the blood —as globules of pus or mercury—it will cause small, circumscribed abscesses, the rest of the liver being healthy. If, on the contrary, the morbid matter be readily diffusible in the blood, all the blood will be vitiated, and diffuse inflammation result, which may or may not be suppurative, according to the quality or concentration of the contaminating matter and the general state of nutrition at the time. In the course of dysentery the liver is very generally disordered, and congestion of it and inflammation that does not go on to suppuration not unfrequently occur.

The admission of this explanation of the relation of abscess of the liver to dysentery, would lead us to expect that abscess of the liver might occasionally be consequent on ulceration of the stomach or gall-bladder—parts which, like the larger intestine, return their blood to the portal vein—and this is found to be the case.

It has been already remarked that in the sixteen cases of abscess of the liver recorded by Andral and Louis, there are three in which the stomach was found ulcerated, without any ulceration being noticed in the intestines or gall-bladder.

In the first of these cases (Andral, *Obs.* 27), the patient, a man about forty-one years of age, died of ulcerated cancer of the stomach. The liver was enlarged, and contained scattered through it a great number of small, firm, red masses, the result, it was supposed, of partial inflammations. In the centre of one of these red masses was an abscess the size of a hazel-nut.

In another of these cases (Andral, *Obs.* 30), the patient, a man about sixty, had presented for a considerable time the symptoms of chronic gastritis—loss of appetite, vomiting, sour eructations, and a sense of weight at the epigastrium. He became sallow, and lost strength and flesh. He was somewhat benefited by milk diet and soothing measures, when, all at once, his pulse became frequent, he fell into a state of prostration, with a brown tongue, and died at the end of some days.

The coats of the stomach, for the breadth of five or six fingers in front of the pylorus, were much thickened; the mucous membrane was ulcerated; and, in place of the underlying coats, there was a uniform gristly substance of a dead white color.

The stomach was united to the liver by bands of false membrane.

The liver was of its usual size. In the left lobe was a cavity the size of a small apple, filled with pus, and lined by a thick and tough membrane. The hepatic tissue surrounding the abscess was in a state of gangrene.

In this case, the abscess of the liver could not have caused the ulcer of the stomach ; but the ulcer may fairly be presumed to have been the cause of the abscess. The abscess had existed for some time. The state of prostration marked the occurrence of gangrene about it.

In the third case (Louis, *Obs.* 4), the patient, a man of fifty, had had for four years disordered digestion, irregular appetite, occasional slight pains in the left hypochondrium, now and then nausea and purging, and frequent alternations of leanness and moderate *embonpoint.* Seventeen days before his admission to the hospital he became much worse than usual, and a set of new symptoms appeared—heat of skin, jaundice, complete loss of appetite, severe pain at the epigastrium, and in the left hypochondrium, and slight oppression. These symptoms continued, and for the last eight days he had, besides, purging and some nausea. He died a fortnight after he entered the hospital.

The liver was somewhat larger than natural, and contained a great number of small abscesses lined by a thin and soft false membrane. Its tissue was softened throughout.

The gall-bladder was small, and obliterated at its neck. The cystic duct contained a gall-stone. The coats of the gall-bladder and cystic duct were much indurated and thickened; the hepatic duct and the ductus communis perfectly healthy.

In the portion of the stomach intermediate to the splenic and pyloric extremities, the mucous membrane was thicker than natural, and presented many deep ulcers three or four lines in breadth.

Here, as in the former cases, we cannot ascribe the ulcers in the stomach to the disease of the liver, but the abscesses in the liver may be fairly attributed to the disease of the stomach. There was likewise, indeed, disease of the gall-bladder and cystic duct; but this, which was of long standing, presented no marks of recent activity, whereas it was obvious that the abscesses in the liver were of recent date.

In another case by Andral (Andral, *Obs.* 32), to which I have already alluded, an abscess of the liver was found associated with *softening* of the mucous membrane of the stomach.

Here, symptoms of disease of the stomach had lasted eighteen months before the patient had any symptoms of disease of the liver. The circumstance that the abscess was not encysted goes to prove that it was of recent date.

In the *Provincial Medical Journal* for December 3, 1842, the case of a man is related who died at the age of forty-eight, with ulcerated cancer of the stomach. The liver contained seven or eight abscesses.

In the *Medical Gazette* for Nov. 24, 1843, there are two cases by Dr. Seymour, where a simple ulcer of the stomach had caused circumscribed abscess of the peritoneum. The patients were young maid-servants. In one, there was a large abscess in the upper part of the right lobe of the liver, which, during life, had burst through the diaphragm into the lung.

I am indebted to the kindness of Dr. Addison for the case of a man who died under his care in Guy's Hospital, in 1849, with ulceration of the mucous membrane of the duodenum, from colloid cancer, involving the head of the pancreas and the contiguous portion of the gut. In the liver, which had no other organic disease, were several phlegmonous looking abscesses, one of which had opened, a few days before death, through the lung.

Ulceration of the gall-bladder or gall-ducts seems just as efficient as ulceration of the stomach in causing abscess of the liver.

I would cite, as a probable example of this, the last case given by M. Louis (Louis, *Obs.* 5). The liver contained from thirty to forty abscesses, varying from the size of a pea to that of a filbert, not encysted, and evidently of recent formation. There was no ulceration of the stomach or intestines, but in the gall-bladder, which contained some small calculi, there were six round ulcers—three superficial and three deep. The mucous membrane of the gall-bladder was three times as thick as it should be.

A case very similar to this is given by Dr. Bright in the first volume of *Guy's Hospital Reports* (p. 630); gall-stones, ulceration of the gall-bladder, numerous abscesses in the liver.

With these cases may be classed one of the cases I had to treat at the Seamen's Hospital.

The patient, aged 33, was brought into the hospital on the 2d of December, immediately on his return from Quebec. At Quebec he had ague, and this was succeeded, three weeks before his admission, by jaundice and pain below the ensiform cartilage. The jaundice continued, but he had gained strength, when, on the 26th of January, just eight weeks after he was brought into the hospital, he was suddenly seized with symptoms of peritonitis, which carried him off in four days.

On the convex surface of the right lobe of the liver was a large irregular abscess, lined by a buff-colored, and moderately firm, false membrane.

The gall-bladder was firmly adherent to the duodenum, and its coats were thickened. Its cavity, which was no larger than a hazel-nut, was filled by a yellow, friable gall-stone, having a firm, dark-green nucleus. The cystic duct was much dilated, and contained a similar gall-stone, the size of a small bean. The common duct was also much dilated, and communicated with the duodenum by an ulcerated opening rather larger than a split pea, about two or three lines from the natural termination of the duct. The hepatic ducts were very large, and were readily traced a long way into the liver. There was no ulceration of the stomach or of the intestines, with the exception of this ulcerated opening in the duodenum, which, as well as the dilatation of the ducts behind and the jaundice, was, no doubt, caused by a gall-stone which had stuck for some time in the common duct, and then passed, by ulceration, into the bowel.

In 1847, a liver, in which numerous small scattered abscesses formed in sequel to disease of the gall-bladder and gall-stones, was presented to the Pathological Society of Birmingham, by Dr. Mackay, and was afterwards sent to me, together with notes of the case, by Dr. James Russel, who was at that time secretary of the Society.

The patient, a lusty woman, 64 years of age, previously in good health, was seized with pain at the pit of the stomach, attended with some fever. The pain yielded to purgatives, but two or three days afterwards recurred with greater severity, attended, as before, with fever, but not with vomiting, or with other signs of the passing of a gall-stone. The epigastrium was now tender, and the liver was found to be enlarged. Leeches and a blister were applied to the side, and purgatives, and afterwards, for two days, calomel and opium were given. At the end of a week, the pain, and tenderness, and fever, had ceased. Jaundice, attended with complete absence of bile in the intestinal discharges, then came on, and continued till her death, which happened three weeks afterwards from gradual sinking, without the occurrence of rigors, or of any other striking symptom, excepting the jaundice. The liver contained numerous small scattered abscesses, evidently recently formed; and other circumscribed portions of its substance were softened, but not yet broken down into abscess. The hepatic duct, just above its junction with the cystic, was blocked up by a gall-stone, the size of a hazel-nut, which was plainly the cause of the jaundice. The gall-bladder was much thickened, and partially ossified;

and a portion of its inner surface was in a state of slough. It contained no gall-stones.

To these cases may be added a case for which I am indebted to Mr. Bowman, and which is given at length in another chapter. A large hydatid cyst opened into the gall-bladder. In a remote part of the liver was a small abscess. There was no ulceration of the stomach or intestines.

In the twenty-nine cases related by Annesley, to which I have so often referred, there are, as I have already remarked, twenty-three in which there were ulcers, or the scars of ulcers, in the large intestine. In four only, of these twenty-three cases, does Annesley notice any morbid change in the gall-bladder or gall-ducts, while he remarks it in three of the remaining six cases.

In one of these three cases (Case 81), the gall-bladder was very small, and seemed to be divided by a stricture in the centre.

In another (Case 93), the common duct was much compressed and obstructed, by enlargement and hardening of the pancreas, which completely enveloped it. On laying open the cystic duct, the mouth of the gall-bladder was found much constricted by a cartilaginous band. The intestines, small and large, were quite sound.

In the third case (Case 126), the gall-bladder completely adhered to the wall of the abscess, and communicated with it. The ducts were impervious, being involved in the adhesive inflammation of the parts that bounded the abscess; and the bile secreted by the liver was either retained in the abscess or discharged by the wound. (The abscess had been opened.) There was no other appearance of disease in any of the viscera.

Abercrombie, in his work on Diseases of the Stomach, &c., has given four fatal cases of abscess of the liver. In two of these cases, to which I have already referred (Cases 93 and 130), there were numerous deep ulcers in the large intestine, but no mention is made of disease of the gall-bladder or gall-ducts, or of gall-stones; in the other two cases (Cases 128 and 129), there were large or numerous gall-stones in the hepatic or common ducts, or in the gall-bladder, but there was no disease of the intestinal canal. In the latter cases, the gall-stones, probably by causing ulceration of the ducts, seem to have taken the place of the ulcerated intestine, in setting up suppurative inflammation of the liver.

The gall-ducts, the gall-bladder, and the capsule of the liver, are nourished by the hepatic artery, and blood flows, not from the portal vein to them, but from them to the portal vein. This circumstance explains how ulceration of the gall-bladder, like ulceration of the stomach or intestines, may cause abscess of the liver, and it also explains the fact, noticed by many physicians who have written on abscess of the liver, that, in this disease, the gall-bladder, the large ducts, and the capsule, are seldom involved. The suppurative inflammation is confined to those parts of the liver that receive blood from the portal vein. The frequent absence of every trace of inflammation of the capsule, in cases of abscess of the liver, has been expressly noticed by Annesley and by Dr. Stokes, as very important in reference to treatment.

Having collected instances of abscess of the liver apparently originating in a vitiated state of the blood brought from the mucous surfaces that feed the portal vein, we require, to complete our catalogue of abscesses of the liver produced by contamination of the portal blood, other instances in which the contaminating matter is brought by the splenic vein. My friend, Mr. Busk, has furnished me with notes of the appearances after death in a case which seems to have been of this kind.

The liver contained a great number of abscesses, about the size of walnuts, containing thick white pus. The intermediate hepatic substance did not seem inflamed. It was pale, firm, and of natural appearance.

The splenic vein was much dilated. The branches by which it arises from the spleen, and all that part of it which runs on the pancreas, were inflamed, and contained a puriform fluid and an irregular deposit of lymph.

A large portion of the spleen was pale, and partially separated as a gangrenous mass from the rest of the organ, which was of a deep red color, and very soft.

There were no ulcers in the intestines; no abscesses anywhere but in the liver.

The most probable supposition is, that the disease in this case originated in the spleen, that the splenic vein subsequently became inflamed, and that the disseminated abscesses in the liver were caused by the noxious matter brought to it by the vein. If this matter were pus, we have another instance of pus brought in large quantity to the portal vein being all arrested in its passage through the liver.

A curious and striking illustration of the principles maintained in the preceding pages is afforded by a case which fell under my care in King's College Hospital, in the spring of 1849, in which scattered abscesses of the liver resulted from the accidental rupture of an hydatid cyst. On account of its singularity, I have not included this case with those of which an analysis has been given above.

The patient, a large and very muscular man, a pugilist, while boxing with the gloves, was felled by a blow from the fist under the right false ribs. He was in good health before, but from that time had continuous pain in the right side, and was never, to use his own expression, *the same man again*. About six weeks after the blow, the pain in the right side became suddenly severe, and this fresh accession of pain was soon followed by headache and nausea, without actual vomiting. He lost his appetite, grew weak and languid, and his bowels became much relaxed. These symptoms persisted, and at the end of two days he noticed that his skin was yellow. The diarrhœa ceased, but the headache and nausea continued, and the jaundice grew deeper. On the 4th of April, five days after the occurrence of the jaundice, and about seven weeks after receiving the blow, he was brought into King's College Hospital, under my care.

At that time he was deeply jaundiced, and complained of severe pain, with much tenderness, in the right hypochondrium. The belly was distended, and the liver was considerably enlarged, extending a hand's-breadth below the false ribs. These symptoms were attended with much fever. The skin was hot and dry; the tongue dry, fissured, and deeply furred; and the pulse above 100. He had no appetite, and much thirst, and felt drowsy, and complained of headache and nausea.

The disease was considered to be active inflammation of the liver, the result of the blow. Leeches were applied to the side, which produced for a short time some alleviation of the pain and tenderness; and he was further treated by salines, and small doses of blue-pill, with occasional purgatives.

The mouth was made sore by the blue-pill, but no amendment took place. The pain and tenderness of the side, the fever, and the jaundice, continued; the liver grew somewhat larger, and the patient often complained much of pain in the right shoulder and down the right arm. The pulse was always rapid, and the tongue dry and furred. Notwithstanding the deep jaundice, the discharges from the bowels were stained with bile.

On the 16th of April, twelve days after his admission to the hospital, the liver extended two or three inches below the umbilicus on the right side, and when the hand was placed there a distinct creaking was felt. On listening there, a rubbing sound, like that of pleurisy, was heard. The other symptoms were just the same as before.

The next morning he was just in the same state: but at 3 P. M. he was found by the clinical clerk very much worse, complaining of great pain at the epigastrium, with an anxious expression, breathing very quickly, with a rapid and very feeble pulse, and bathed in a cold, clammy sweat. He gradually sank, and died at 10 P. M.

On examination, the liver was found greatly enlarged; extending on the right side as low as the umbilicus. Its surface was covered with soft lymph, but there were no marks of peritonitis elsewhere in the belly.

On raising the liver, a clot of blood was found in the epigastric region, and on withdrawing this, I pulled out with it a large hydatid cyst, which must have escaped from its sac, entirely or in part, before death. The cyst was collapsed, and contained no small hydatids.

The sac from which the cyst came was situated on the under surface of the liver, between the right and left lobes, was as large as a shaddock, and was full of clotted blood. Its walls were unusually thin for a hydatid tumor of that size. In the substance of the liver were a great number of abscesses, varying in size from a small pea to a large walnut, the pus of which had an orange or yellow tinge. All these abscesses were in the neighborhood of the hydatid cyst, and in the upper portion of the liver between the cyst and the diaphragm. There were none in all the lower portions of the right lobe.

Interspersed with these abscesses were small spots, some having a yellow tinge, others of a dark brown.

On examining sections of the liver under water, it was evident that the morbid change, which ended in suppuration, had commenced in the lobules. In the first stage of disease the lobules were of a dark brownish color. In a subsequent stage they had a deep yellow tinge, which continued until they were broken down by the suppurative process, when the yellow tinge was communicated to the pus. (See plate iii. fig. 1.) The hepatic and portal canals and vessels, as far as could be ascertained, were in a healthy condition.

A microscopic examination of the lobules (in making which I had the assistance of my friend, Dr. Johnson) confirmed the inpression which had been given by inspection with the naked eye.

1. In many of the lobules, whose color and general appearance were natural, the hepatic cells had their usual characters: they were of the normal size, their nuclei were distinct, and they had the usual appearance of granular biliary matter and oil-globules, little, if at all, exceeding the healthy standard.

2. In the dark-brown lobules the cells appeared to be more crowded, as if from a process of rapid cell-formation; and they were, many of them, smaller than in the healthy lobules. In addition to this, many of them presented an unusual appearance: they were remarkably opaque, and seemed to be filled with solid matter, which in some cells had a glistening, whitish appearance (without any oil or biliary matter). In these cells no nucleus was visible.

3. In the lobules, which had a decided yellow tinge, some cells had the appearances described above: others contained a large amount of deep yellow biliary matter, and there was a quantity of the same matter free (not contained in cells) and mixed with pus-corpuscles and oil-globules.

In the larger abscesses the pus was more abundant in proportion, being mixed with yellow biliary matter, oil-globules, and amorphous particles, which were probably the débris of hepatic cells and of broken-down tissue.

From the history of the case, and from the situation of the abscesses in the neighborhood of the hydatid tumor and in the upper portion of the liver between this and the diaphragm, there can be no doubt that the series of changes above described resulted from the injury done to the hydatid tumor. The probable explanation of these changes is, that the hydatid cyst was ruptured by the blow, or by blood afterwards effused into the sac which contained it, and that the proper fluid of the cyst was then gradually absorbed and carried with the portal blood to the lobules. It there led to a modification of the secreting cells, by which an effort was made to eliminate it, and subsequently to the suppurative process.

It may at first seem improbable that such serious mischief should be caused by the fluid of an hydatid cyst, which is limpid and colorless as the purest water, and which, on chemical analysis, is found to consist of little more than water holding common salt in solution. But, as will be seen in a subsequent chapter, this fluid, simple as it may seem, is very irritating to particular tissues. When by the bursting of an hydatid tumor, it is effused into the peritoneal sac, it sets up peritonitis almost as severe and as rapidly fatal as that which results from the bursting of the gall-bladder or of an abscess.

An old encysted abscess of the liver may also give rise, through ulceration of the walls of its sac, to a fresh crop of scattered abscesses. My attention has been called to a case which, if I am not mistaken, was of this kind.

A circumstance strongly confirmatory of the view I have taken of the different sources of abscess of the liver in the cases that have been adduced, is, that not more than one of these probable sources existed in the same subject. Where the abscess could be traced to a blow or to suppurative inflammation of some vein that returns its blood immediately to the vena cava, there were no ulcers in the stomach, intestines, gall-bladder, or gall-ducts. When ulcers were found in the intestines, by which the occurrence of abscess in the liver could be explained, there were no ulcers in the stomach or gall-bladder. When the stomach was ulcerated, there were no ulcers in the intestines or in the passages of the bile. When there were ulcers in the gall-bladder or gall-ducts, there were none in any part of the intestinal canal.

It is not, perhaps, every form of ulceration of the stomach and intestines that gives rise to abscess of the liver. I have never seen abscess of the liver noticed in conjunction with ulcerated intestine, in fatal cases of typhoid fever. This fact is very striking when we consider how prevalent and fatal typhoid fever is; how generally it is attended with extensive ulceration of the bowels; and how attentively all the morbid appearances in this disease have been observed and recorded, of late years, in this country and in France.

Abscess of the liver is not noticed in any of the cases (ten in number) of ulceration of the duodenum after burns given by Mr. Curling in his paper in the *Med. Chir. Trans.*, for 1842. It is very rare in conjunction with ulceration of the intestine in phthisis. In two of the cases given by Andral, in which abscess of the liver was associated with ulceration of the intestines, there were tubercles in the lungs, and the ulcers were probably of tuberculous origin. But these form an insignificant proportion in the immense number of fatal cases of phthisis with ulcerated intestines in which the morbid appearances have been observed and recorded. It is also rarely consequent on simple ulcer of the stomach. The only instance I have met with of this sort is the case already cited from Dr. Seymour.

Abscess of the liver seems to occur chiefly in conjunction with the sloughing ulceration in acute dysentery and with chronic ulcers, attended with thickening and induration of the submucous areolar tissue. In the latter cases, the inflammation of the liver occurs on some exacerbation of the gastric or dysenteric symptoms. It occurs also occasionally in conjunction with ulceration resulting from cancer.

The causes that have here been assigned for abscess of the liver will, I believe, be found to apply to a great majority of cases—at least, of the cases that are met with in this country. There will remain, then, if I am right in my conclusions, but few cases that require us to admit the agency of other conditions.

Yet various other conditions have been very confidently assigned as causes of suppurative hepatitis.

Among these may be mentioned—

1st. Inflammation of the duodenum. Great importance was attached to this presumed cause by Broussais and his followers. Broussais, having remarked that the lymphatic glands in the vicinity of ulcerated mucous membranes are often enlarged and inflamed, and dwelling on the known sympathy between some secreting glands—the lachrymal, the salivary—and the adjacent mucous membranes, was led to generalize, and to assign inflammation of the duodenum as the most frequent cause, indeed, as almost the only cause, of inflammation of the liver. This opinion is not borne out by facts. In most of the cases collected by Andral and Louis, and in those observed by myself, the condition of the duodenum was noticed, and in hardly one did it present any trace of disease. Ulceration or organic disease of the duodenum may, no doubt, cause abscess of the liver, like similar disease of other parts which transmit their blood to the portal vein, but such disease is very rare in the duodenum.

2d. Another cause assigned for hepatitis is spirit drinking. But this produces adhesive inflammation and induration of the liver, not suppurative inflammation and abscess. Notwithstanding the great prevalenee of the habit of gin drinking among the lower orders in this metropolis, years often pass away without a single case of abscess of the liver being admitted into a large London hospital. Not one was received into King's College Hospital for five years from its establishment.

3d. A third cause confidently assigned by Annesley and many other writers, is congestion of the liver. Congestion of the liver, as we have seen, may result from some mechanical impediment to the flow of blood through the chest, or from an unhealthy state of the portal blood.

Congestion of the former kind certainly does not produce suppurative inflammation of the liver. Abscesses of the liver are never met with as a consequence of the congestion caused by the organic diseases of the heart so common in our hospitals; and in not one of the cases recorded by Louis, or Andral, or Annesley, could the abscesses be attributed to this condition. When congestion results from noxious matter in the blood, it may, as the cases before referred to sufficiently testify, be followed by abscess; but in such cases the abscess is the result, not of the mere state of congestion, but of the inflammation which the noxious matter excites. A particular injury, and probably a particular unhealthy state of the blood, may cause either congestion merely or suppuration, according to the state of the general health. Congestion may also result from injury of the nervous system, and in unhealthy states of the system this may go on to suppuration. Bernard states, as the result of his experiments,[1] that division of the sympathetic nerve in the neck of a healthy rabbit causes vascular fulness (congestion) of the corresponding side of the head; but that if the rabbit be weak or unhealthy, it immediately causes inflammation and suppuration of that side of the head.

4th. In India great influence is attributed to the heat of the climate in causing inflammation and abscess of the liver. A hot climate, no doubt, deranges the functions of the liver, and causes increased secretion of bile, which often is irritating in quality and produces inflammation of the gall-ducts and intestines, and in this indirect way it may lead to suppurative inflammation of the substance of the liver. It may perhaps also lead directly and without such intervention to suppurative inflammation and abscess; but I feel persuaded that it does so far less frequently than is generally imagined, and that the notion had its origin in the prevalence of *dysentery*, which we have seen to be a frequent cause of abscess in many tropical climates. The heat of our own summers or of those of France never brings on abscess of the liver, which is very rare in the civil hospitals of London and Paris. Sailors employed in the trade to the west coast of Africa are exposed to heat perhaps as great as those in the trade to India, and suffer much more in health, but they are not equally liable to abscess of the liver or to dysentery.

Men employed in japanning and other processes in the arts are often exposed to heat much greater than that of India, and their health suffers in consequence, yet we never find them coming into our hospitals with abscess of the liver.

5th. Another condition brought forward to explain the frequency of abscess of the liver in India is remittent or intermittent fever, or more correctly the malaria that produces these fevers. It seems established that in some of these fevers the liver, like the spleen, becomes congested and much enlarged in consequence, and in yellow fever and the severe forms of remittent fever it is much and permanently damaged in its secreting element; yet it may be doubted whether suppurative inflammation of the liver takes place in these cases without ulceration of the stomach or gall-bladder or intestines, which so often occurs in some climates in the course of the severe forms of marsh fever. During the time I was visiting

[1] Bernard, Leçons, 1855, p. 352.

physician to the Seamen's Hospital, I had continually to treat men in the most deplorable state from fever caught on the west coast of *Africa*, but none of these men had abscess of the liver.

Louis, in his elaborate account of the yellow fever, which he was sent by the French Government to observe at Gibraltar in 1823, says he constantly found the liver of a pale slate color from anemia, but without any marks of inflammation.

Annesley, indeed, notices abscesses in the liver among the morbid appearances of the remittent fever of India, but he also notices ulceration of the intestine. (*Annesley*, vol. ii. p. 456.) Sir G. Blaue, in his account of the Walcheren fever, remarks that the liver was occasionally the seat of abscess; but here, as in India, the fever was associated with dysentery. It is probable that in both cases the abscesses occasionally found in the liver were the consequence of the dysentery and not the immediate effects of the fever.

It may be, however, that in some parts of India a peculiar malaria—aided perhaps by the heat of the climate, and, as regards the English residents; by habits of life unsuited to it[1]—produces abscess of the liver independently of ulceration of any part of the mucous surface that returns its blood to the portal vein. We know that marsh-fevers differ very much in type, and damage different organs in different seasons and climates, and even according to different degrees of concentration merely of the poison by which they are produced. The question once asked will soon be answered by men practising in India, who in general show the most praiseworthy zeal in collecting facts and adding to our knowledge of all subjects connected with medicine.

Having considered the causes of suppurative inflammation of the substance of the liver, we may proceed to the *changes of structure* resulting from it.

[1] It is a remarkable fact that in the Indian army abscess of the liver occurs in much higher proportion among the English affected with dysentery than among the natives. This circumstance has been generally attributed to the difference of diet in the two classes. The English in India live as freely as they do in this country, while the native Indian soldiers eat no animal food and drink no wine, but subsist almost entirely on vegetable food and milk. I have been informed by Dr. J. Jackson, who practised at Calcutta with much distinction for twenty-five years, that among the natives of Bengal who have adopted the European manner of living abscess of the liver is not uncommon, and that in most instances the inflammation in the liver has come on during the course of dysentery.

The earliest perceptible changes in the appearance and texture of the liver from suppurative inflammation, involving its substance, are uniform redness and softening. These were the earliest changes observed by Cruveilhier in his experiments of injecting mercury into the mesenteric veins of dogs. When the dogs died before sufficient time had elapsed for the formation of pus, the mercury was found strewed through the liver, and the hepatic tissue around each globule was of a deep red color, and softened. In the human subject, when abscess of the liver proves speedily fatal, the hepatic tissue about the abscess is generally of a bright red, and softened.

This preliminary stage is, however, of very short duration. The inflammation soon passes, in some cases in a few days only, to suppuration and abscess. As suppuration takes place, the inflamed substance becomes yellowish, and of course still softer than before. At first the pus is disseminated through the lobules, the outline of which can still be distinguished; but the pus-corpuscles become rapidly more and more abundant, the softened tissue breaks down, and an abscess is formed.

The state of yellow softening, or purulent infiltration, is therefore very transitory, and, in consequence, is seldom observed, except for a distance of two or three lines, about a recently formed abscess.

Such are the more obvious and striking changes. Microscopic examination of the diseased lobules would, doubtless, from the first, show, in most cases, some morbid change in the secreting cells.

The inflammation we are considering commences in the lobular substance of the liver, and is often confined to it; the capsule of the liver, the trunks of the vessels and of the ducts, being perfectly healthy. But if the inflamed part reach the surface of the liver, adhesive inflammation of the capsule is generally set up in the portion immediately above it, and coagulable lymph is poured out, which causes permanent adhesion between that portion of the liver and the parts with which it is in contact. This adhesive inflammation is usually of small extent, being confined to the portion of the capsule immediately above the abscess. It sometimes happens, too, when the portion of the liver inflamed reaches a trunk of the hepatic vein, that inflammation is set up within the vein. In two instances in which abscesses had formed in the liver after amputation of the leg, I found one or two branches of the hepatic vein blocked up by soft fibrin; and in each, I ascertained that an abscess reached the vein, where it ceased to be obstructed by the fibrin. Backwards from this point, all the twigs were blocked up that went to form the obstructed branch. It would seem that the abscess, reaching the thin coat of the vein, had set up inflammation within it (just as it sets up inflammation of the capsule at parts where it reaches the surface), and that the vein, being blocked up at that point by the effused fibrin, all the twigs that went to form it became obstructed in consequence.

I have never found a branch of the portal vein inflamed in such cases, but Dr. James Russel, of Birmingham, has sent me notes of a case in which abscesses formed in the liver and other parts after amputation of the leg, and in which he found lymph and pus in a branch of the portal vein contiguous with one of the abscesses.

The branches of the hepatic vein are perhaps more apt to become inflamed secondarily, in this way, than those of the portal vein, from their coats being thinner, and from their not being surrounded, like the branches of the portal vein, by areolar tissue.

Abscesses of the liver sometimes attain an extraordinary size. In one instance, I estimated the quantity of matter in an abscess of the liver at two quarts. A case is related by Annesley, in which an abscess in the liver contained ninety ounces of matter; and Dr. Inman, of Liverpool, has sent me an account of one still more extraordinary, that fell under his own observation, in which the quantity of matter was found by measurement to be thirteen pints.

The matter in a hepatic abscess is usually white or yellowish, and is free from odor, unless when it is in close proximity to the lung, whence it sometimes becomes decomposed and fetid, from the admission of air.

Many of the old writers describe the pus of abscess of the liver as being generally red or claret-colored, but this description is incorrect. In all the abscesses of the liver that I have examined, the pus was white or yellowish, just like that of a phlegmon. The error of those who have described it as being reddish resulted, perhaps, from their having met with a case in which the abscess opened into the lung, and in which the pus, in its passage through the lung, became mixed with blood and broken down pulmonary tissue. They describe the matter *expectorated*, and not the matter contained in the abscess. It is not very uncommon for an abscess of the liver to open into the lung. Several instances of the kind have fallen under my own notice, and in all of them the matter expectorated was a dirty-red, or brownish pus. The reddish color of the pus was acquired in its passage through the lung. The matter in the abscess was yellowish or white.

Rokitansky states that in old abscesses of the liver there is always an appreciable quantity of bile mixed with the pus. I did not remark this in any of the dissections I made at the Seamen's Hospital; perhaps from my attention not being directed to it.

In cases that have proved speedily fatal, the abscess is bounded simply by red and softened hepatic tissue; but in others it is lined by a false membrane or cyst. The structure of this cyst varies very much in different cases—depending in some degree, perhaps, on the general condition of the patient, but chiefly on the date of the abscess, and on its size. In small abscesses, and in abscesses recently formed, the pus is surrounded by a layer of albuminous matter, a line or two in thickness, resembling concrete pus, and beyond this the hepatic tissue has its natural texture; while in old abscesses of large size the cavity is bounded by a dense gray substance, like cartilage, three or four lines in thickness; and the hepatic tissue for a line or two even beyond this is pale and condensed, obviously in consequence of pressure exerted by the abscess upon it.

The following seems to be the mode in which these cysts are produced. At first, the pus becomes circumscribed by a layer of concrete albuminous matter. The abscess then acts as a foreign body, causing pressure on the surrounding parts, and an inflammatory action which leads to the effusion of plastic lymph. This lymph, becoming firm and more or less organized, forms the cartilage-like layer described.

When an abscess in the liver has become thus isolated by a firm cyst, it may, especially if it be of small size, remain a long time without further change; but in most cases, after being, perhaps, some time stationary, it grows larger, apparently through secretion of fresh matter from the inner surface of the now organized cyst. By the pressure exerted on it by the distending force, the cyst may become ulcerated, and in this way, as well as by mere distension, the abscess may grow larger. It would seem that, by the process of ulceration, a gall-duct imbedded in the cyst, or lying on it, may bo opened, and a small quantity of bile become mixed with the pus. Rokitansky thus accounts for the bile which he constantly found mixed with the pus in old abscesses of the liver. He says, the large gall-ducts about the abscess break down by the spreading of the suppuration, and open obliquely into the cavity on the *distal* side, but only exceptionally, and in very large abscesses, on the side towards the intestine.

When an abscess of the liver in its first formation, or by its subsequent growth, reaches the surface of the liver, it may have various issues. The abscess may burst into the cavity of the peritoneum, causing inflammation of that membrane, which proves speedily fatal. But this seldom happens. In a great majority of instances, when the matter gets near the surface of the liver, adhesive inflammation is set up in the portion of peritoneum immediately above it, and lymph is poured out, which glues the liver to adjacent organs—to the abdominal parietes, the diaphragm, the stomach, the duodenum, the colon, according to the seat of the abscess—and the matter is discharged, not into the peritoneal sac, but outwards, or into the lung, or pericardium, or pleura, or the different portions of the intestinal canal just specified.

Livers containing abscesses are found of all shades of color that can be produced by different degrees of congestion, and by differences in the quantity of oil and in the quantity and color of the biliary matter retained in the cells; but they are seldom indurated from interstitial deposit of fibrin. The inflammation which terminates in abscess, and that which leads to effusion of fibrin and induration, or cirrhosis, are not different in degree merely, but in kind. Abscesses are never found in the *hob-nail* livers of the gin-drinking population of our large towns; and it happens seldom, and then, I believe, only by coincidence, that there is much induration of the liver in persons who return from India with abscess of this organ.

We may now consider the *symptoms* of suppurative inflammation of the liver.

In most works on medicine these have been described as being much more uniform than they really are. A picturesque group is sketched, which it seems very easy to identify; but in actual practice it is far otherwise. The physicians who have had most experience in this disease confess their inability, in many cases, to distinguish it from other diseases of the liver; and, in some, even to pronounce that the liver is the seat of disease at all. Here, as in the diseases of other internal organs, our diagnosis will be much aided by knowledge of the circumstances under which the disease arises: knowledge which will make us observant of symptoms that would otherwise escape our notice, and will enable us to interpret them rightly.

The symptoms are most in accordance with the descriptions usually given, when the inflammation is caused by a blow, or some direct injury from without. The injury is usually inflicted on the convex surface of the liver, and then the local symptoms are well marked. There are pain and tenderness in the region of the liver, and a sense of fulness and resistance under the false ribs, from increased size of the organ. The liver becomes enlarged, and if the abdomen be flaccid and the intestines empty, its edge can be felt some inches below its natural limit. The secretion of bile may be defective, or its flow through some of the ducts impeded, and the patient be jaundiced.

In addition to these symptoms, which may be called *special*, from their pointing to the liver as the seat of disease, there soon appear, as in simple inflammation of other organs, the general symptoms of inflammatory fever: the pulse is frequent and full; the skin hot; the tongue furred and yellowish; appetite is altogether absent or much diminished. The patient is thirsty, and there is occasionally vomiting of bilious matter, while the urine is scanty, high colored, and deposits a red sediment.

These general symptoms, together with the special symptoms—pain and tension in the region of the liver, and jaundice—occurring after an injury to the side, and perhaps, in the absence of evidence of disease of the lung or pleura, are sufficient to characterize suppurative inflammation of the liver.

But, as before remarked, the liver is so well shielded by the ribs, that the disease is seldom caused in this way. It occurs much more frequently after injuries done to other parts of the body, and after surgical operations, from suppurative inflammation of some vein, and the consequent contamination of the blood by pus.

In such cases, the general symptoms do not aid us in detecting it. There is already high fever, which rapidly assumes a typhoid character—the consequence of the contamination of the whole mass of blood, and of the various local inflammations to which this gives rise.

We can only infer that abscesses are forming in the liver by the occurrence of *special* symptoms—pain in the region of the liver, and jaundice—in the midst of the general disorder. But these special symptoms do not exist in all cases. There may be no jaundice; and pain, even, may be wanting, or the typhoid state into which the patient falls may prevent his distinctly perceiving or expressing it. In such cases, the abscesses in the liver can be discovered only after the death of the patient.

In the same way, when inflammation of the liver occurs during the acute stage of dysentery, or on the recurrence of acute symptoms in chronic dysentery, the general symptoms do not aid us in discovering it, because they are fairly attributable to the primary disease. The diagnosis must be founded on local symptoms chiefly —pain and tenderness referable to the liver, tension in the right hypochondrium, and jaundice. Our knowledge of the connection between the two diseases enables us to attach due importance to these symptoms, and to ascribe them to their actual cause. Pain and tenderness in the region of the liver, slight increase in its volume, and jaundice, which, in other circumstances, might excite little alarm, and be attributed to their most frequent cause—inflammation and obstruction of the gall-ducts—when they occur in the course of dysentery, will lead us to dread suppurative inflammation and abscess.

But these special symptoms are far indeed from being all present in every case; and in some cases they are entirely wanting.

On the 2d of October, 1839, a Lascar, 62 years of age, was admitted into the Seamen's Hospital, with general emphysema and catarrh. He complained only of weakness, but sweated at night, and had hectic fever, which led to the suspicion that he had miliary tubercles. He grew weaker, and died of the catarrh on the 12th of November. While in the hospital he made no complaint of pain or tenderness in the right hypochondrium, had no vomiting, no diarrhœa, no jaundice—not a symptom to lead me to suspect that his liver was diseased. On examination, an abscess, containing more than a pint of matter, was found in the substance of the liver. The abscess was bounded by a moderately firm cyst, and the hepatic tissue for a line or two beyond this was pale and condensed. The rest of the liver was healthy, and the capsule presented no marks of having been inflamed. The stomach and small intestines were sound. In the large intestine there were numerous scars, traces of former dysentery, but no actual ulcers. The lungs were extremely emphysematous, and the bronchial tubes choked by mucus. There were no other marks of disease.

My friend and former pupil, Dr. Inman, of Liverpool, has sent me notes of an interesting case, in which abscesses of the liver occurred in consequence, it would seem, of dysentery, without any symptom immediately referable to the liver. The patient, a woman 45 years of age, was admitted into the Liverpool Infirmary, on the 21st of June, 1843, in a state of extreme weakness, from bad living and from constant diarrhœa, which had then lasted nine or ten weeks. The diarrhœa came on without urgent symptoms, and was unattended by griping or tenesmus. The stools were occasionally tinged with blood. The belly was drawn in, and not tender on pressure. She died on the 12th of July. There was extensive ulceration of the large intestine from the ileo-cæcal valve to the rectum. The stomach, the small intestines, the kidneys, and the spleen, were healthy. The liver was larger than natural, and near the lower surface of the right lobe were three abscesses, containing in all about twenty ounces of pure yellow pus. The abscesses were not encysted, and their walls were rough and jagged. There were no marks of inflammation of the capsule of the liver. The lungs were œdematous; otherwise healthy. In the account he sent me, Dr. Inman observes: "No pain in the side or shoulder had been noticed, no vomiting, nor any other symptom that led to the suspicion that there were abscesses in the liver. The abscesses were discovered by accident in the examination of the body."

Andral, Abercrombie, and indeed all writers who have published a series of cases of suppurative inflammation of the liver, have noticed the same fact—that, occasionally, in this disease, the patient has no symptoms immediately referable to the liver.

Annesley says: "The supervention of abscess of the liver" (in dysentery) "is often not manifested by symptoms of a decided nature." "The formation of matter may commence and terminate without the appearance of any of those signs on which the inexperienced are taught to rely." In another place he says: "When the disorders of both viscera are nearly coeval, the inexperienced observer may not detect the presence of biliary derangement until the disease is hastening to a fatal termination, and unequivocal signs of abscess are present. In cases of this description, the violence of the dysenteric symptoms absorbs the whole attention of both patient and practitioner, and the complication is overlooked."

The presence or absence of the symptoms directly referable to the liver depends chiefly on the *situation* and *extent* of the part of the liver inflamed. These symptoms are, as before remarked, fulness of the right hypochondrium, from enlargement of the liver; pain or tenderness; and jaundice.

The degree of enlargement must evidently depend in some measure on the *extent* of the part inflamed. If only a small portion of the liver be inflamed, the inflammation, though attended with considerable distension of vessels, may run through all its stages without producing any enlargement of the organ discoverable by touch. But in this kind of inflammation there is seldom, I believe, much increase in volume even of the part inflamed. Enlargement of the liver is much more common in adhesive inflammation—that is, in inflammation which terminates in effusion of coagulable lymph, and causes permanent induration, or cirrhosis. This latter kind of inflammation, at least when produced by spirit-drinking, usually involves the entire organ, and, apparently by causing an interstitial deposit of lymph, often much increases its size; while suppurative inflammation is generally limited to a small part of it, and before pus is formed, even this part may be little increased in volume.

The circumstance that suppurative inflammation is generally partial serves also to explain the occasional absence of *jaundice*. A portion only of the liver is inflamed, and as any part can perform its function independently of the rest, the sound parts may be adequate to free the blood from the principles of bile.

The presence or absence of *pain* seems to depend not so much on the *extent* as on the *situation* of the portion inflamed.

As long as the inflammation is confined to deep-seated parts and is not sufficiently extensive nor attended with sufficient congestion to cause enlargement of the liver and stretching of its capsule, there is little or no pain. The substance of the liver, like that of the lungs and other parenchymatous organs, is little susceptible of pain. The sharp and severe pain that frequently attends inflammation of those organs has its seat in their fibrous or serous covering.

The occasional absence of symptoms directly referable to the liver is not then so inexplicable as might at first appear. It is satisfactorily accounted for by the circumstance which dissection has already disclosed to us, that suppurative inflammation is generally partial, and often involves only the *substance* of the liver, the natural sensibility of which is slight.

When suppurative inflammation involves all the secreting substance of the liver there is deep jaundice, and the patient dies from oppression of the functions of the brain. A case which seems to have been one of this kind is given by Andral (*Clin. Med.*, iv. p. 381).

When an abscess in the liver has become encysted, if small and deep-seated, it causes but little constitutional disturbance, and, provided it remain stationary, the patient may enjoy even tolerable health for years. I had clear proof of this in the case, to which I shall again refer, of my late colleague Mr. Lawson, consulting surgeon to the Seamen's Hospital, who for ten years before his death had undoubtedly his liver studded with abscesses, but was still competent to all the duties of his profession. If, however, the abscess be large, the health is usually much broken. Even when there is neither pain nor tenderness there is yet some degree of fever, the pulse is frequent, there are night-sweats, the patient does not recover strength, and not unfrequently the urine deposits a pinkish sediment. The complexion, too, has in most cases lost its natural clearness, and is sallow or muddy.

But besides the general symptoms of inflammatory fever and the special symptoms, pain and tension in the right hypochondrium and jaundice, which occur in well-marked cases of suppurative inflammation of the liver, and which, when found in conjunction with the circumstances in which suppurative inflammation is known to arise, are perhaps sufficient to characterize it, there are some other symptoms occasionally observed, which cannot be referred to either of the preceding heads, and which frequently continue after the feverish symptoms are past. These symptoms are pain in the right shoulder, vomiting, a short dry cough, and permanent rigidity of the muscles of the abdominal parietes, but especially *of the right rectus muscle.*

Pain in the right shoulder has long been noticed—indeed, from the time of Hippocrates—as an attendant on hepatic disease, and considerable importance has been attached to it as a sign of hepatic abscess. M. Louis, in his paper on *Abscess of the Liver*, states that none of his patients (they were five in number) had any pain in the shoulder, and he hesitates to believe that this symptom really belongs to disease of the liver. He conjectures that when present it may depend on concomitant disease of the lung or pleura. Nearly the same opinion has been expressed by M. Andral.

Pain in the right shoulder is, indeed, far less frequent in cases of abscess of the liver than is generally imagined, but it existed in five of the fifteen cases I had to treat at the Seamen's Hospital, and in some of these cases there could be no doubt that the pain in the shoulder was dependent on the disease of the liver.

In one of these five cases there was a small abscess on the convex surface of the right lobe, and the peritoneum covering the abscess adhered for the space of a shilling to the reflected layer of the peritoneum. There were some old adhesions of the lung to the pleura costalis, but no trace of recent pleurisy. Both lungs were pale and perfectly sound.

In another of these cases, in which the abscess was on the convex surface of the liver and formed a prominent tumor, the pain of the shoulder was so severe as to cause the patient to moan. The pain continued extremely severe for a long time, and at length *was relieved on our opening the abscess.*

In a third case, where the abscess likewise formed a prominent tumor, the patient complained of an aching pain in the right shoulder, extending to the shoulder-blade and up to the right side of the neck.

In a fourth case, pain in the shoulder varied in intensity with pain in the right side. When the side was easy, the shoulder was easy also. The two pains were evidently related. In this case there were five or six abscesses of various sizes in the liver; one opened into the lung; another was on the convex surface of the right lobe.

In the fifth case, the abscess was single, and was likewise situated on the convex surface of the right lobe. There was no recent inflammation of the lung or pleura.

In two of these cases, the pain in the right shoulder continued for months; and in all of them it was associated with pain in the region of the liver. In all the cases there was an abscess on the convex surface of the right lobe, and adhesions had formed between the peritoneum covering this abscess and the layer of peritoneum reflected over the diaphragm or abdominal parietes.

These cases tend to bear out a statement made by Annesley, that pain of the right shoulder is a sure indication that the disease is in the right lobe; and they explain how it happened that pain in the right shoulder was supposed to be so much more frequently associated with abscess of the liver than it really is. Pain in the right shoulder occurs chiefly in those cases in which the abscess is situated on the convex surface of the right lobe.[1] Now, before the practice of opening bodies had become general, it was only when the abscess was so situated, and when it formed a prominent tumor, that its existence was detected. The physicians of those times, therefore, observed pain in the shoulder in a large proportion of the cases in which they discovered an hepatic abscess; whereas the frequent dissections made of late years have taught us that abscess is more frequently seated deep in the substance of the liver than on its surface, and that pain of the right shoulder is more frequently absent than present.

The pain is usually described as a gnawing, aching pain, about the top of the shoulder. There is no swelling or redness of the shoulder, and the pain is not much increased by pressure—sometimes, indeed, it is relieved by holding or pressing the shoulder—*but it is often increased by pressure on the liver.* The pain is, in fact, as it has always been represented to be, a *sympathetic* pain, like the pain of the knee from disease of the hip.

This sympathetic pain in the shoulder is occasionally felt in other diseases of the liver. It now and then occurs in cancer of the liver, and in cases of hydatid tumor, and it may even be produced by a tumor compressing the liver from without. It was complained of by a man who was admitted into King's College Hospital under my care in April, 1843, with aneurism of the abdominal aorta. The man died suddenly from bursting of the aneurism, between four and five weeks after his admission. The aneurism, which sprung from the side of the artery opposite the origin of the cæliac axis, formed a tumor as large as a man's head immediately behind the liver. It had partially destroyed the bodies of the first, second, and third lumbar vertebræ, and had very much flattened the liver. The tissue of the liver was quite healthy, and the capsule presented no marks of ever having been inflamed.

The cough and the vomiting are symptoms of the same kind. Irritation of the liver, like irritation of the stomach, produces a

[1] Andral gives a case (t. iv. obs. 32) where there was pain in the right shoulder, with abscess on the under surface of the right lobe.

short, dry, *sympathetic* cough; and, like irritation of most of the abdominal viscera, it may occasion vomiting.

M. Louis has not only thrown discredit on pain of the shoulder as a symptom of hepatic abscess, but has advanced similar opinions respecting the vomiting and cough. The *vomiting* he supposes to arise from inflammation of the mucous membrane of the stomach, and the *cough*, to be the consequence of bronchitis.

I have had several opportunities of satisfying myself that the opinion of this eminent pathologist on these points is incorrect; and that the cough and vomiting, so frequently observed in abscess of the liver, do not depend on any disease of the lung or stomach, but are, what I stated them to be, *sympathetic* disorders, depending solely on irritation of the liver.

In the autumn of 1837, a sailor, 29 years of age, was admitted into the Seamen's Hospital immediately on his arrival from Calcutta. He was much emaciated, and stated that he had been ill thirty days of fever, and that during the last ten days he had vomited everything he had taken. His belly was much drawn in, and the parietes were extremely rigid, but there was no tenderness on pressure. He was somewhat thirsty, but afraid to drink, on account of the vomiting immediately excited by doing so. My impression was that his disease was gastritis, and I prescribed for him accordingly. The symptoms increased, and at the end of a fortnight he could be got to take little besides toast and water, which he sipped rather than drank. He died about a month after his admission to the hospital. The stomach was found apparently sound, but the liver was the seat of a large abscess, the presence of which had not been even suspected.

It has been mentioned that in this case, although there was no pain or tenderness, the abdominal parietes were constantly in a state of rigidity. I remarked the same condition in several of the other cases. In one of them it was very striking; the abdominal parietes were hard like board, especially on the right side, with the skin loose over them.

Rigidity of the right rectus muscle was, I find, noticed by the late Mr. Twining, and considered by him, and by some other surgeons in India, as one of the surest indications of deep-seated abscess of the liver. Like the other symptoms with which it is here associated, it is a purely sympathetic affection. It is now and then met with in other diseases besides abscess of the liver. I observed it in a case of long continued jaundice from closure of the common duct, which is related in another chapter, and also in a very striking degree in a case where a cancerous ulcer of the stomach had eaten into the liver, to which the stomach adhered. It is noticed in a case of inflamed gall-bladder, published by Dr. Graves, of Dublin, to which further reference is made in a subsequent chapter.

These sympathetic affections—the pain in the right shoulder, the vomiting, the cough, the rigidity of the abdominal muscles—are of very doubtful import in the early stage of suppurative inflammation while there is yet much fever; but when they exist after the acute stage has passed, and the fever has subsided, and, at the same time, present the characters above noticed—when the pain is seated about the top of the shoulder, is unattended by redness or swelling, and is not much increased by pressure on the shoulder, but by pressure on the side—when the cough is short and dry, and cannot be explained by the condition of the lung—when the vomiting occurs *immediately* after food or drink has been taken, which is a general character of sympathetic vomiting—when, in fact, these symptoms have the characters of *sympathetic* affections, they are strong indications of the existence of an hepatic abscess.

The symptoms that have now been enumerated are almost the only symptoms of suppurative inflammation of the liver, or of its termination—abscess—while the abscess is confined to the substance of the organ.

But, when the abscess is large and near the surface, it may, according to its situation, discharge itself in various ways. If situated on the outer surface of the liver, it may either burst into the cavity of the peritoneum, or, by means of adhesion, make its way through the abdominal parietes; if it be situated on the upper part of the liver, in contact with the diaphragm, it may perforate the diaphragm and burst into the sac of the pericardium or the pleura, or adhesions may form between the lung and the portion of diaphragm covering the abscess, and the abscess may open into the lung and be discharged through the bronchial tubes; if the abscess be near the edge, or on the under surface of the liver, adhesions may form between the peritoneum covering it and the stomach, duodenum, or large intestine, and the matter be discharged through the intestinal canal.

There will, of course, be a variety of symptoms indicative of these several results.

If the abscess burst into the cavity of the peritoneum, there will be sudden accession of pain, vomiting, and all the symptoms of peritonitis from perforation. The patient will speedily fall into collapse, and survive but a few days at most.

If, however, the matter escape by *oozing* merely, it may not become diffused over the surface of the peritoneum, so as to excite general peritonitis. It will spread over the liver, and will be limited by adhesions so as to form a circumscribed abscess in the cavity of the peritoneum. This mode of termination is noticed by Cruveilhier, and happened in two of the cases that fell under my own observation in the Seamen's Hospital.

If the abscess open into the stomach, there will be sudden vomiting of purulent matter; if into the intestines, sudden diarrhœa, with discharge of pus; and, in either case, the occurrence of these symptoms will be attended by subsidence of the palpable tumor, if any exist.

If the abscess perforate the diaphragm, it may burst into the cavity of the pleura, and suddenly set up extensive suppurative pleurisy; but this seldom happens. In almost all cases in which the abscess is making its way through the diaphragm, it excites inflammation of the pleura immediately above it, and adhesion, which is sometimes singularly limited, takes place between the diaphragm and the lung. The abscess then opens into the lung, and the matter is discharged through the bronchial tubes. When this happens, it is marked by very characteristic symptoms—by a new train of stethoscopic phenomena, which it is, perhaps, unnecessary to detail, and by the sudden expectoration of a dirty red or brownish puriform matter. The peculiar color of this matter, which has been already noticed, arises from the pus, in its passage through the lung, becoming mixed with blood and broken down pulmonary tissue. There is no matter like it expectorated in any disease of the lung itself, and I believe that its appearing is pathognomonic of abscess of the liver, or, at least, of abscess perforating the lung.

I observed it in several instances in the Seamen's Hospital, and more than once was led by it to detect an abscess in the liver, of which I had previously no suspicion. When the abscess is large, this matter may continue to be spit up for a great length of time.

It generally comes up very easily, in some cases by mouthfuls, almost without effort on the part of the patient.

When an abscess of the liver opens into the intestines, or into the lung, all the matter may be discharged, the cavity may close up, and the patient recover.

In 1847, I was consulted by an officer in the Indian army, in whom, eight years before, an abscess of the liver had burst through the lung. Symptoms, which led to the inference that he had abscess of the liver, came on while he was suffering from dysentery, in 1839. About three months after their occurrence, while on the deck of a ship, he was suddenly taken with spitting of a mahogany-colored matter, and, in the course of the day, brought up as much as a pint. The spitting continued for three weeks (the matter gradually diminishing in quantity, and losing its dark color), and then ceased. From that time he had occasional pain in the side, but no other illness referable to the liver, and when I saw him, his recovery from the abscess seemed to be perfect.

At the Seamen's Hospital, I met with another instance, in which a man, who had all the symptoms of abscess of the liver discharging through the lung, so far recovered that he left the hospital apparently well. But such a happy result is very rare, except when the abscess is small or recently formed. In the majority of other cases, the patient dies, exhausted by protracted suppuration and hectic.

The protracted suppuration depends on the nature of the walls of the abscess. The hepatic tissue, and the hard gristly substance that always surrounds an old abscess of large size, cannot contract so as to close the cavity, which must consequently continue to be filled with pus. The case is analogous to those cases of old empyema, in which the lung is condensed and irrecoverably bound down against the vertebral column. In such cases, the fluid, if serous, continues to be absorbed, as long as the contraction of the side, the encroachment of the opposite lung, the dilatation even of the bronchial tubes of the compressed lung, continue to diminish the pleural cavity of the diseased side; but when all these means have reached their limit, and the cavity can be made no smaller, an end is put to the absorption of the fluid. It is a physical impossibility that a drop more of the fluid can be absorbed. In the same way, in old abscesses of the liver, if the hardened tissue about the abscess cannot contract so as to close the cavity, the cavity must continue to be filled by pus.

It is, then, to the unyielding nature of the walls of the cavity that we must ascribe the protracted suppuration, and the fatalness of hepatic abscess, even in cases in which the free discharge of the pus would seem to promise a more favorable issue. The fatalness does not result from the matter being discharged through the lung. I have met with several cases in which the abscess opened through the abdominal parietes, and all of them, with one exception, to be presently mentioned, proved fatal; so that it seems doubtful whether such an opening is more favorable than one into the intestine or lung.

The abscess, if large, may discharge through more outlets than one. In one of the cases I treated at the Seamen's Hospital, the abscess discharged first through the lung, and afterwards through the abdominal parietes also. The reason of this is, that from its sides not collapsing, the abscess is not emptied through the first opening.

It has been supposed by some medical men in India, that the pus in an abscess of the liver may be absorbed and eliminated, *as pus*, in the urine. But this notion is evidently erroneous. Pus-globules, from their large size, cannot directly enter the bloodvessels or escape from them. The matter in the urine supposed to be pus, was probably a deposit of phosphates. During the severe constitutional disorder that attends suppurative phlebitis, there is often a sediment of this kind in the urine—having to the naked eye much the appearance of pus, but under the microscope, showing, instead of pus-globules, beautiful phosphatic crystals.

The *treatment* of suppurative inflammation of the substance of the liver is very unsatisfactory.

When the inflammation is caused by phlebitis consequent on a wound or injury of the head or limbs, the whole mass of venous blood is contaminated by pus, suppurative inflammation is likewise set up in many lobules of the lungs, perhaps in some of the joints, and, it may be, in various other parts of the body; and the patient soon falls into a typhoid state, which bleeding and other lowering measures would only make worse. The inflammation thus excited passes rapidly on to suppuration, and we have little, if any, power to arrest it.

The chief objects of treatment should be to prevent, where this is possible, the passage of any more pus into the blood from the injured part, and to support the strength of the patient.

When suppurative inflammation of the liver is caused by a blow, the lungs and other organs do not suffer as in purulent infection of the blood: neither are they thus implicated when it is induced by ulceration of the stomach, or intestines, or gall-bladder, since, in these cases, the noxious matter, whatever it may be, which excites the inflammation, is detained in the liver, or drained off through it. Here, the strength of the patient is not so profoundly sunk, and we may hope, by means of depletion, especially by local bleeding, to control the inflammation, and limit its extent; and, by rendering the abscesses smaller, to protract, at least, the patient's life. In some cases we may, perhaps, by active measures employed early, prevent matter from forming; but we have no evidence that this can be done when the inflammation is caused by pus and is the consequence of inflammation of one of the veins that return their blood to the portal vein.

In this country, mercury has generally been resorted to, when the local symptoms have led to the suspicion that the liver was diseased; but, I fear, with no benefit. It has been well observed by Abercrombie: "In the liver diseases of this country mercury is often used in an indiscriminate manner, and with very undefined notions as to a certain specific influence which it is supposed to exert over all the morbid conditions of this organ. If the liver be supposed to be in a state of torpor, mercury is given to excite it; if in a state of acute inflammation, mercury is given to moderate the inflammation and reduce its action."

This indiscriminate use of mercury has resulted from its unquestionable efficacy in some derangements of the liver, and from the difficulty of distinguishing the different disorders of this organ. In doubt as to the real nature of the malady, the practitioner is naturally anxious to give his patient the chance of a remedy that occasionally produces marked benefit; but often, in doing so, he aggravates the disorder it is his object to relieve.

This misapplication of mercury will continue until the various diseases and derangements of the liver are better discriminated, and practitioners have ascertained those in which mercury has a curative influence. There can be no doubt that much of our uncertainty as to the action of this and other medicines arises from our confounding under the same name, and treating in the same manner, diseases that result from different conditions and are essentially different in their nature.

Mercury seems, on many grounds, to be peculiarly unsuited to the disease we have been considering—suppurative inflammation of the liver.

One objection to its employment in this disease is the short time allowed for its action. When the inflammation is consequent on a wound or injury, and also, in all probability, when it occurs in the course of dysentery, it passes on to suppuration in two or three days; and when suppuration has once taken place, and abscess has formed, it is agreed by most practitioners who have had experience on the subject, not only that mercury does no good, but that in whatever quantity it be given it seldom produces its usual constitutional effects. Annesley says: "There can be no doubt that the system will not be brought under the full operation of mercury, or that ptyalism will not follow on the most energetic employment of this substance, where abscess exists." He repeats this opinion again and again, and even considered resistance to the action of mercury a proof that abscess had formed in the liver. It is only, then, before suppuration has taken place that mercury can do any good, and during this time, from the presence of high fever, the system is with difficulty affected by it.

When abscesses have formed and become encysted, the time for active treatment by medicine has of course passed away. The wisest course then is, I believe, merely to regulate the bowels by rhubarb, or rhubarb and aloes, to recommend habits of strict temperance, and, where the circumstances of the patient allow, residence in a mild climate, and other measures that tend to improve the general health. If the complexion be sallow or dusky, the nitro-muriatic acid, as recommended by practitioners in India, will often be productive of benefit. Whenever there is reason to infer, from increase of pain and fever, that fresh inflammation is set up within the cyst, and that the abscess is growing larger, blood should be taken from the side by leeches or cupping, or a blister should be applied there.

Many physicians have recommended that abscesses of the liver should be opened; but there is much danger in the practice.

One source of danger noticed by Annesley, Dr. Stokes, and many other writers, is the difficulty of distinguishing an hepatic abscess, and our liability to mistake a distended gall-bladder for an abscess. Such a mistake is almost immediately fatal to the patient. A distended gall-bladder is seldom adherent to the abdominal parietes, and if it be punctured, the bile escapes into the cavity of the peritoneum, the patient is seized with vomiting, falls rapidly into a state of collapse, and generally dies at the end of a few hours. Two cases of this kind are alluded to by Dr. Stokes in the fifth volume of the *Dublin Hospital Reports*, and many others are on record. This source of danger may, however, be avoided by attention to the situation and character of the tumor. The tumor formed by a distended gall-bladder is globular, and circumscribed, and hard, and equally resisting in every part, while the tumor from abscess is more diffused, and is soft and fluctuating at its summit, while its base is hard and resisting.

A source of far greater danger is the circumstance, which has been before noticed, that the inflammation which leads to abscess is often confined to the substance of the liver and does not involve its capsule. As the abscess approaches the surface, adhesive inflammation of the peritoneum immediately above it usually takes place, and a small quantity of lymph is poured out, which causes adhesion between the wall of the abscess and the parts with which it is brought into contact. These adhesions are often of very small extent. Sometimes they do not form at all, and, as I have before remarked, the abscess bursts into the cavity of the peritoneum, causing speedy collapse and death. By opening an abscess of the liver before adhesions have formed, we may be directly instrumental in bringing on this fatal issue—the pus may escape into the sac of the peritoneum, and the patient die in a few hours, obviously in consequence of the operation.

It is, therefore, very important, before opening the abscess, to make out whether the liver adheres to the abdominal parietes or not. This may sometimes be done, when the liver is large, and the abdominal parietes are thin, by feeling the edge of the liver, or some prominent part of its surface, and marking the place of this with a pen on the surface of the belly. If the liver be adherent to the abdominal parietes the line or spot so marked will correspond to the edge or prominence of the liver in all positions of the body. If it be not adherent, the liver will slide along the wall of the belly when the patient draws a deep breath or changes his posture; the liver will fall, for example, towards the left side when he turns from his back over to that side, and the line or spot will no longer correspond to the edge or prominence in question.

When there is a circumscribed œdema, or a slight blush on the skin, over the abscess, we may be sure, not only that the liver is adherent, but also that the abscess is making its way to the surface.

When, on the contrary, the skin has its natural appearance and color, and other signs that the liver is adherent are wanting, if we thrust a knife into the abscess, we run the risk of discharging the matter into the peritoneal sac.

Dr. Graves has ingeniously recommended a mode of proceeding by which he supposes this danger may be obviated. It is: not to open the tumor at once, but to make an incision across the most prominent part of it through the abdominal muscles, so as to reach the peritoneum, without dividing it, and to fill up the wound with a pledget of lint. The object of this is to excite circumscribed inflammation of the peritoneum, which may produce adhesion between the reflected layer of the peritoneum and the layer covering the abscess. The abscess may then be opened, or be allowed to open of itself. I have tried this mode of proceeding twice, with unsatisfactory results, and have come to the conclusion that it is very inadequate to the purpose.

But in opening an abscess in the substance of the liver, there is another, and greater, and more unavoidable source of danger, which has not been noticed by the writers to whom I have referred. It is, that the solid hepatic tissue cannot readily collapse, so as to close the cavity when the abscess is opened. When, then, a free opening is made, even into a recent abscess, air almost necessarily enters the cavity, and, from the sudden removal of pressure, or, it may be, from the manipulation employed to empty the cavity, violence is done to the walls of the abscess, and there is often some degree of hemorrhage from them. Air and blood thus become mixed with the pus in the abscess, decomposition takes place, and the air, or the decomposed pus, sets up fresh inflammation of the inner surface of the sac. This causes, of course, a fresh accession of fever, and of other constitutional disturbance, and if the abscess be large, a profuse, and fetid, and continuous discharge, which may soon exhaust the strength of the patient.

The secondary inflammation thus excited by the presence of air, or by the decomposed pus, may even lead to gangrene, and speedily destroy life. This happened in one of the cases that fell under my care in the Seamen's Hospital. An abscess that pointed outwardly was opened, with considerable temporary relief to the pain which the patient suffered in the side and shoulder. But the discharge soon became fetid and dark, of the color of coffee-grounds, and at the end of a week the patient died. The walls of the abscess, and the hepatic tissue immediately around them, were found in a state of gangrene. A similar case is noticed by Cruveilhier. (*Anat. Path.*, liv. 40.)

In consequence of the dangers of this secondary inflammation, it is, I think, generally best, when an abscess of the liver projects at the side, to allow it to open of itself. The prominent part should be poulticed, and the matter be allowed to escape in the poultices, but should not be squeezed or pressed out. Nature performs the operation better than the surgeon. When the abscess opens of itself, it is usually by a very small aperture, like those in worm-eaten wood, which never closes, and the matter gradually oozes out as the sac contracts. No air gets mixed with the matter of the abscess, and no violence is done to its walls; and, consequently, no fresh inflammation is set up. The discharge is very gradual, and as small in quantity as it can be. There is less shock to the system, and less drain from it, than when the abscess is freely opened by the knife. The advantages of this proceeding were well shown in the following case, which fell under my care through the recommendation of my friend, Dr. Paget, of Cambridge:—

A country gentleman, about 60 years of age, whose health had been impaired by asthma, from which he had suffered for 25 years, had an attack of typhoid fever, in November, 1846. At the same time, two of his children also had the fever, which was of the kind common in the neighborhood of Cambridge, and which is attended by ulceration of Peyer's glands. From that time he had more or less pain or uneasiness in the region of the liver, and, in the spring of 1848, had the side repeatedly blistered on account of it. When he first consulted me, on the 19th of January, 1849, the liver was enlarged or pushed down, and over the right lobe, just to the right of the epigastric region, was a prominent tumor, as broad as the palm of the hand, which both Dr. Paget and myself took to be an abscess of the liver, making its way to the surface.

It was recommended that the tumor should be poulticed, and that the abscess should be allowed to open of itself.

On the 25th of February, I received a letter from him, telling me that this had happened. He says:—

"On the 15th inst., you gave it as your opinion that the swelling in my side would probably break at the end of a week, or before a fortnight. I now beg to inform you that, on Saturday morning, we discovered that a moderate quantity of matter had discharged during the night, and it still continues slowly running from two very small apertures that might almost be compared to the pores of the skin. The quantity we could not well ascertain, it was so much mixed with the poultice; but some had escaped down the side. Whenever it is fresh dressed, we observe always a mixture of matter. During the day I have four changes.

"I think your directions at our last interview were to continue the poultices, and this we shall do, unless I hear from you to the contrary.

"I feel convinced you have arrived at the result we could have desired, with the least possible suffering to myself.

"I feel, perhaps, a little languid, but my general health and spirits are good."

The pain and tenderness of the side, and the fever, which had existed previously, soon disappeared, and the general health improved much; but an oozing of matter from the side continued. In October, 1850, the discharge ceased, doubtless from the channel becoming blocked up; and matter collected again, so as to form a tumor, which pointed two or three inches higher up than the original tumor. This tumor, like the former, was allowed to open of itself, and from that time there was a slight oozing of matter from the second aperture (which did not cause more disturbance of the health, or more inconvenience, than would be caused by a small issue) till the beginning of 1853, when the drain ceased, and no further annoyance from the side was felt.

Since the abscess first broke, the asthma has several times recurred, as before.

From what I have seen and read of hepatic abscess, it seems to me that the proportion of recoveries has been just as great, if not greater, when the abscess has opened into the lung or the bowel, as when it has made its way through the side; and I can only explain the circumstance by the fact that, when the abscess has pointed at the side, it has seldom been allowed to open of itself.

When the abscess is large, and has existed long, its walls are thick and unyielding, and it has, in consequence, still less disposition to close up. When an abscess of this kind opens of itself, either outwardly or into the intestine or lung, matter continues to be discharged, and the patient generally dies, worn out by the protracted suppuration. When the abscess is opened by the knife, the same thing of course happens, and the patient dies the earlier for our meddling.

In India, it seems now to be a common practice to thrust a long exploring needle into the liver, where the presence of an abscess is suspected; and, now and then, perhaps, the disease may be cured in this way. A single abscess may be opened, when it is of moderate size, and before its walls are too thick and firm to fall together, and the cavity may be closed up. But there are many objections to the practice, that to me seem quite decisive against it. First, there is the danger of hemorrhage, and of setting up fresh inflammation by the mechanical injury thus done to the liver. This danger may, perhaps, be small for a single puncture, but if the abscess be deep-seated, it may not be hit at the first thrust. Again, from the difficulty of distinguishing the different diseases of the liver, if the operation be commonly adopted, it must often be performed where there is no abscess at all. It will readily be imagined that much mischief may be done in this way. Often, too, there is more than one abscess. This was the case in thirteen of the twenty-nine cases recorded by Annesley, and in a still larger proportion in the cases collected by Andral and Louis, and myself. We can hardly hope to reach all the abscesses, and, unless we do, we cannot cure the patient. Then there is the danger that has been before alluded to, of letting the matter escape into the sac of the peritoneum, and setting up peritonitis, that may prove speedily fatal. An occasional instance of success will, I fear, be a poor set-off against the cases in which the operation has done mischief, or failed of doing good.

Hitherto, we have considered only suppurative inflammation originating in the lobular substance of the liver. There are several other forms of suppurative inflammation of this organ, but they are much more rare.

1st. One of these is where the inflammation originates in the areolar tissue in the portal canals, and where the pus, instead of forming a circumscribed abscess, is diffused through the areolar tissue that surrounds the portal vein, and the accompanying artery and duct. A case of this kind is given by Cruveilhier.

A professional flute-player, of intemperate habits, after long anxiety, fell into a state of extreme weakness, attended with feverishness, for which he sent for Cruveilhier, on the 18th of December, 1818. His face was then pale and thin; he had distaste for food, a short dry cough, and a slow fever, with evening exacerbations.

Cruveilhier examined the chest and abdomen, without discovering the cause of illness. The symptoms continued, the patient grew thinner, the tongue became very dry and brown; and, at length, the patient fell into a typhoid state, and died on the 5th of February. On examination, pus was found diffused through the areolar tissue surrounding the branches of the portal vein, in the substance of the liver. The lobular substance of the liver was perfectly healthy. There were also small abscesses along the vessels in the meso-colon and meso-rectum. The state of the intestines is not mentioned.

2d. Another form is where suppurative inflammation is set up in the capsule of the liver, or in the peritoneum covering it. This may take place without suppurative inflammation of the substance of the liver, and, at first, without inflammation of the rest of the peritoneum. But, when pus has formed on the surface of the liver, it becomes diffused over the surface of the peritoneum, and causes general and rapidly fatal peritonitis, just as when discharged by the bursting of an abscess. A case of this kind is given by Andral (*Clin. Med.*, iv. 310). It would seem that in such cases the material cause of the inflammation is conveyed by the arterial blood.

3d. A third variety of suppurative inflammation, is where the inflammation originates in the portal or hepatic veins. This variety is so important that I shall consider it in a separate chapter.

4th. A fourth variety is where suppurative inflammation occurs in the gall-bladder or ducts, without similar disease in the secreting substance of the liver. This, too, is so important that I shall speak of it in a separate chapter.

5th. There is still another variety, where suppurative inflammation is set up in the interior of an hydatid cyst, converting it into an abscess. This, considering the rareness of hydatids in the human liver, is not of unfrequent occurrence. Two instances of it have fallen under my own notice. Three are recorded by Andral, and two or three by Cruveilhier. The fragments of hydatids were found floating in pus. The observations of Cruveilhier render it probable that, in most of such cases, the suppurative inflammation is set up by the entrance of bile into the cyst. These cases will be again referred to in a subsequent chapter on hydatids of the liver.

SECT. II.—*Gangrenous inflammation—Appearances sometimes mistaken for gangrene—Circumstances in which gangrene of the liver really occurs.*

THE infrequency of gangrene of the liver has been remarked by Annesley, Dr. Stokes, and many other writers. Annesley states that he did not meet with a single instance of gangrene in all the subjects he examined with abscess and other diseases of the liver, and supposes that medical men have often mistaken for gangrene, changes that occurred after death. I have little doubt that Annesley is right in this opinion. If the abscess be recently formed, and not encysted, and the body be examined after the matter in the abscess has become partly decomposed, the hepatic tissue immediately surrounding the abscess will be found blackened by the sulphuretted hydrogen formed by decomposition of the pus, and will thus present very much the appearance of gangrene. In the month of July, 1837, I met with a striking instance of this, in a man who died, under my care, in the Dreadnought, with a recently formed abscess of the liver, and whose body was examined *forty* hours after death. The hepatic tissue about the abscess was black and ragged, just as it would be from gangrene. Where the patient has died in a low typhoid state, and decomposition is unusually rapid, this change of color may occur much sooner after death, and in colder weather, and, of course, be still more likely to be mistaken for gangrene. It will, however, here, as in other cases, be associated with a greenish color of the skin of the belly and neck; or with the presence of gas in the veins; or with some other changes characteristic of decomposition. A black stain is often found on that part of the surface of the liver which touches the intestine, and is produced in the same way by the intestinal gases, which, after death, permeate the coats of the bowel.

In persons who die of suppurative peritonitis, the whole surface of the liver soon acquires a black color, which extends a line or two into its substance, the deeper, the longer after death the body is examined. Now and then, in cutting across a liver, a black stain of the same kind may be seen in the portions of liver in contact with the gall-ducts, produced, no doubt, by permeation of sulphuretted hydrogen, or other gases, through the coats of the ducts.

When an abscess is old and bounded by thick and dense false membrane, this change in the color of the surrounding hepatic substance is less likely to take place after death, and as an effect of mere chemical change; and, consequently, a blackish-green color is here a surer sign of gangrene.

In the last chapter, mention is made of a case which fell under my care, in the Seamen's Hospital, where gangrene of the liver resulted from opening an abscess, and reference is given to a similar case noticed by Cruveilhier.

An instance of gangrene occurring about an old abscess, which has also been referred to in the preceding chapter, is given by Andral; the only instance, he tells us, in which he had then met with gangrene of the liver. The patient, a laboring man, about 60 years of age, was much emaciated, in consequence of an extensive chronic ulcer of the stomach. The gangrene, or death of the part, was probably the result of defective nutrition. It occurred around the abscess, just as a bruise-mark or ulcer occurs in the place of an old scar in scurvy, because the vitality of that part having been previously impaired, it gives earlier tokens of defective nutrition than the sound parts.

The following case, for which I am indebted to Mr. Busk, is the most striking instance of gangrene of the liver I have met with, and offers besides many points of great interest.

CASE. *Mortification of the toes from cold—Removal of the dead parts—Severe rigors, followed by typhoid symptoms—Death on the sixth day—Gangrene of the liver, the lung, and the spleen; necrosis of the thyroid cartilage; ulceration of the pharynx; pus in the shoulder-joint.*

A Scotchman, 35 years of age, was admitted into the Seamen's Hospital, the 14th of January, 1841, with the extremities of the two great toes, and of several other toes, in a state of gangrene, from exposure to cold in coming up channel, after a voyage to the West Indies. He had good health while in the West Indies, but, with the rest of the crew, had drunk rum to excess in the voyage home.

There was little appearance of inflammation, and but little pain in the feet, and he was otherwise in good health—spare, muscular, and rather florid.

In a few days, under the use of warm fomentations, the dead parts began to separate from the living, and on the 25th of January, the separation was nearly complete at the junction of the second and last phalanges, which were then removed, sufficient flaps being left to cover the bones. The day after this little operation he had rigors, followed by incessant vomiting and great general disturbance. The rigors recurred very frequently, and the vomiting continued incessant. No pain or tenderness could be detected in any part. In a day or two he became jaundiced, and expectorated rusty-colored, viscid matter. The motions were clay-colored. The tongue was dry and brown.

On the 29th, several joints, especially the right shoulder, were painful and tender, but he had no pain or tenderness of the abdomen or chest. The following day, mild delirium; finally, stupor, and death on the 1st of February (the 6th day from the rigors).

The body was inspected twenty-four hours after death.

The body was lean, muscular, universally rigid, jaundiced, with dark purple mottling on the back and on the sides of the neck and ears.

Head. The dura mater on the outside looked healthy. Its inner surface was minutely vascular, and covered by a thin film of fibrinous matter, of a bright yellow color, and presenting many minute spots resembling ecchymoses. On examination, these spots were found to be entirely in the effused matter. The cerebral arachnoid was also covered, but over a smaller surface, by a similar film of transparent, yellow, gelatinous-looking fibrin, which, however, was not vascular, and but very slightly opaque. There was a small quantity of liquid of a bright yellow color in the cavity of the arachnoid, and also some colorless fluid beneath it. The vascularity of the arachnoid and the film of fibrin were alike on the two sides, and were confined to the upper surfaces of the hemispheres. At the base of the brain there was no unnatural vascularity, and no lymph effused.

The cerebral substance, when sliced, presented large bloody points, more numerous in the back part of the brain, but otherwise it looked healthy, and it had its natural consistence. There was a very small quantity of colorless liquid in the lateral ventricles.

Chest. Both lungs were everywhere united to the side by firm old tissue.

The upper and front part of the right lung was congested, but still crepitant, and slightly infiltered with reddish frothy fluid. The lower and back part of the lung was more solid, and gorged with thin red fluid; and in the midst of the lower lobe, which was quite solid, was a portion, the size of an orange, completely gangrenous. The gangrenous part was of a pale ash color, mottled by infiltration of white pus, and had the extremely offensive odor of gangrene of the lung. This dead portion was separated by a well-defined line from the surrounding pulmonary tissue, which was of a deep purple color, solid and friable. Many other portions of the lung were quite solid, and beginning to lose their color, and others were in the first stage of inflammation, but none had exactly the usual appearance of pulmonary purulent deposits.

The left lung was in a similar state, but less advanced.

Both lungs had a most disgusting smell.

The mucous membrane of the right ventricle of the larynx was ulcerated, and of a deep purple color. The mucous membrane of the air-passages was injected throughout, the color becoming deeper in the small tubes. There was a large ragged abscess outside and in front of the thyroid cartilage, which was bare and carious.

The pericardium contained a large quantity of red fluid, and the right auricle and ventricle were filled with very fluid blood, and a few yellowish flakes of fibrin. The valves and the lining membrane of the heart were perfect and unstained. The blood in the large vessels was dark-colored and fluid, with small, soft coagula. No pus-globules could be distinctly observed in the blood examined by the microscope.

Digestive organs. The mucous membrane of the pharynx presented one or two small superficial ulcers or abrasions, covered with a thin fibrinous effusion, and was of a deep purple from minute vascularity. The deep color ceased on a level with the upper edge of the thyroid cartilage. The mucous membrane of the œsophagus was pale and healthy.

The stomach was not examined.

The intestines, small and large, were healthy throughout, without any enlargement of either Peyer's patches or the solitary glands. The fecal matter was of a pale clay color.

The liver was large and closely united to the under surface of the diaphragm by firm old tissue. On the outside it was not discolored, and presented no marks of recent inflammation. When it was cut into, *numerous* ragged cavities of various sizes were found, containing hepatic substance in a state of complete gangrene, and reduced in many of them to a semifluid, ash-colored, flocculent matter, separated by a very defined line from the surrounding substance, which, in immediate contact with the gangrenous portions, was of a deep greenish slate color. In other spots less completely disorganized, the hepatic substance was of a pale ash color, apparently quite dead, but the lobular structure could be plainly seen; thus proving clearly that there was little or no deposit of foreign matter. Other portions again, alike in size and shape, were of a deep purple, and slightly softened; and this probably the first step in the changes leading to the complete disintegration first described.

The coats of the large veins, where they came in contact with the gangrenous portions, partook in the change, in consequence of which their inner surface had a mottled appearance, the dead portions being of a dull yellowish-white, separated from the healthy part by a very delicate red line.

The inner surface of the vein was not roughened, or otherwise altered, either in the dead or living parts, and had no lymph on it, either adherent or free; but in some of the larger veins pus was found. Several small, gangrenous spots of the liver were found, which had a small vein in their centre, and there the coats of the vein in all their circumference were dead and discolored.

The gangrenous portions of the liver were horribly fetid, but still less so than those of the lung.

The gall-bladder contained a small quantity of thick, viscid bile.

The spleen was closely united to all the surrounding parts by firm old tissue. Its middle portion was reduced to a grumous pulp. Nearer the surface, its substance was firmer, and of a dark purple color, and had the smell of gangrene.

The kidneys were healthy and pale.

The right shoulder-joint was filled with thick, fetid pus.

In this case, the existence of gangrene, both in the liver and in the lung, was clearly shown by the defined line surrounding the gangrenous portions.

The source of the mischief here was, no doubt, the gangrene of the toes produced by cold. The man was in the prime of life, of spare habit, muscular, florid, and in good health at the time of the frost-bite. The case shows us what a serious thing a small patch of gangrene in any part of the body may become.

The dissemination of the gangrenous masses—the existence of a number of them *isolated and at a distance from one another*—proves that the septic agency was conveyed by the blood. The noxious matter thus disseminated, destroyed the vitality of the tissues on which it acted most strongly.

The chemical theory of these septic changes is now well known. All parts in which they are taking place, have a tendency to affect other parts brought into contact with them, with the same mode of transformation. The case just related—and it is by no means a solitary one—offers one of the most interesting illustrations of this theory in the whole range of pathology. But whatever be the explanation adopted, the fact is certain, and it is one of extreme importance, that gangrene of the extremities, or of any part of the surface of the body, produced by cold, by pressure, or in any other way, has a tendency to infect other and remote parts of the body with the same change.

The occasional occurrence of gangrene in remote parts of the body in low fevers, after sloughing of the skin of some one part has been caused by pressure, was particularly noticed by Dr. Graves, in his remarks on a case in which gangrene of the lung was consequent on sloughing of the sacrum thus caused.

The patient, a man, twenty-four years of age, died in Sir Patrick Dun's Hospital, the twenty-ninth day after the first appearance of confluent smallpox. Dr. Graves says: "It is probable that this case would have terminated favorably had not extensive gangrene of the sacrum taken place, to which the nurse did not direct my attention until it was of an alarming extent. It was first pointed out to me on the eighteenth day, at which time he labored under hoarseness and bronchitic symptoms, unattended, however, by any difficulty of respiration. In the course of a few days, however, dyspnœa came on; the wheezing in his chest increased, and seemed to accelerate the period of death, which appeared, to all those who had witnessed the progress of the case, to be the result of constitutional prostration, induced by the external gangrene. On dissection, two large and two smaller gangrenous sloughs were detected in the right lung. The gangrenous portions of the pulmonary tissue were insulated, being separated from the surrounding substance of the lung by a whitish membrane, apparently formed of coagulated lymph. The question here occurs, whether these internal gangrenes were a consequence of the external one, or whether they were the result of the same fatal constitutional derangement that predisposed the external parts to become gangrenous from pressure? The former supposition seems the most probable; at the same time, we must admit that gangrene often takes place, in fever, in external parts not liable to pressure, as, for instance, the soles of the feet. It is to be observed, however, that I never knew such parts to become gangrenous, *except after some other portions of the integument had mortified, evidently in consequence of pressure.*" (*Clinical Medicine*, p. 781.)

In the case I have before given, there can be no doubt that the gangrene of the liver and lungs was caused by the gangrene of the toes. There was no other influence acting to produce it.

M. Dance published a case in many respects similar, where gangrene of the spleen was consequent on gangrene of the uterus.

In another chapter, I shall relate a case sent me by Dr. Inman, of Liverpool, and interesting on several accounts, in which gangrene of the lung was consequent on gangrenous sloughing of the vagina.

Cruveilhier (Liv. xxxvii. pl. 2, p. 3) has given a case where gangrene of the gums and cheek was consequent on gangrene of the uterus from cancer.

I might, if it were needful, adduce many other instances, showing that gangrene of one part, produced by some cause acting only on that part, has a tendency to cause gangrene in other parts remote from it, and not subject to the same influence. It is in this way, in effect of gangrene of some other part, that true gangrene of the liver is most frequently produced.

SECT. III.—*Adhesive inflammation of the capsule, and of the substance of the liver—Cirrhosis—Other forms of inflammation of the substance of the liver.*

ADHESIVE, or plastic inflammation, that is, inflammation which causes effusion of coagulable lymph, may, as we have seen, be set up around an abscess in the liver. When the process of suppuration is over, the pus, collected into a cavity, becomes bounded by a layer of soft albuminous matter. Around this, again, coagulable lymph is effused, which becomes firm and tough, and more or less organized, and thus forms a cyst for the matter. It has already been shown that the texture of the cyst varies chiefly with the date of the abscess, and with its size. In small, and in recently formed abscesses, the walls of the cyst are soft and thin; whereas, in large abscesses of long standing, the matter is usually bounded by a substance three or four lines in thickness, having the look and the toughness of cartilage.

The adhesive inflammation is here limited to the immediate vicinity of the abscess, because it is excited by the abscess, and because the lymph poured out there cannot be diffused through the substance of the organ.

When the abscess is near the surface of the liver, it sometimes sets up adhesive inflammation of the peritoneum covering it, and lymph is poured out, which unites the peritoneum above the abscess to the parts—the diaphragm, the abdominal parietes, the stomach, the colon—with which it happens to be in contact.

The adhesions thus formed are often of very small extent. The wall of an abscess on the convex surface of the liver may adhere to the diaphragm, or to the abdominal parietes, in a space no larger than a shilling. From this, and other circumstances, many writers have inferred that the peritoneum is less liable to adhesive inflammation than the pleura. But such does not seem to be the case. The adhesion is limited, because the irritation that excites it is limited, and because the matter poured out does not become diffused over the surface of the membrane.

Under similar circumstances, adhesions of the pleura may be of equally small extent. In a case in which an abscess of the liver discharged through the lung, I found that the space in which the lung was adherent to the portion of the diaphragm covering the abscess was not larger than a shilling. Where small circumscribed abscesses form in the lungs from contamination of the blood by pus, the lungs are now and then found adherent to the pleura costalis in a great number of points, corresponding to superficial abscesses, without any diffuse inflammation of the pleura. In the same way adhesive inflammation of the pleura, from the presence of tubercles, is often of very small extent.

When lymph is effused in greater quantity on the surface of the liver it causes adhesion of greater extent; and if any of the lymph fall down among the intestines, it may glue adjacent folds of the intestine together.

When an abscess excites adhesive inflammation of the *substance* of the liver, the lymph can never be diffused in this way. It all remains where first deposited, immediately around the abscess, and forms a cyst for the matter.

An hydatid tumor in the liver, like an abscess, may excite adhesive inflammation in the substance of the liver about it, or on the capsule and peritoneum above it; but it does not always do so, and in consequence an hydatid cyst, like an abscess, may burst into the sac of the peritoneum.

Adhesive inflammation of the surface of the liver now and then occurs also over cancerous tumors. The lymph effused in such cases is usually in very small quantity and transparent, and the false membranes found uniting the liver to the diaphragm and the adjacent organs are, in consequence, very white, and thin, and filmy —passing merely from the summits of some of the prominent cancerous masses to the opposite surface of the peritoneum. But, over cancerous tumors on the liver, inflammation, even to this extent, is the exception and not the rule. Cancerous tumors seem never to cause effusion of fibrin, and consequent induration, in the substance of the liver; and the liver may be enormously enlarged and much deformed by them without any inflammation of its capsule.

Small miliary tubercles are occasionally found in great numbers in the livers of persons dead of phthisis. I have never met with an instance in which they seemed to have caused adhesive inflammation of the substance of the liver, and have met with only one instance in which they had excited inflammation of its capsule. The rarity of marks of inflammation of the liver in conjunction with a tubercular deposit is remarkable, considering the tendency tubercles have to set up inflammation of the different tissues of the lung. In the livers of monkeys, dead of phthisis, masses of white tuberculous matter as large as a small bean are often met with; and not unfrequently, as in cancer in the human subject, some thread-like false membranes pass from some of the superficial tumors to the opposite surface of the peritoneum.

Adhesive inflammation of the capsule of the liver of much greater extent than that set up by the local causes that have been just mentioned occurs very frequently in this country, among the lower orders in large towns, in conjunction with deep-seated adhesive inflammation of the liver, especially where this involves chiefly the areolar tissue in the large portal canals.

Deep-seated adhesive inflammation of the liver produces different effects, according to the parts it principally involves. Sometimes the lymph is effused almost exclusively into the areolar tissue in the portal canals of considerable size, and if the person die long after this has occurred, all the considerable branches of the portal vein are surrounded, in some places to a distance, it may be, of half an inch, by a tough fibrous tissue, which by its contraction has drawn in and puckered the adjacent portions of the liver. The rest of the liver may be little, if at all, altered in texture, and may be readily scraped away from these indurated portions. The main branches of the vein are pervious, but many of the small twigs that spring from them are obliterated. The parts of the liver which these twigs supplied are atrophied, and the liver is proportionally reduced in bulk. Where such parts are near the surface, the capsule is somewhat drawn in and puckered. Together with these changes, there are usually, if not always, thick false membranes on the capsule of the liver, or extensive adhesions, by means of old tissue, between the liver and adjacent organs. Usually, too, there are old false membranes on the surface of the spleen, and marks of adhesive inflammation of other parts—especially the pericardium and the pleura.

I have several times met with this form of disease in persons who had drunk hard of spirits. It comes on with well-marked symptoms of inflammation of the liver—pain in the side, vomiting, fever, and perhaps jaundice. These symptoms subside after a time, but the patient does not regain his former health. The liver has been permanently damaged; part of its secreting substance becomes atrophied from closure of the small portal veins; and it is no longer adequate to its office. The patient has difficult digestion, looks sallow, and does not recover his former strength.

In other cases of deep-seated adhesive inflammation of the liver, the lymph is not effused solely, or chiefly, in the large portal canals. The fibrous tissue is not found about the large branches of the portal vein especially, but about the small twigs that separate the lobules. All the substance of the liver is rendered tough by this new fibrous tissue, which, when the liver is sliced, is seen to form thin lines between small irregular masses of lobules. At the parts on the surface of the liver which correspond to these lines, the capsule is drawn in, so that the surface has a "hob-nailed" appearance. The tissue of the liver is paler than natural, from the presence of this white fibrous tissue, and from its containing but a small quantity of blood; and it is often yellowish from accumulation of biliary matter in the cells. When such is the case, a section of the liver has the grayish and yellow color of impure beeswax, and, in consequence, the disease has been called by the French *cirrhosis*.

In other cases, again, the quantity of this adventitious fibrous tissue is much greater, and by its contraction the lobular substance of the liver is drawn into round nodules, which being of a deep yellow color from accumulation of biliary matter, are in strong contrast with the gray fibrous tissue between them. This state has been described by Abercrombie, who says the yellow matter of cirrhosis is sometimes in small nodules, like peas, dispersed through the substance of the liver. He adds, "A case is described by Clossy, in which the structure of the liver was wholly constituted of a congeries of little firm globules, like the vitellarium of a laying hen; it occurred in a boy of fifteen, who had immense ascites. In a case by Boismont, these nodules were as large as peas, and the liver was much diminished in size; the case was chronic with ascites. The French writers have a controversy whether the cirrhosis, or yellow degeneration of the liver be a new formation, or a hypertrophia of the yellow substance which they suppose to constitute a part of the structure of the liver in its healthy state. No good can arise from such discussions, as it is impossible to decide them." (*Diseases of the Stomach, &c.*, 2d edition, p. 369.)

The disease is seldom met with in this degree, and as the changes of structure are very remarkable, I venture to subjoin the following case, in which this condition of the liver is more fully described.

CASE. — *Spirit-drinking — Jaundice — Vomiting of blood — Ascites and œdema of the legs — Extreme degree of cirrhosis.*

Gilbert Campbell, æt. 40. was admitted into King's College Hospital, under my care, the 16th of June, 1843. At the age of thirty he became a commercial traveller, and continued so seven years, during which he drank hard of wine and spirits. The last three years he had been a commission agent, and had drunk much less, his chief beverage being ale.

He had very good health till he became a commercial traveller, but from that time had frequently pain in the stomach and vomiting after excess in drinking. In the month of February, 1841, when travelling to Birmingham, he became jaundiced. The jaundice went off in about a fortnight, and after that he had no particular ailment, till the summer of 1842, when he was laid up two or three weeks with gout in the left foot. This was his first attack of gout, and he had no return of it. In addition to these ailments, he had for several years suffered from stricture of the urethra, and from a winter cough. Lately, has had occasional bleeding from the nose.

He followed his usual occupations till three weeks before his admission to the hospital, when he was taken in the street with vomiting of blood. The vomiting recurred several times during the day. He thinks he brought up, in all, as much as four quarts of blood, and was very faint in consequence. Two days afterwards he noticed that his belly was swelled, and in a day or two more he had also swelling of the ankles.

When he came into the hospital he had a sallow, cachectic look, his conjunctivæ were yellowish, his skin hot and dry, his mouth parched, his lips chapped and bleeding. His legs and thighs were very œdematous, but there was no œdema of the hands or face. The belly was much distended with fluid, but it was not painful or tender, and his chief complaint was of a sense of tightness across the loins. The cutaneous veins of the belly were not enlarged.

Pulse 100, regular, tolerably full.

Inspirations, twenty a minute. He had some cough, and spat up viscid mucus. No pain of the chest. A soft, systolic bellows-sound was heard at the base of the heart and along the arteries.

The urine was of natural color, clear, of sp. gr. 1015, free from albumen.

His intellect and his senses were unimpaired, and he slept well.

The following day he complained more of the feeling of tightness across the loins, and, as he had passed but little water, the physician's assistant imagined the bladder was distended. A catheter was introduced in consequence, but only a small quantity of urine was drawn off. The operation was very difficult, on account of the stricture, which was found to be a close one. It was followed by considerable bleeding from the urethra; and for three or four days afterwards some blood came away before the urine each time he passed it.

From this time to the 26th of August no striking change took place. The pulse ranged from 96 to 114. The appetite was uncertain and the bowels were irregular. He vomited the day after the catheter was passed, but at no other time. He had now and then some bleeding from the nose and from the gums. His skin was hotter than natural, and his tongue was generally dry and somewhat glazed, but he did not complain much of thirst. The urine was always clear, and free from albumen, and its sp. gr. ranged from 1015 to 1022. He had, throughout, the same sallow, cachectic look as at first.

At the end of this time the cutaneous veins of the abdomen had become much enlarged, and the ascites, which had been gradually increasing, was enormous. The legs, too, were enormously swelled, and the scrotum and penis were very œdematous. He complained much of the sense of distension and of pain in the loins. The belly was then tapped, and twelve pints of serous fluid were drawn off.

The fluid had a sp. gr. 1013; and according to my friend Dr. Miller, who made an analysis of it, contained in 1000 parts—

Water	966.95
Albumen	22.51
Salts and extractive matter	8.54
	998.00

It contained phosphates of lime and magnesia; chlorides of potassium and sodium; sulphate of potash and free soda; a trace of iron, and a trace of silica, but not a trace of urea.

After the tapping, he was for some time much more comfortable, but the ascites came on again; and by the 18th of September, had reached its former degree. He suffered much from the great œdema of the penis and scrotum, and to relieve this some punctures were then made in the legs. The discharge from the punctures was very profuse, and the œdema of the scrotum and of the legs diminished. The skin about the punctures in the left leg became red and painful, symptoms of sinking came on, and he died on the 26th.

On his admission to the hospital he was put on milk diet, which, with a few *extras*, was his diet throughout, and he was ordered a saline draught with nitre and henbane. On the 21st of June he was given, in addition, two grains of calomel with a quarter of a grain of opium, three times a day, till the 26th of June, when, the mouth being sore, the calomel was ordered to be taken only occasionally. The mouth was kept sore till the 3d of July, without any benefit. The medicines he had been taking were then left off, and he was ordered instead to take a diuretic draught, containing three grains of iodide of potassium, three times a day, and to rub in over the liver some compound iodine ointment every night.

This treatment was continued till the beginning of August, without producing any appreciable change in his condition. It was then left off, and afterwards he took only a simple diuretic mixture, with a saline purgative now and then, when the bowels were confined, or when he felt unusual distension.

The body was examined thirteen hours after death.

The legs were very œdematous, and on the skin about the punctures in the left leg were some vesications, as if from commencing gangrene. There was no œdema of the hands or face.

The abdomen contained a large quantity of straw-colored serous fluid.

The liver was small, and weighed only two pounds and eleven and a half ounces. Its under surface was whitened by a very thin false membrane, and its upper surface had an opaline tint, apparently from an extremely thin false membrane extended over it. It was united to the diaphragm by a few threads of false membrane near the suspensory ligament, but had no other unnatural adhesions. Its edges were rounded, and its surface was roughened by the projection of small, round nodules. When sliced, it was found to be generally pale, from containing but little blood, and the cut surface had a mottled appearance from being thickly studded with roundish bodies, varying in size from the smallest perceptible to that of a small pea, and contrasting in color with the intervening substance, the color of the round bodies or nodules being yellow in various shades, from pale yellow to brown ; that of the intermediate substance being pale without any yellow tint. The rounded bodies were pretty uniformly distributed throughout the substance of the liver. They were not generally larger or more numerous deep in its substance than near the surface.

The matter of these round yellow nodules, examined under the microscope, showed a mass of the nucleated cells of the liver tinged yellow. Some cells were yellow throughout ; in others, there was a spot of yellow about the nucleus, or rather about the centre of the cell, while the portion near the circumference had its usual appearance. The quantity of yellow matter in the cells was greater the deeper the color of the nodule from which they were taken. Some cells from the lighter colored nodules, or from the substance about them, had no yellow tint, and were perfectly natural. Some cells contained a good deal of oil, in globules, which was very unevenly distributed ; the cells in some portions containing little, in others much.

The gray substance intermediate to the nodules was tough, and seemed a modification of white fibrous tissue. It was opaque, and had a confused granular appearance under the microscope. When a drop of acetic acid was placed on the specimen under the microscope, it became much more transparent, and exhibited a great number of distinct granules.

The gall-bladder and gall-ducts, as far as they could be readily traced, and the portal veins, seemed quite healthy.

The gall-bladder contained olive-colored bile, so viscid that it could be drawn out in threads.

The spleen was rather large, and its surface was mottled with white, by a very thin coating of contracted lymph. Its substance was tolerably firm, and of its natural color.

There were no marks of inflammation of the peritoneum investing the stomach and intestines. The mucous membrane of the stomach was healthy, and nowhere softened. There was some thickening and induration of the submucous areolar tissue, forming a ring, not above two lines in breadth, about the pylorus. No thickening of the areolar tissue in other parts of the stomach.

The coats of the intestines were pale, and those of the small intestine were thin ; but the mucous membrane was healthy throughout.

The ascending and the transverse portions of the large intestine were much distended with gas.

The kidneys were quite healthy.

The cavity of the left pleura contained a considerable quantity of serous fluid, and on the lower lobe of the left lung, and the corresponding part of the pleura costalis, there was a thin coating of recently effused lymph. The lower lobe of the lung was compressed by the liquid, but the lung was otherwise healthy. The right lung was united to the pleura costalis by a few threads of old false membrane, but presented no other marks of disease.

The heart was small, and the pericardium and valves were quite healthy. The aorta was healthy.

The brain was not examined.

The right branch of the portal vein was injected for me by my colleague, Mr. Simon. The size did not flow freely, and the left lobe of the liver was not at all colored by it. The larger of the nodules in the right lobe were, however, colored by the size, and, under the microscope, the capillary vessels in their interior were seen to be injected.

I could not discover that any portal veins of a size to be readily traced were obliterated.

In this case, the appearance of the liver corresponded exactly to the description given by Abercrombie of one form of cirrhosis, where the yellow matter is dispersed through the substance of the liver in small nodules like peas, or, to take the comparison of Clossy, as in the vitellarium of a laying hen.

An examination through the microscope showed at once that this yellow matter was the original lobular substance of the liver, which was drawn into these round nodules by the adventitious tissue between them.

The nodules were empty of blood, and tinged with bile from the impediment the new tissue caused to the entrance of blood by the portal veins, and to the escape of the bile through the ducts. The adventitious tissue (which had much the appearance of false membrane at an early stage of organization) was formed, no doubt, from coagulable lymph.

The small size and weight of the liver, notwithstanding the existence of this new tissue, shows to what an extent the original lobular substance of the liver had shrunk. It is worthy of remark, that notwithstanding this great atrophy of the lobular substance, there was no decided jaundice.

In the winter of 1850, I met with another instance of the same kind, in which the disease existed in still higher degree, and caused deep jaundice. The patient was a man, sixty-four years of age, who for great part of his life had been in the habit of drinking enormous quantities of gin. The liver was very small and very tough, and its surface was roughened by the projection of small round nodules. When sliced, the cut surface presented a mottled appearance, from being studded with very small, roundish bodies, the largest no bigger than a small pea, which were of various shades of yellow, and which, in consequence, were in strong contrast with the intervening substance, which had no yellow tinge. These variously colored nodules were all that remained of the original secreting substance of the liver. The gray intervening substance, to which the liver owed its toughness and great part of its bulk, was mainly composed of adventitious tissue.

Some conception of the degree of atrophy which the proper structure of the liver had undergone, may be formed from the fact, that although the man was of very large frame, the whole organ weighed only thirty-seven ounces, and only a small portion of it consisted of the original hepatic substance.

Atrophy of the lobular substance of the liver may result, as we have seen, from mere passive congestion, long continued; it may result also from spirit-drinking, without the aid of inflammation, through the direct influence which the spirit has in lessening the vitality and the power of reproduction of the liver-cells; it may result, in like manner, from the action of many other poisons, and, I believe, from depressing mental emotions, and whatever else is capable of long impairing its secreting function—and the texture of the liver may be altered in consequence; but the ordinary appearances in cirrhosis, and the remarkable changes above described, are mainly the consequence of adhesive inflammation in the areolar tissue about the small twigs of the portal vein, by which serous fluid and coagulable lymph are poured out. The serous part of the effusion gets absorbed, and the lymph contracts and becomes converted into dense fibrous tissue, which divides the lobular substance of the liver into well-defined masses, gives great density and toughness to the organ, and by compressing the small twigs of the portal vein and the small gall-ducts, and thus impeding the flow of blood and the escape of bile, induces great atrophy of the original hepatic tissue, and causes the grayish and yellowish tints which a section of the liver presents.

The appearance and consistence of the liver is sometimes further altered by the supervention of what is termed "the fatty degeneration;" in other words, by an accumulation of oil globules, in the cells and between the cells, in the lobular substance. This interstitial deposit of oil swells out the lobules, or the small defined masses of lobules into which the liver is divided, and thus makes the liver still more nodulous, or more coarsely granular, and at the same time renders the lobular substance softer, so that it can be more readily scraped away from the fibrous tissue, and of a paler yellow than it otherwise would be.

In the chapter on suppurative inflammation of the substance of the liver, it was remarked that where the inflammation results from contamination of the portal blood, the capsule of the liver, and the peritoneum covering it, are often exempt from disease; that it is only when the abscess approaches the surface that adhesions form between the liver and adjacent organs; and that even in such cases the adhesions are often of small extent, being limited to the portion of peritoneum covering the abscess.

In adhesive inflammation of the liver, brought on by spirit-drinking, the physical cause of the inflammation is likewise brought by the portal blood, and the capsule is not primarily affected. In some cases, even of hob-nail liver, the peritoneum covering the liver presents no trace of disease, and the capsule has its natural appearance, and can be readily stripped off. In other cases the capsule is hard to remove, and frequently there is an extensive false membrane on the surface of the liver, or there are tufts of newly-formed tissue, uniting the liver to adjacent organs.

In the form of disease before described, where the newly formed fibrous tissue is found in great quantity, but solely or chiefly in the portal canals of considerable size, false membranes on the surface of the liver are perhaps constant, and are certainly, in most cases, much thicker than in ordinary hob-nailed, or granular liver, where the new fibrous tissue is more interstitial.

The size of a liver in a state of cirrhosis is very variable. The lymph effused into the areolar tissue of the portal canals, from which all the changes result, of course tends, at first, to augment the size of the liver; and if much of this lymph be poured out at once, the liver may for a time be much enlarged. But, by degrees, the serous part of the effusion is absorbed, the lymph contracts, and the organ again diminishes in bulk. When this happens, the diminishing bulk of the organ is not owing simply to the diminishing bulk of the lymph itself. The lymph, in contracting, compresses the portal veins, and impedes the passage of the blood to the secreting substance of the liver, diminishing its vascularity, and, consequently its bulk. Many small branches of the portal vein it entirely obliterates, *and, by so doing, causes complete atrophy of the portions of the liver which these branches supplied.*[1]

It is to the contraction of the lymph itself, and to the diminished vascularity of the organ, and to the complete atrophy of portions of its secreting substance, that the shrinking of the liver is owing.

Dr. Bright says that, in some cases, he has been able to follow distinctly the enlargement of the liver early in the disease, and its gradual diminution afterwards. On account of the slowness of the change, and the difficulty of ascertaining the exact size of the liver, we can seldom obtain this direct evidence of the fact. But if adhesions have formed between the liver and adjacent organs, we may frequently assure ourselves that the liver has greatly shrunk, by simply inspecting the bands of adhesion.

Some time ago, in a case of advanced cirrhosis, I found a band of areolar tissue, some inches in length, uniting the liver to the spleen. The adhesion must have taken place when the organs were in contact, and the band have been drawn out as one or the other contracted.

In another case of advanced cirrhosis, I found the convex surface of the liver united to the diaphragm by tufts or bands of false membrane, an inch in length. The parts of the liver at which these tufts were inserted were *hollow or depressed*, and when all the tufts were divided the surface of the liver was very uneven. Here, as in the case in which the liver and spleen were united, the adhesions must have taken place when the surfaces were in contact, and the bands have been drawn out as the surfaces receded from each other. In both cases, these tufts or bands were evidence of the contraction of the liver, after adhesions had formed. The degree of contraction being different in different parts, the surface of the liver becomes uneven.

[1] See remarks on adhesive inflammation of the portal vein in a subsequent chapter.

The small gall-ducts, like the branches of the portal vein they accompany, are compressed, and perhaps sometimes completely obstructed, by the new fibrous tissue—and such obstruction is, as will be shown further on,[1] an additional cause of atrophy of the lobular substance—but the mucous membrane of the gall-bladder and of the larger ducts is generally healthy. The outer coats of the gall-bladder are sometimes found thickened, and the gall-bladder contracted, from the deposition of lymph, which has subsequently become organized or contracted; but this change, like the adhesions of the capsule of the liver, which are generally found along with it, seems to be secondary;—the consequence of inflammation propagated from the deep-seated tissues.

If the inflammation of the capsule be extensive, and much lymph be poured out, some of this may fall among the intestines, and cause adhesion of contiguous folds.

The coagulable lymph poured out in inflammation of a serous membrane seems to cause adhesive inflammation and effusion of lymph of the same kind at every part of the membrane to which it may be mechanically transferred. In this way, perhaps, cirrhosis may lead to adhesive inflammation of the entire surface of the peritoneum. In persons who have died of ascites, apparently the result of cirrhosis, the entire surface of the peritoneum investing the liver and intestines has now and then been found covered by a dense false membrane. I have met with one or two instances of this kind, and some others are recorded by Dr. Bright in his Hospital Reports. It is possible that in some such cases adhesive inflammation of the peritoneum was the primary disease, and that the diminished size and increased firmness of the liver, and obstruction to the circulation through it, were caused by the contraction of the dense false membrane upon it.

The bile found in the gall-bladder in persons dead of cirrhosis presents various appearances. Often it is thin or serous, and of an apricot or orange color (Andral, *Obs.* 21); in other cases, where the change in the texture of the liver seems just the same, it has its natural appearance (Andral, *Obs.* 18). Sometimes it is inspissated, and of a dark olive.

In consequence of the impediment to the passage of the portal

[1] See cases of complete obstruction of the common gall-duct related in a subsequent chapter.

blood through the liver, the intestinal veins which feed the vena portæ are found distended, and, when there is no false membrane on the peritoneum, the minute veins in those parts of the peritoneum to which the blood gravitates are seen beautifully injected and varicose. It now and then happens in such cases that the coats of the intestine are œdematous; and in a case related by Andral there was œdema of the coats of the gall-bladder. In a subject examined by Carswell, the trunks and branches of the portal vein were found blocked up by fibrinous coagula. The condition of the liver is described by Carswell, and represented in (plate 2, fasc. *Atrophy*) his work on Morbid Anatomy.

With such evidence of impediment to the passage of the portal blood through the liver, we might expect that the spleen would always, or generally, be congested and enlarged in cirrhosis. But it is not found to be so. The appearance of the spleen does not indeed seem to be much modified by the existence of cirrhosis. It may be of natural size and appearance (Andral, t. iv. *Obs.* 18); or small and soft (Ib., *Obs.* 17); or small and firm (Ib., *Obs.* 19).

How is this to be accounted for?

The skin, without exhibiting any other striking change, is almost always dry and unperspiring; and sometimes remains so when the cirrhosis becomes complicated with tuberculous disease of the lung or other conditions that usually induce free sweating. Spirit-drinking, which is the most common cause of cirrhosis, injures the texture of the skin, and seems, as it does with the liver, to impair the nutrition and impede the development of its secreting cells, and thus to lessen its secreting power.

Morbid changes are often found in the kidneys and other organs in persons dead of cirrhosis—produced in part by the habits of life that caused the cirrhosis, in part by the unhealthy state of the blood and the unusual stress on other secreting organs, especially the kidneys, which necessarily result from defective action of the liver and skin. The most common of them are the small serous cysts on the surface of the kidneys, atheromatous disease of the arteries, and marks of slight adhesive inflammation on the surface of the heart. No such changes, however, are peculiar to cirrhosis, or so constantly accompany it that they can be considered essential, or that they need be specified in a general description of the disease.

Causes.—There are perhaps various conditions capable of producing, or that may help to produce, the different forms of adhesive inflammation of the substance of the liver under consideration, but the most common and most powerful cause in this country, indeed the only cause whose influence is apparent, is spirit drinking. These forms of disease are in consequence most frequent in large manufacturing towns, among the poorer classes, many of whom spend great part of their earnings in gin; and for this reason the granular and the hob-nailed liver, known to the French as cirrhosis, has been familiarly termed by English practitioners, the *gin-drinker's* liver.

The liver is more liable to inflammation from spirit-drinking than other organs, because the spirit when absorbed by the blood-vessels of the stomach is at once conveyed to it, without change, and without undergoing further dilution than by admixture with the portal blood from other sources: whereas, before it can reach other organs, it must filter through the liver, where much of it may be retained, or excreted, or changed by the chemical affinities there at work, and must, besides, be still further diluted by diffusion through the whole mass of venous blood that is returned from the rest of the body.

The influence of spirituous liquors in causing cirrhosis depends not merely on the quantity of alcohol drunk, but on its degree of dilution and on the times at which it is taken. It is well known that *spirit*-drinkers are the especial victims of cirrhosis, and that wines and malt liquors have little tendency to produce it. Now, in wine and malt liquors the alcohol exists in a state of mere admixture with their other constituents, and there can be little doubt, therefore, that the more injurious effects of ardent spirits on the liver depend mainly on the circumstance, that the victims of spirit-drinking not only drink large quantities of spirits, but often drink them "neat," and when the stomach is empty—so that the alcohol is rapidly absorbed and conveyed to the liver with comparatively little dilution. In wine and beer the alcohol is already largely diluted, and the beverages, when drunk to excess, are usually drunk at, or soon after meals, when the alcohol is still further diluted with the other contents of the stomach.

Some interesting observations on the effects of poisoning by alcohol were published a few years ago by Dr. Percy, in an Essay which obtained one of the gold medals annually given in the University of Edinburgh. Dr. Percy found that, in dogs poisoned by alcohol he could recover alcohol from the blood, the brain, and various other organs, but, as might have been expected, in greatest quantity from the liver.

The inflammation of the *areolar tissue* in the portal canals is probably owing to the diffusion of alcohol through it from the portal veins. We can readily fancy such diffusion taking place, if we consider how readily alcohol permeates animal membranes and tissues. This property of alcohol, and the readiness with which it mixes with water, also explain the circumstances noticed by most pathologists, that in cirrhosis the *whole* liver is changed in structure, and the different parts of it generally in pretty equal degree.

If globules of mercury or of pus find their way into the veins that feed the vena portæ, they become arrested at particular *points* in the lobules of the liver, and excite at each of those points circumscribed inflammation and abscess, while the rest of the liver may continue healthy; but alcohol, mixing readily with water, becomes equally diffused through the whole mass of portal blood flowing through the liver, and the inflammation it excites involves in consequence the entire organ.

There are various circumstances that seem to favor the action of alcohol in producing cirrhosis. One of them is obstructed circulation through the lungs or heart. This, by lessening the activity of respiration, causes the alcohol in the system to be expanded more slowly, and, by retarding the course of the blood in the capillaries of the liver, it may cause the alcohol mixed with the blood to have greater effect on the tissues. M. Becquerel, in an elaborate paper on Cirrhosis, published in the *Archives Générales*, in 1840, states that the heart was diseased in twenty-one out of forty-two cases of cirrhosis of which he has given an analysis; and that in these cases the heart was diseased before the liver. But he also states that in thirteen of these twenty-one cases the cirrhosis was at what he calls the first degree, and gave rise to no symptoms, or to very trifling symptoms. It is perhaps fair to infer that in some of these cases M. Becquerel mistook for the first stage of cirrhosis the nutmeg appearance of the liver produced by partial congestion of the capillaries.

If we exclude these doubtful cases, there still remain a considerable number in which some disease of the heart was found associated with the disease of the liver, and, if we may credit M. Becquerel, was antecedent to it. M. Becquerel, indeed, maintains that disease of the heart, by producing long-continued congestion of the liver, is, of itself, the most common cause of cirrhosis. But it is far more probable that obstructed circulation through the chest has no *direct* influence in causing the disease, and that it contributes to it only by giving greater effect to the influence of alcohol and other efficient causes. There is no reason to believe that mere passive congestion of other organs has any direct influence in causing active inflammation of them; and disease of the heart would surely lead to œdema of the legs and general dropsy, before it would cause extravasation of the fibrin of the blood into the substance of the liver.

The frequent association of disease of the heart with this disease of the liver, however, may be in part accounted for by the great prevalence of disease of the heart, from rheumatism and other causes, among the lower classes in our large towns, who are the chief victims of spirit-drinking; and also by the fact that this destructive habit has a tendency to produce disease of the heart and large bloodvessels, as well as of the liver.

Another condition that favors the influence of alcohol in producing cirrhosis is a hot climate. In cold countries ardent spirits may be drunk with impunity, sometimes perhaps with benefit, in quantities that would be very injurious in hot countries. The reason of this is, that in cold countries the alcohol is rapidly expended in keeping up the temperature of the body. When it has once passed into the general circulation, its carbon and hydrogen combine with the oxygen absorbed in the lungs, and are then exhaled in the form of carbonic acid and water. In hot climates, where respiration is less active, the alcohol accumulates more in the system, and has a more injurious effect on the tissues. It is well known that in India, and in other tropical countries, hard drinking produces the most baneful effects. It must be remembered, however, that alcohol has *always* to pass through the liver before it can be consumed in the respiratory process. It has thus an immediate effect on this organ, which is in a great measure independent of climate, and readily produces fatal disease of it even in the coldest countries. Coldness of climate, indeed, may indirectly lead to greater frequency of the disease we are considering, by causing a more general desire for ardent spirits, and thus inducing a freer consumption of them. Cirrhosis is more common in England and Scotland than in France.

There are, perhaps, various other conditions that give greater effect to habits of intemperance in inducing disease of the liver. A congested state of the liver, from whatever cause, or a feverish state of the system, in all probability disposes to it.

The influence of ardent spirits in producing cirrhosis accounts for the fact that the disease is more common in men than in women, and much more common in persons above the age of thirty than below it.

Cirrhosis is occasionally met with in some of our domestic animals. Dr. Carswell has given a drawing of a portion of a cow's liver in which this disease existed. He states that the cow had ascites, but says nothing of the food upon which it had been kept. I have found the same disease in the liver of a pig.

It is also sometimes met with in temperate persons—so that there must be other causes for it besides spirit-drinking. There may be other substances, among the immense variety of matters taken into the stomach, or among the products of faulty digestion, which, on being absorbed into the portal blood, causes, like alcohol, adhesive inflammation of the liver. What these substances are is as yet, however, only matter of surmise.

In a considerable proportion of the published cases of cirrhosis there was organic disease of the stomach: and in many of those published by Andral—the most detailed to which I can refer—the illness seems to have commenced with vomiting and purging, which was followed, after some time, by ascites. Many cases seem certainly to show that the disease is occasionally produced by some product of faulty digestion, or by some errors of diet other than the undue consumption of ardent spirits.

This inference is strongly borne out by the experience of practitioners in India. Adhesive inflammation of the liver, leading to enlargement and induration of it, and consequently to chronic derangement of its functions, is a common form of hepatitis in that country, and seems to result in part from the use of alcoholic drinks, which are the more injurious from the heat of the climate, in part from the large quantities of curries, and of hot spices of various kinds which the English in India consume.[1]

[1] I have pleasure in referring the reader who is desirous of information on this point, to the admirable treatise by Dr. Parkes, "On the Hepatitis and Dysentery of India."

Symptoms.—Cirrhosis usually comes on very insidiously; and when the inflammation does not involve the capsule of the liver, the symptoms are in most cases few and obscure, until the lymph effused in the substance of the liver has caused impediment to the flow of the portal blood and to the secretion and escape of bile. Some enlargement of the liver, a dull pain in the right hypochondrium, and disordered digestion, are the chief symptoms in the early stages, and some of these even may be wanting, or be so slight as to escape our notice.

In some cases, however, the onset of the disease is more sudden, and the symptoms at first are more striking and more indicative of active inflammation. The patient has fever, with loss of appetite, perhaps occasional vomiting, and, it may be jaundice, and his urine is high colored and charged with lithates. There is much pain and tenderness in the region of the liver, and the liver is readily felt to be enlarged.

The disease begins in this way when much lymph is effused at once and the inflammation involves the capsule of the liver.

When the acute symptoms are subdued by treatment, or subside of themselves, the patient follows his usual occupations, and presents only the slight tokens of disease before mentioned. But he finds that he gradually grows weaker and thinner, his appetite is uncertain, his skin becomes dry and rough, and his complexion sallow and earthy.

After the lapse of some weeks, or months, or years—according to the quantity of lymph first effused, the success of the treatment then adopted, and the subsequent habits of the patient—the fibrin poured out has become so contracted and is in such quantity that the free passage of the blood through the liver, and perhaps also the free escape of bile from it, is prevented. There then occur a different train of symptoms, which are so characteristic that there is seldom much difficulty in detecting the disease.

The belly becomes enlarged by a dropsical fluid, which collects, without pain or tenderness, in the peritoneal sac, and gradually increases so as to cause great distension of the belly, and often, by impeding the movements of the diaphragm, much difficulty of breathing. In some cases this dropsy of the belly is followed by œdema of the legs, but there is no œdema of the hands or face, unless there be likewise disease of the heart or kidneys.

At the same time the veins on the surface of the belly grow

larger, and the patient becomes liable to hemorrhage from the stomach and bowels. This enlargement of the superficial veins of the belly shows clearly that the current of the portal blood is impeded, and is very characteristic of cirrhosis.

The complexion is sallow and earthy, or of a slightly greenish cast, and the skin is almost invariably dry and rough.

The appetite is uncertain and often entirely gone; the skin is hotter than it should be; the patient has occasional thirst; the tongue is slightly furred; the lips are frequently redder than natural, and contrast strongly with the pale and sallow face; digestion is painful or disordered, often attended with heartburn and sour eructations; and the urine is almost always scanty and high-colored, and generally throws down a deep-red, sometimes a pinkish, sediment of lithate of ammonia.

There is likewise tendency to hemorrhage from the nose and other parts in which there is no particular stress on the vessels. Small purpuric spots often appear on the face or forehead, sometimes on the distended belly; and if the patient be cupped, ecchymosis is apt to take place about the punctures.

When ascites has once occurred, it persists; the patient continues to lose flesh and strength, and after the lapse of some months, or perhaps a year or two, dies, usually from gradually increásing exhaustion.

In some cases, when the patient is much reduced, death is hastened by the occurrence of colliquative diarrhœa, or by the drain from the system caused by tapping, to which recourse is had to relieve the distress of breathing, or the other evils occasioned by the great distension of the belly.

The intellect and senses are usually free from disorder to the last.

It will readily be seen that the most distinctive symptoms in the advanced stage of cirrhosis result from obliteration or compression of the small twigs of the portal vein, and the consequent obstacle to the circulation in the liver. The blood in the portal vein cannot pass through the liver with its usual freedom, the veins that go to form the portal vein become, in consequence, distended, and various effects are produced.

1st.—The most striking of these is *ascites*, or dropsy of the belly, which is an immediate effect of the distension of the veins that return the blood from the peritoneum. In consequence of this distension, the serous part of the blood transudes through the vessels, or absorption by those vessels is less active than it should be, and serous fluid—of much less density, however, and containing much less albumen, than the serum of the blood—collects in the peritoneal sac.

Ascites constantly exists in the advanced stages of cirrhosis, and is the more important as a distinguishing sign of this disease, because it occurs in few other diseases of the liver. In abscess of the liver, in hydatids of the liver, in the fatty liver, in diseases of the gall-bladder and gall-ducts, the course of the blood is not impeded, or is not sufficiently impeded to cause ascites. Ascites is, however, not unfrequently produced by cancerous masses in the liver, but here the dropsy seldom attains the degree that it does in cirrhosis. It may likewise be produced by obliteration of branches of the portal vein, which is found now and then the only morbid change in the liver—very seldom, however, to such extent as to produce this effect. Ascites occurs also in what has been termed scrofulous disease of the liver, but this disease also, at least in the degree requisite to produce dropsy, is very rare. So that in most of the cases in which considerable dropsy of the belly depends on the liver it depends on cirrhosis.

The dropsy in many cases is confined to the belly, which may be enormously distended with fluid, while there is no œdema whatever of the face or arms, or even of the legs. Frequently, however, together with ascites, there is œdema of the legs, but unless there be some disease of the heart, or of the kidneys, the œdema of the legs is always consecutive to the ascites. This circumstance may be readily explained. An obstacle to the flow of blood through the liver acts at first almost exclusively on the portal system of bloodvessels. It has no direct effect on the general circulation, except through the anastomoses between the hæmorrhoidal veins, and the branches of the internal iliac vein. It causes, therefore, little direct impediment to the return of blood from the legs. The œdema of the legs, observed in some cases of cirrhosis, not only comes on after the ascites, but is caused by it, and is the effect of compression of the vena cava, and of the iliac veins by the fluid distending the peritoneal sac.

Another effect of permanent obstruction to the flow of blood through the liver is a constantly congested state of all the vessels of the intestinal canal, which often gives rise to piles,[1] and not unfrequently to hemorrhage from the stomach or bowels. The distension of the vessels, although frequently productive of hemorrhage, does not, except perhaps in advanced stages of the disease, cause any drain of serous fluid through the mucous membrane. The serous part of the blood does not anywhere escape from *mucous* or from *synovial* membranes, as it does from serous membranes and in the areolar tissue, from mere passive distension of the bloodvessels. Instead of there being a flux from the bowels in cirrhosis, the natural secretions of the mucous membranes are lessened, and the bowels are sometimes confined throughout the whole course of the disease. When hemorrhage takes place it is seldom that much blood is vomited or discharged from the bowels at once. The blood escapes in small quantities, by oozing from the unbroken surface of the mucous membrane, which may continue for many days, or even weeks, in succession. If the stomach be the seat of hemorrhage, the patient during this time has constant pain at the epigastrium, and may vomit daily a small quantity of blackened blood, which is generally mixed with mucus, or in very small distinct coagula. But it often happens that the extravasated blood passes out of the body unnoticed. Too little is poured out at a time to cause vomiting. It is therefore voided by the bowels, and in its passage through them gets mixed with other matters, and is, besides, so much altered that it is no longer recognized as blood.

The blood of the portal system, when thus impeded in its course through the liver, finds another passage to the heart through the superficial veins of the belly, chiefly by means of the anastomoses between the hæmorrhoidal branches of the inferior mesenteric vein and branches of the internal iliac vein; and these superficial veins,

[1] The disposition to piles that results from the obstructed circulation through the liver is most probably increased by the scanty secretion of bile. It is well known that piles are especially frequent in persons in whom, from any cause, the action of the liver is defective. The bile probably tends to prevent the occurrence of piles by its purgative action, and by some more special influence exerted by the *taurine*, which, together with the coloring matters and the cholesterine of bile, is voided by the bowel, and which contains more than 25 per cent. of sulphur, one of our best remedies for piles.

in consequence of having to transmit an increased quantity of blood, grow rapidly larger and longer.

When adhesions form between the surface of the liver and the abdominal parietes, they become organized and traversed by numerous vessels, which can be readily injected from the hepatic artery,[1] and which establish additional channels between the capsular branches of the portal vein, and the superficial veins of the trunk. It is very common in cases of advanced cirrhosis to see large cutaneous veins on each side of the belly and chest. Generally they are most marked on the right side, and become larger at the hypochondrium, but can be traced upwards from the flank. More than once, however, I have seen a large vein emerge abruptly immediately below the right false ribs, and pass up, in a varicose condition, over the chest.

Blood likewise finds its way to the heart circuitously by means of anastomoses between the capsular branches of the portal vein and branches of the phrenic vein. These indirect channels are also often increased in number by means of adhesions between the liver and the diaphragm. Such adhesions, then, so far answer a good purpose that they favor the return of blood to the heart, and lessen the distension of the portal veins.

The sallowness of complexion so generally observed in cirrhosis most probably results chiefly from the impediment to the escape of bile from the lobules and through the small bile-ducts, which the indurated tissue in the portal canals occasions—an impediment of the existence of which there is often sufficient evidence in the unequal biliary congestion of the lobules found after death.

A sallow, jaundiced complexion is much more constant in cirrhosis than in abscess of the liver, but the jaundice is seldom decided, and, even in advanced stages of the disease, the discharges from the bowels are colored by bile.

The change in the complexion takes place gradually, as the contraction of the effused lymph impedes more and more the secretion and escape of bile. Dr. Bright, speaking of such cases, says, "The change from the natural color is usually gradual; and the yellow tinge of the conjunctiva often precedes for some weeks any more decided indication. In time, however, the bronzed appearance of the forehead, or the darkened areola of the eye, bespeak the ap-

[1] Kiernan, Phil. Trans., 1833.

proaching change; and a jaundice, bearing the lighter tints, from a saffron suffusion to a fainter or more decided lemon hue—still, however, liable to considerable fluctuation—establishes itself over the whole body."

The sallow cast of the complexion in the advanced stage of cirrhosis depends, like the ascites, on an organic change in the texture of the liver, which does not admit of remedy. When the effused lymph has become organized, it forms part of the living tissues, and is incapable of removal. The sallowness, then, like the ascites, although it may vary somewhat in degree, never disappears when it has once come on at this stage of the disease.

When observing the complexion, we must take care not to be misled by the permanent bronzed appearance of the face, so common in persons who have been much in hot climates, which is produced by mere exposure to the sun, without any disease of the liver. In such persons, the skin of the chest, and parts covered by clothing, have their natural healthy tint.

We must also take care not to be misled by the sallowness of the face, that results from mere deficiency of red globules in the blood. The sallowness thus produced is readily distinguished by the circumstance that the conjunctiva is of a bluish-white and pearly, while in that which results from deficient secretion of bile, the conjunctiva is more decidedly yellow than the skin.

The emaciation and the loss of strength that occur in cirrhosis, may depend, in part, on direct injury to the stomach and other organs caused by the habits of life that induce cirrhosis; but they are, no doubt, mainly owing to atrophy of the lobular substance of the liver, and to the impediment which the disease creates to the passage of blood through the liver, and to the escape of bile from it. The obstructed circulation impedes the absorption of water and other nutritive substances by the veins of the stomach and intestines; keeps the mucous membrane of this portion of the intestinal canal, and the glands associated with it, in a permanent state of congestion, and thus enfeebles the digestive power; and when the obstruction is so great that blood is diverted from its appointed channel, it must tend directly to produce an impure condition of the blood. That part of the portal blood which does not pass through the liver, but finds another way back to the heart, cannot be freed from the principles of bile, and be otherwise purified, as it should be, and must, therefore, contaminate to a certain degree the whole mass of blood with which it is mixed.

Impediment to the escape of biliary matter from the lobules, and through the small bile-ducts, impairs nutrition directly, by causing a deficiency of bile in the intestinal canal, and a bilious impregnation of the blood; and it has a more remote injurious effect, by being an additional cause of atrophy of the lobular substance.

Destruction of the lobular substance of the liver tends to impair nutrition, by rendering the secretion of bile defective, and thus deranging the work of the intestinal canal, and, by leading directly to an unhealthy and impoverished condition of the blood, which, in consequence of this destruction of the lobular substance, is imperfectly filtered in the liver, and does not undergo there, to their full extent, those reparative changes which the action of the healthy liver causes. Whenever, from any cause, much of the lobular substance of the liver is destroyed, a state of anemia results.

The loss of flesh and strength, then, like the ascites and sallow complexion, depends, in great measure, on changes of structure which we cannot remedy; and although it may be hastened by lowering treatment, or other causes, and may be in some degree stayed by judicious measures, it is, of necessity, when the disease has attained a certain degree, constantly, though slowly, progressive.

Diagnosis.—In the early stage of cirrhosis, the symptoms are often few, and present no distinctive, and, to common eyes, no alarming characters, so that it is only by considering the circumstances in which they arise that we are led to perceive their true significance. Slight shallowness of complexion, a dull pain, or some degree of tenderness in the right hypochondrium, with occasional feverishness, in a person above the age of thirty, who has been long in the habit of drinking spirits to excess, are almost conclusive evidence of the existence of cirrhosis, even before there is any direct proof that the circulation through the liver is impeded. The symptoms in themselves may be slight, but knowledge of the habits of the patient enables us to regard them as tokens of organic disease. Here, as in so many other cases, it is only by knowing the causes of the disease, or the circumstances under which it usually occurs, that we become watchful of its earliest tokens, and learn to interpret them rightly.

When, by the progress of the disease, the course of the blood through the liver is so impeded as to cause ascites, the diagnosis is much more easy; because ascites from other conditions is generally associated with a train of symptoms different from that of cirrhosis, and does not occur especially in spirit-drinkers.

The conditions, besides cirrhosis, that most frequently give rise to persistent ascites are, great enlargement of the spleen, chronic peritonitis, and malignant disease of the liver or omentum.

When ascites results from enlargement of the spleen, the superficial veins of the belly are enlarged, the complexion may be somewhat sallow, there may be occasional hemorrhage from the stomach or bowels, and there is usually, as in cirrhosis, slow and progressive loss of flesh and strength. But the disease may generally be distinguished from cirrhosis by its not occurring especially in spirit-drinkers, by the perspiring or moist state of the skin, and by the existence of a large tumor in the left side of the belly, which, from its form and position, and from the notches on its anterior edge, is readily recognized as the spleen. The course of this disease is often different from that of cirrhosis. The ascites, after having attained a high degree, and lasted a considerable time, may entirely disappear, and although the spleen remains large, the patient may regain health enough for his former pursuits. Now and then, however, the ascites persists and attains the highest possible degree—preventing the descent of the diaphragm, and causing terrible distress—the loss of flesh and strength continues, and the disease destroys life just in the same way as cirrhosis. After death, no cause for these symptoms may be found, except a firm, fleshy, and enormously enlarged spleen.[1]

When ascites results from chronic or adhesive peritonitis, it is attended with wasting of flesh, and the urine, as in cirrhosis, is usually high-colored and highly charged with lithates. But in chronic peritonitis there is not the sallow look of cirrhosis, and there are pain and tenderness all over the belly, with hectic fever and sweating—symptoms which are usually wanting in the advanced stages of cirrhosis.

[1] It may be that in these cases the liver is diseased as well as the spleen. The ascites may depend on obliteration of some branches of the portal vein, and may gradually disappear as the requisite freedom of circulation is restored through other channels.

Again, in peritonitis the fluid poured out is seldom so abundant as in cirrhosis. The belly may be as much distended, but this is owing in great part to the intestines being distended by gas—which they always are in peritonitis.

The ascites, too, does not persist as it does in cirrhosis. If the fluid be serous, it soon becomes absorbed. There is not the same impediment to the absorption of the fluid in peritonitis as in pleurisy. In cases of pleurisy, when the lung has been much compressed, and is irrecoverably bound down by false membranes, the fluid in the cavity of the pleura, even if serous, cannot be absorbed faster than the space it occupies can be filled up by the contraction of the side and the encroachment of the opposite lung. When these means have attained their limit, it is physically impossible that a drop more of the fluid can be absorbed; and consequently a collection even of serous fluid may remain in the cavity of the pleura for years. But in peritonitis there is no such impediment to the absorption of the fluid. The abdominal parietes can continue to fall in so as to close up the cavity occupied by the liquid. The obliteration of this cavity is further aided by flatulent distension of the bowels. When the fluid is absorbed, the folds of intestine, which are united to each other and to the parts with which they have been brought into contact, are always distended with gas. The abdomen is large, and gives out a tympanitic sound on percussion.

Moreover, in peritonitis, even when there is much fluid in the sac of the peritoneum, the sense of fluctuation derived from percussion is usually much less distinct than in ascites from disease of the liver. In peritonitis, contiguous loops of intestine are glued together, and the fluid is contained in pouches, so that the shock communicated by percussion is propagated through it less perfectly than when it is contained in a single cavity.

We are still further guided in distinguishing the two diseases by knowledge of the most common circumstances in which they respectively occur. Cirrhosis, as we have seen, is rarely met with in persons of temperate habits, or under the age of thirty. Chronic peritonitis occurs at all ages, without any marked relation to particular habits of life, and in grown-up persons is almost always dependent on the presence of tubercles, which are deposited in the lung as well as on the peritoneum. If there be no evidence of the presence of tubercles in the lung, we have strong presumption that the fluid in the peritoneum is not the result of chronic inflammation of that membrane.[1]

Cancer of the liver has also, in some cases, many points of resemblance with cirrhosis. The patient may have the same sallow look as in cirrhosis; there may be some degree of ascites, with loss of strength, disordered digestion, and scanty, high-colored, and turbid urine; and the disease occurs at a time of life when cirrhosis is common.

But in cancer of the liver the ascites seldom attains the degree it has in cirrhosis. The fluid is seldom in sufficient quantity to render the walls of the belly tense. In cancer, too, as the disease advances, the liver always grows larger, and, in most cases, where the cancerous tumors so obstruct the circulation through the liver as to cause ascites, the liver can be felt extending far below its natural limits. In the advanced stages of cirrhosis, on the contrary, the liver shrinks, and is generally smaller than in health. In cancer, there is usually hectic fever with *sweating;* in cirrhosis, the skin is dry and rough.

The diseases may be still further distinguished by considering the previous habits of the patient. Cancer has no marked dependence on particular modes of life, and is perhaps as common in the higher classes as in the lower. Confirmed cirrhosis, on the contrary, is rare in the higher classes, and is seldom met with in any class, except among those who have been long in the habit of drinking spirits to excess.

Cancer of the *omentum*, like cirrhosis, may cause great ascites, with very distinct fluctuation and enlargement of the superficial veins of the belly: and the thickened and uneven omentum may form a tumor at the epigastrium, which, being indistinctly felt through the liquid, may be taken for a large and nodulous liver.

The disease may be distinguished from cirrhosis by the greater emaciation and *more rapid* wasting; by the higher degree of fever; by the absence of jaundice or sallowness; by the more diffused pain in the belly; by the perspiring skin; and, it may be, by want of clear evidence of spirit-drinking.

[1] Many of the distinguishing marks of cirrhosis here noticed were pointed out by M. Becquerel, in the elaborate paper in the Archives Générales before referred to.

I have also known ovarian dropsy, where the fluid has been contained in a single thin cyst, mistaken for ascites, supposed to result from cirrhosis. The following circumstances sufficiently distinguish the two diseases:—

1. Ovarian dropsy does not occur especially in spirit-drinkers, and in this disease the skin is not generally dry and sallow, and the superficial veins of the belly are not generally enlarged, as in the advanced stages of cirrhosis.

2. In ovarian dropsy the fluid is contained in a cyst, which is in contact with the walls of the belly in front, and pushes the intestines into the epigastric and lumbar regions; so that, in any posture of the patient, the front part of the belly, from the pubis upwards as high as the tumor rises, is dull on percussion, and there is resonance only along the epigastric region, and, on strong percussion, in the lumbar regions: whereas, in ascites, the intestines usually float to the surface of the liquid, and, when the woman is lying on her back, there is usually resonance on percussion in the umbilical region, which is then uppermost, and dulness in the epigastric and lumbar regions, which are below the surface of the liquid.

3. A pouch of an ovarian tumor occasionally extends into the pelvis; and its firm, elastic surface may be felt in the vagina.

Treatment.—From what has been already said of the nature of cirrhosis, it is quite clear that it is only in the early stage of the disease that we can materially benefit the patient. During this stage, while the inflammation is active, it may perhaps be in our power to lessen the amount of effusion, and, before the lymph effused has become organized, even to cause its removal by absorption. But when lymph has been thrown out in large quantity, and when it has become organized, or is otherwise incapable of removal, and has already by its contraction caused much impediment to the flow of the portal blood and materially impeded the elimination of bile, medical treatment can be only palliative. It is, therefore, of the utmost importance that the disease should be detected early, in order that we may be able to obviate such serious and irremediable effects. But, as we have seen, the detection of the disease in its early stages is sometimes very difficult, as the symptoms are then often slight and equivocal, and it is only by considering the previous habits of the patient that we are led to perceive their real significance. In the person of a spirit-drinker, pain and tenderness in the region of the liver should never be neglected, especially if associated with some degree of fever.

At the commencement of the disease the most efficient remedies are—cupping, or leeches, over the liver; cooling saline purgatives, such as sulphate of magnesia or bitartrate of potash; iced drinks; and a very low diet. While there is much tenderness, and some degree of fever exists, nothing produces so much relief as the local abstraction of blood. It must not be forgotten, however, that hard drinkers bear bleeding ill, and care must be taken not to push this remedy too far. Delirium tremens, or other alarming disorder, may be the consequence of its rash and inordinate employment. When bleeding is not considered safe, much benefit may be derived from the application of a blister.

When the fever has abated, and the liver is still large, mercury and iodide of potassium are the medicines from which most benefit may be expected. Blue pill may be given in moderate doses, so as slightly to affect the mouth; or iodide of potassium may be given internally, and the iodine ointment be rubbed into the side.

At the same time we should endeavor to prevail upon the patient to give up his pernicious habit of drinking. We may infer, from the slight degree of fever and the slight pain that often attend the early stages of cirrhosis, that the lymph is thrown out, not all at once, from a single attack of inflammation, but by little at a time, in successive attacks, of which no one is sufficiently severe to cause serious illness. The mischief is done gradually, under the gradual and repeated operation of the cause. By changing the habits of the patient future attacks may be prevented, and the disease be stayed before it has produced fatal organic changes.

Very often our powers of persuasion will fail. The patient will pursue his ruinous course in spite of all our warnings. Often, too, from the insignificant character of the early symptoms, and from general disregard, among the laboring classes, of ailments that do not stop them from working, advice is only sought after the occurrence of ascites. And then the disease has proceeded so far as to be in great measure beyond the power of remedy.

The presence of ascites proves that there is already a mechanical obstacle to the passage of the blood through the liver, and this obstacle we can seldom succeed in removing. The case is analogous to that of stricture of the intestine from the contraction and organization of lymph effused under the mucous coat, or to that of disease of the valves of the heart. There is a permanent mechanical impediment to the due performance of the functions of the organ. The disease will most inevitably, sooner or later, prove fatal.

At this time, that is, after the occurrence of ascites, we can do little good, and may do much harm by bleeding, and other measures that much lessen the power of the heart. It not unfrequently happens, indeed, that, after the disease of the liver has existed a long time, and without any recent aggravation of it, the ascites comes on suddenly or increases suddenly, when by loss of blood or any other cause the power of the heart is much lowered. It must be remembered that there is an impediment to the current of blood through the liver, and that one of the agents to overcome this impediment is the muscular power of the heart.

Even at this stage of the disease, if there have been any recent inflammatory action in the liver, and there be lymph within it that can still be absorbed, good may result from small doses of blue pill or iodide of potassium, which may be given in conjunction with mild diuretics. If diuretics be given alone they generally fail of effect, because when, from cirrhosis or any other condition, much ascites exists, the liquid in the peritoneal sac compresses the kidneys, and prevents their action. The influence of this pressure is made very manifest by the operation of tapping. It is almost constantly found that when by tapping the liquid in the belly is withdrawn, there is a more abundant secretion of urine, and that the quantity of urine again diminishes as the liquid in the belly collects again. This circumstance shows how important it is, in disease of the heart, to get rid of dropsy before much fluid collects in the peritoneal sac to impede the action of the kidneys.

When the cirrhosis is in high degree, a flow of urine, however copious, will not remove, or even very much reduce, the ascites. Of this I had clear proof in a patient admitted into King's College Hospital in the winter of 1840. He was a broker's porter, had drunk hard of spirits, and had long suffered occasional pains in the right hypochondrium. A month before his admission to the hospital he noticed that his belly was much swelled, and soon afterwards swelling of the legs came on. At the time of his admission he had great ascites, striking enlargement of the superficial veins of the belly, and other symptoms of the advanced stage of cirrhosis.

On further inquiry, we learnt that he had also diabetes. He had a craving appetite, with great thirst, and passed daily from ten to twelve pints of urine, which was of light amber color, transparent, and of sp. gr. 1040—1045: containing no albumen, but a large quantity of sugar. He remained in the hospital rather more than a month, when he died of phlegmonous erysipelas of the right thigh.

Notwithstanding the large quantity of urine passed daily, there was not the slightest diminution of the ascites. The belly was enormously distended to the last. After death the liver was found very large and hob-nailed, and united to the diaphragm and to the abdominal walls by bands of adhesion of long standing. The gall-bladder was filled with bile, of a pale orange color. All the capillary vessels in the posterior part of the peritoneum, to which the blood had gravitated, were beautifully injected and varicose. The heart was small, and had no other mark of disease than a white spot on its outer surface. The kidneys were healthy.

In a few instances, after mercury and diuretics have failed, I have seen the ascites removed for a time by hydragogue purgatives. A good purgative of this class is an electuary made by mixing cream of tartar and jalap in equal parts with confection of senna, and it is best given, as are all medicines of similar action, in a single dose in the morning before breakfast, as it then, besides the drain it causes from the coats of the bowel, only sweeps away the refuse of digestion, whereas, if it be given in divided doses during the day, it sweeps away the food that has been digested, but the nutritious particles of which have not been absorbed. It sometimes happens, especially in hard drinkers, that a disposition to nausea exists in the morning, and the medicine is then best given at night. The action of hydragogue purgatives is much increased by giving them in a concentrated form, and by restricting as much as possible the quantity of liquids consumed by the patient.

In many instances hydragogue purgatives, like diuretics, fail to remove the ascites, and they may do much harm by weakening the patient, when his assimilating powers can scarcely maintain his actual position. If they be given at unseasonable times, and when the patient is much reduced in flesh and strength, they cause great prostration, render the tongue dry and brown, and, by lowering the force of the circulation, tend to increase the ascites rather than diminish it.

It sometimes happens that the ascites, by impeding the descent of the diaphragm, causes great distress of breathing, especially in asthmatic and emphysematous persons, or when the breath is already shortened by catarrh. This distress may be relieved for a time by letting out the fluid by tapping. After the operation the patient draws his breath more freely, and feels as if a weight were taken off his chest. Usually, owing to pressure being removed from the kidneys, he makes more water after the operation than he had been making before. But this relief is in most cases only temporary. The fluid accumulates again in the belly, and, after a time—varying, according to the degree of obstruction, from a few days to three or four weeks—reaches its former amount.

The operation should never be had recourse to unless the difficulty of breathing, or the other evils that result from distension of the belly, are very distressing; for the ascites speedily returns, and the operation has consequently the effect of withdrawing a large quantity of serous fluid from the vessels. By repeating the operation frequently, the system may in this way be completely drained of the serous part of the blood. The patient will fall into a state of great prostration, with complete loss of appetite, and with a dry and brown tongue—and will die much sooner than if nothing had been done.

In the advanced stages of the disease considerable comfort may often be given to the patient by the judicious employment of sedatives.

Suppurative inflammation of the liver and adhesive inflammation, the forms of inflammation hitherto considered, leave permanent traces—collections of pus and contracted fibrin—that may be readily discovered after the death of the patient. But there are probably various morbid states of the secreting substance of the liver, which, in the latitude usually given to the term inflammation, should be comprehended under this title, in which, as in erysipelas of the face, and in the affection of the joints in rheumatic fever, the fluids poured out during the inflammatory process become again absorbed, leaving no permanent traces, or only such traces as cannot well be distinguished. In such cases, the nature of the morbid process can be judged of by the symptoms only, unless the patient happen to die during the acute stage of the malady, and while its effects are still present.

Such a morbid process in the liver often occurs in pneumonia of the right lung, perhaps from the heat developed in the seat of the neighboring inflammation. The patient is sometimes jaundiced, and, if the disease prove speedily fatal, the upper part of the right lobe of the liver is found softened and much altered in texture. This change in the condition of the liver was noticed by Abercrombie, who has described it under the term—*simple "ramollissement" of the liver.* He says: "This consists of a broken-down, friable, and softened state of a part of the substance of the liver, without any change of color. It is, in general, most remarkable on the convex surface, extending to a greater or less depth; it is accompanied by a separation of the peritoneal coat at the part, and sometimes there appears to be a loss of substance, as if a portion had been torn out, leaving a ragged irregular surface below. The softened portion has commonly so far lost its consistence that the finger can be pushed through it with very little resistance; and in some cases the affected part is infiltrated with sanious or puriform fluid, not collected into abscesses, but mixed irregularly through the substance of the softened part. This appearance we have every reason to consider as the result of inflammation. It is found in combination with abscess or other marks of inflammation, and I have very often observed it on the upper surface of the liver in connection with extensive inflammation of the right lung. In these cases there was not, in general, any symptom indicating that the liver was affected. Mr. Annesley states that this appearance is frequently met with in India, in persons who have died rapidly from cholera or dysentery."

I have often met with this softening of the part of the liver next the diaphragm, in cases of extensive inflammation of the right lung, but have never found pus in the softened portion. I imagine that suppuration takes place seldom, and that in almost all those cases in which the patient recovers from the pneumonia the liver regains its natural texture.

It is probable that inflammatory disease of other adjacent organs, and especially of the right kidney, sometimes causes a similar change in the texture of the liver, now and then terminating in the formation of pus. Among the cases of abscess of the liver published by Andral, there is one (*Clin. Med.*, iv. obs. 29) in which it is, I think, probable that the inflammation originated in this way.

It certainly, however, very rarely happens that inflammation of the right lung or kidney causes abscess of the liver by the heat developed during the process of inflammation. If this excite any morbid process that can be comprehended under the term inflammation, it is such as to leave, in general, no permanent traces.

Dr. Graves has remarked that symptoms indicative of inflammatory action in the liver—enlargement of the liver, with pain or tenderness, and jaundice—sometimes come on during the course of scarlatina.

In one of his clinical lectures (*Clinical Medicine*, p. 569), he refers to two cases of this kind that happened in the same week in the Meath Hospital. One of these patients, a little boy, was seized with scarlatina in a very severe form, with high fever, and a brilliant eruption all over the body. After two days he had evident symptoms of disease and enlargement of the liver. The other patient was a young man, who had scarlet fever of a milder form. "On the third day he likewise got inflammation of the liver, but was cured by general and local antiphlogistic treatment."

Dr. Graves states that in persons whom an attack of scarlatina has left in a feverish condition, he has often found the liver in a state of *inflammation*—as proved by the benefit derived from local antiphlogistic measures—but inflammation "of rather a chronic character, without any of that remarkable pain and tenderness which characterize acute hepatitis." He considers that this condition of the liver retards and prevents convalescence.

My own observation confirms that of Dr. Graves. I have met with several instances in which enlargement of the liver has come on, and more than one in which jaundice has come on, soon after the disappearance of the rash in scarlatina; but I have never had an opportunity of inspecting the liver in a case of this kind. It is most probable that the disease of the liver is analogous to the disease of the kidney, which so often occurs in scarlatina, after the disappearance of the rash; and that the enlargement of the liver results from rapid development and shedding of the secreting cells, caused by the elimination of some noxious matter through the gland.

This occasionally happens both in the kidney and in the liver, in the course of typhoid fever. In the winter of 1846, a young man, about twenty years of age, who had led a sober life, and had not previously exhibited any signs of liver disease, was admitted at King's College Hospital, under my care, with typhoid fever. The fever was not very severe, and he was convalescent from it, and about to leave the hospital, when he died, almost suddenly, from erysipelatous inflammation of the larynx (cynanche laryngea). The liver was enlarged, and presented a curious mottled appearance, from being studded with small irregular white masses, which, to the naked eye, looked very much like small masses of tuberculous matter, but which, on microscopic examination, were found to consist of hepatic cells. The cells were opaque, and contained a good deal of granular matter, and about the normal quantity of oil. I had, some time before, observed a similar appearance of the liver, where death had occurred during convalescence from fever.

SECT. IV.—*Inflammation of the veins of the liver—Suppurative inflammation of the portal vein—Adhesive inflammation of the branches of the portal vein—Inflammation of the branches of the hepatic vein.*

Inflammation of the veins of the liver.—Inflammation in veins, as in other textures, may be *suppurative*, that is, it may lead to the formation of pus: or it may be *adhesive*, and lead only to the effusion of coagulable lymph, which blocks up and obliterates the vein. But in the inflammation of veins that leads to the formation of pus, coagulable lymph is usually poured out, as well as pus; and the pus does not fill all the inflamed portion of the vein, but is interrupted, here and there, by plugs of fibrin, or coagulated blood, so as to form a string of abscesses along the vein.

Inflammation of the trunk of the vena portæ is of very rare occurrence. From being so deep-seated, this vein is not liable to wounds or other injuries—the most common causes of inflammation of other large veins.

The following case, published by M. Lambron in the *Archives Générales de Médecine*, for June, 1842, is the most complete case of the kind I have found recorded. Inflammation of the trunk of the vena portæ was here caused by a fish-bone, which passed through the pyloric extremity of the stomach and the head of the pancreas and stuck in the superior mesenteric vein.

The patient, a man 69 years of age, was admitted into the hospital *La Pitié*, on the 4th of June, 1841. For some weeks he had been suffering pain in the stomach, with occasional nausea, and his bowels had been much confined. On account of these ailments, a week before his admission, he took a grain of tartar emetic, which produced no amendment.

The day he entered the hospital, he was seized with shivering and nausea, and on the following night he slept ill.

On the morning of the 5th, he was carefully examined. His pulse was nearly natural, and his breathing quite tranquil. His tongue was white, he had some degree of nausea, and his bowels were confined. He complained of constant uneasiness, with paroxysms of pain, which he compared to very severe cramp, in the right hypochondrium, but pressure on that part gave hardly any pain. The liver and the spleen were of natural size. The other functions seemed duly performed. (Wine-lemonade; low diet.)

The 6th and 7th of June he had no rigors. The pain in the right hypochondrium was very severe, but there was no tenderness. The tongue was covered with a whitish coat, there was some nausea, and the bowels were still costive. (A grain of tartar emetic; veal broth; julep.)

On the 8th he suffered still more, and the skin and conjunctiva had become slightly yellow.

On the 11th the jaundice was more marked, and the urine, as tested by nitric acid, contained bile. The pain in the right hypochondrium persisted, with exacerbation from time to time. About f℥vj of blood were taken from the side by cupping.

On the 12th, the pain was less, but he had nausea, and in the evening a shiver, followed by heat and sweating. His tongue was dry, and covered with a blackish coat. Hiccough, and some greenish liquid evacuations. Pulse, 96. The spleen was not perceptibly enlarged. (Quinæ sulphat. gr. iij.)

On the 13th he was nearly in the same state. Some rigors occurred during the night, but they were not succeeded by a hot stage, and the sweating was less profuse than before. Occasional hiccough. Pulse, 80. (A blister was applied to the stomach; the quinine was continued.)

The rigors and the hiccough continued to recur.

On the 15th the fits, like those of ague, recurring more or less regularly, and not yielding to sulphate of quinine, the hiccough, the jaundice, the pain in the right hypochondrium, the absence of disease in other parts of the body, and the nearly natural size of the spleen, led to the inference that the disease was *hepatic phlebitis.*

The 17th the patient was in a typhoid state. The 18th he was a little better, and the jaundice less marked.

The 24th he felt better, and asked for something to eat. In the evening, he was seized with violent shivering, with fever, but now the different stages were confounded, and he shivered while his body was covered with sweat. The urine contained much less bile.

The 25th the fever had not ceased, and seemed likely to become continued. The skin was covered with sweat. The tongue, which had been moist for some days before, had become again dry; and the pain, which had ceased for five or six days, came on again.

The 26th and 27th the shivers recurred, with occasional hiccough, the fever became remittent, the pulse was firm and tolerably full, but the patient was much depressed.

The 28th and 29th he sank lower and lower, and became slightly delirious. Pulse 104, small, and compressible.

He died in the night of the 29th.

The body was examined thirty hours after death. All the tissues were slightly jaundiced. There was no serous fluid in the abdomen. The liver was of a natral size, and of a dark, greenish-yellow, or bronze color. It adhered, at some points, to the diaphragm, but its investing membranes were otherwise healthy. The gall-bladder was of natural size, and had also formed some adhesions to contiguous parts. It was filled with bile, which had all the characters of ordinary bile. The gall-ducts were healthy.

The trunk of the vena portæ contained a sanious fluid, with some flakes of pus.

On tracing the mesenteric roots of the vein, a fish-bone, the size of a large pin, was found stuck into the trunk of the superior mesenteric vein. The bone, implanted in the head of the pancreas, transfixed the vein from above downwards, and from before backwards. At the point where it was pierced by the bone, the mesenteric vein was blocked up by false membranes, which adhered firmly to its inner coat. The false membranes extended from the mouths of the small veins which come directly from the upper part of the duodenum to the orifice of the splenic vein, becoming less and less firmly adherent. Below this obstruction, the roots of the mesenteric vein contained some fibrinous coagula for an extent of some inches, but were otherwise healthy.

The splenic vein was healthy, but contained some reddish fluid like that in the portal vein, from which it had probably flowed into the splenic vein after death.

The trunk of the portal vein was not closed, but was narrowed by false membranes adhering slightly to its coats, which were only a little thickened. It contained pus mixed with blood, and, at some points, pus like that of an abscess. The hepatic divisions of the vein were some of them filled with the same reddish liquid ; their coats being in some parts healthy, in other parts inflamed, thickened, and coated by false membranes. Others contained only clots of blood, which extended to very small ramifications of the vein. Other branches again were perfectly healthy.

The liver contained no abscesses, but its tissue about the transverse fissure was very soft. In parts of the liver supplied by those branches of the portal vein that remained healthy, there was no change of texture. The lobules, of a greenish-yellow color, were distinct, and the interlobular spaces, as well as the intralobular vein, were red from the blood they contained.

In the parts supplied by those branches that were filled with coagula, the lobules were likewise distinct, but were less red at their margins and centres. Lastly, in the parts supplied by the branches of the vein that contained pus and were inflamed, the form of the lobules was still preserved, but the interlobular tissue was very soft, and the divided intralobular veins seemed empty of blood, and gaping.

The hepatic veins were quite healthy, and contained very little blood.

On the posterior wall of the stomach, near the pylorus, was a brownish spot, corresponding to one end of the fish-bone, and on the inside, at the same spot, there was a slight depression capable of lodging the head of a pin. It was clear that the bone had passed through the stomach at this spot, pierced the head of the pancreas, and, going still onwards, had stuck into the mesenteric vein, and caused all the subsequent disorder.

The kidneys, the spleen, and the intestines, were healthy. In the right lung there was some degree of hypostatic pneumonia, but neither lung contained anything like an abscess.

The heart was large, and contained some clots. The right ventricle contained a fibrinous clot, which extended into the pulmonary artery.

This case is very simple. The inflammation of the vein was caused by a mechanical injury, and there was no other disease to interfere with or to mask its effects. The vein most probably became inflamed on the 4th of June, when the patient first shivered. The pain at the stomach and the occasional nausea he had some weeks previous, were most likely caused by the fish-bone then passing through the stomach and pancreas. After the 4th of June the symptoms were just those which might have been expected. There were frequently-recurring rigors, followed by heat of skin and sweating, and, after a short time, typhoid symptoms—as in suppurative inflammation of other large veins—while the pain in the region of the liver, the nausea, the hiccough, the jaundice, and the absence of marked disorder of other organs, showed that the liver was the chief seat of the local disease. The deep situation of the vein explains the absence of tenderness.

In the following case, for notes of which, as well as an opportunity of examining the parts after death, I am indebted to Mr. Busk, the inflammation of the portal vein had a different origin, and led to somewhat different results, but was marked by nearly the same train of symptoms. I cannot describe the case better than in Mr. Busk's own words:—

May, 1844.

I have sent you what I think you will consider a very interesting specimen. It was procured from a man who died last Sunday, after an illness of seven weeks. He was a patient of Mr. Sherwin's, and I have seen him frequently for the last six weeks. His case was extremely obscure, but I surmised from the first that we should find suppuration in the liver.

He was a very robust man, an engineer in the dockyard at Woolwich, and had never been out of England, and was of very sober, temperate habits, married, with one child. Had always enjoyed good health, with the exception of occasional pain in the abdomen, which was not considered of any importance till his last attack. He never had ague.

Seven weeks ago he was seized rather suddenly with severe pain in the abdomen, which obliged him to keep his body bent forward, and he had a severe rigor. I saw him about a week afterwards, and he had then the appearance of great depression. He complained of severe, but only occasional, pain in the epigastric region, predominating on the right side. The pain was not increased by pressure. It did not appear to be of a piercing character, but was attended with a feeling of extreme sinking and distress, and relieved by morphia. It recurred several times a day at irregular intervals, and about twice in twenty-four hours he had a severe rigor, followed by most profuse sweating. There was no distension of the belly, and no enlargement of the liver could be detected on the most careful examination, nor was there any tenderness in the hepatic region.

When I first saw him the evacuations from the bowels were light-colored and very fetid, but he was not jaundiced. Soon afterwards, however, he became jaundiced, and the urine contained bile. The jaundice went off in a few days, and the evacuations became of natural color and consistence. At the same time the urine lost the bile, and threw down a very copious lateritious sediment, which continued to the last. The jaundice passed off suddenly, and the change in the character of the evacuations was preceded by a copious discharge of nearly pure bile.

The symptoms continued with little change to his death. He gradually sank, becoming much emaciated. He never vomited, and had a great desire for oysters, which were almost his whole support.

On examination of the body the lungs were found perfectly sound.

The peritoneum contained several pints of straw-colored serous fluid, mixed with flakes of coagulable lymph; and the stomach, transverse colon, and great omentum were all glued together by soft lymph.

The liver was large, and extended to the left side. Its convex surface had a coating of puriform matter, and was of a dark color. On raising the anterior margin, it was found that the concave surface, including the portal fissure and behind it, was adherent to the stomach and surrounding parts: and on separating the adhesions, the substance of the left lobe was found to be occupied by numerous abscesses, which were bounded externally by the adhesions and by the wall of the stomach. The upper surface of the left lobe was closely adherent to the diaphragm, and in the middle of this portion of the diaphragm there was a circular space, about the size of a shilling, having a semi-gangrenous appearance, opposite to which, on the upper surface of the muscle, the base of the lung was firmly adherent, and pus was deposited in its substance. On detaching the liver from the other parts, a very large collection of thick pus was found in the portal fissure. Pus could be pressed out in great quantity from the dilated portal vein, and was also deposited in the areolar tissue surrounding it. The whole of the left lobe was occupied by innumerable abscesses of all sizes, so as to resemble a coarse sponge filled with pus. In most of these abscesses the pus was thick and white, but in a few it was of a bright yellow. There were also numerous abscesses, some of them of considerable size, in the right lobe.

The portal canals, in the left lobe especially, were thickened, white and firm; and, as far as I could ascertain, the gall-ducts were healthy. I have no doubt the abscesses were connected with branches of the portal vein. In a portion of the surface of the liver which I have sent you, near the fissure in the anterior margin, you will observe a chain of small abscesses, apparently following the course of a vessel, and showing in a very striking manner the real nature of the disease.

The gall-bladder was distended by a very pale mucous fluid, and, like the ducts, was perfectly healthy.

The spleen was of natural size, and except two small superficial abscesses on that part of the surface which bounded an abscess beneath the liver, was quite healthy.

The pancreas was healthy.

The splenic and superior mesenteric veins were healthy, but immediately after their junction the vena portæ was extensively ulcerated, and what remained of its inner surface was covered by a buff-colored false membrane. The tissue in which this part of the vein was lodged was indurated and black; and immediately in contact with the vein were large and suppurated mesenteric glands. The whole mesentery was much thickened, and the glands much enlarged, and in a state of suppuration.

I have sent you the mesentery with the pancreas and duodenum, and as much as I could get of the vena portæ, and of the splenic and superior mesenteric veins. You will see the commencement of the diseased part of the vena portæ, and its apparent connection with the suppurated glands, which I am inclined to believe were the origin of the inflammation of the vein.

The stomach and intestines were carefully examined throughout, and no morbid appearances were found in them.

The kidneys were pale and quite healthy.

The origin of the disease in this case is very obscure. The most probable supposition is, that the man had long had disease of the mesenteric glands (perhaps the result of fever), which caused only the occasional pain in the belly to which he had been subject, till an abscess in one of these glands burst into the trunk of the portal vein, and occasioned the inflammation of the vein and the consequent disease of the liver of which the man died. The inflammation of the vein came on, no doubt, seven weeks before death, when he was seized suddenly with such severe pain in the belly, and had, for the first time, a severe rigor. After this the symptoms were very like those in the case before related; and the frequent recurrence of rigors, followed by profuse sweating, together with the sense of sinking and general distress, the pain in the right epigastric region, and the jaundice, were enough to justify the opinion Mr. Busk at once formed, that the liver was the seat of suppuration. The formation of pus in the areolar tissue about the portal vein was perhaps consequent on ulceration of the vein. From there having been no vomiting, and no tenderness of the belly, at least at first, it would appear that the general inflammation of the peritoneum was likewise consecutive to inflammation of the vein, and that it occurred but a short time before death.

In January, 1853, I visited, in consultation with Dr. Gull, a lady in whom suppurative inflammation of the portal vein appears to have resulted from ulceration of the gall-ducts caused by the irritation of a gall-stone. The symptoms of inflammation of the vein were very like those in the cases before related, but the malady was much more protracted—irregular aguish attacks, most probably arising from partial suppurative phlebitis, having continued to recur for seventeen months before death. For the following notes of the case, which presents many points of interest, I am indebted to the kindness of Dr. Gull:—

Mrs. P——, aged thirty. married, and the mother of three children, was in good health until three years ago, when she had an illness supposed to be due to the passage of gall-stones. It was attended with much pain at the epigastrium and jaundice. The irritation was so severe as to give rise to symptoms of local inflammation, for which leeches and mercurials were prescribed. After two or three weeks, convalescence took place, but she was never again in her former good health. She remained, however, free from any particular ailment until seventeen months before her death. Being then at Scarborough, in October, 1851, she began to have aguish attacks, which recurred at irregular intervals, varying from a few days to a week. These attacks were generally attended with pain about the liver, and a degree of jaundice often very decided. After these symptoms had lasted for eight months, I saw her in consultation with Mr. Ingoldby. The skin was then icteric, *the spleen large*, and the right lobe of the liver extended down to the crest of the ilium.

The infusion of calumba with ammonio-citrate of iron was prescribed, and the patient went for change of air to Guernsey, where she remained many weeks. The result was a great improvement in the general health, and a less frequent return of the aguish paroxysms. These, however, still continue to recur, but with much irregularity as regards both their intervals and type—sometimes returning after two or three days, and sometimes being absent a week: sometimes the chills and shivering were decided and prolonged, and at other times transient, and followed by considerable sweatings.

On her return from Guernsey, in the autumn of 1852, I was again called to see her by Dr. Rooke. The spleen was then smaller than it had been three months before. The liver appeared in the same state, the right lobe extending downwards to the crest of the ilium.

The same plan of treatment was persevered in, and she was ordered to take an ounce of the "mistura ferri composita" twice a day, and three grains of the neutral sulphate of quinine in a pill every night at bedtime.

After a short time the aguish paroxysms became regular in their returns, assuming a quartan type, and the general health continued to improve greatly. Unfortunately, towards the end of the year, her health became again seriously impaired by anxiety and watching, and her spirits depressed by the death of one of her children. I was now a third time called to see her. She had then passed several sleepless nights, and her nervous system was greatly depressed. Sulphuric ether and camphor were prescribed with extract of lettuce at night, with direct benefit, but the amendment was of short duration, for in a few days very severe symptoms, like those caused by the passage of a gall-stone, came on, and were soon followed by deep jaundice. After thirty-six hours the pain subsided, and the bile reappeared in the stools. In the first of these containing bile, a laminated gall-stone was found, of the size of half an almond. The jaundice gradually subsided as the bile flowed freely into the intestine, but at the same time the aguish paroxysms returned with greatly increased severity, and at intervals more irregular than before. This exacerbation of all the symptoms began on the 8th of January, 1852. The shiverings were intense, and attended with a remarkable tendency to collapse—the pulse becoming scarcely perceptible at the wrist, and very rapid. This state would last from twenty to thirty minutes, and be followed by a short stage of reaction, which would be often interrupted by a return of the shivering and collapse, and then a most profuse perspiration would break out, which lasted until the cold stage returned again; this sequence of events would be repeated three or four times in the twenty-four hours. In the intervals, when such occurred, there was complete apyrexia; the respiration was natural, and the pulse 100. As this state of things continued, the spleen, which had been decreasing in size, became greatly enlarged. From day to day the case was carefully watched, in the hope that some indications of an abscess making its way to the surface might be discovered. There was no tenderness at any part, but a slight uneasiness at the epigastrium and about the region of the gall-bladder. The urine was abundant, high-colored, but free from purpuric or lateritious deposits. The bowels were relaxed—the evacuations containing a large amount of bile. There was no sickness or nausea: the stomach retained well all the nourishment given. The expression of the face was placid, the eye bright, the pupil dilated.

The remedies employed were quinine, opium, and wine. The symptoms remained unchecked, and the patient was seen by Dr. Addison, and subsequently by Dr. Budd—all agreeing as to the existence of suppuration either in or about the liver. It was determined that nothing was to be done beyond supporting the powers of life and allaying irritation. At the end of January, diarrhœa came on, with an inclination to the typhoid state. The rigors continued, but with less frequency, though equally severe, and with no local signs of an advancing abscess. In the beginning of February jaundice returned, but with only slight pain at the epigastrium. This jaundice continued till death. As soon as the bile ceased to flow into the intestine, the diarrhœa, which had been hardly kept in check by opium and astringents, such as infusion of catechu and decoction of logwood, was at once arrested, and marked constipation followed. Two days before death a slight pain was complained of in the lower part of the right side of the chest, and on auscultation a well-marked friction-sound was heard there. In the night of the next day the patient complained of a sudden increase of the pain, fell into a state of collapse—with symptoms of rupture of the peritoneum—and died in nine hours.

Post-mortem.—When the abdomen was opened, the peritoneum was found covered with recently effused lymph. On the convexity of the right lobe of the liver, was a slough of the peritoneum over an irregular abscess, surrounded by gangrenous liver-substance, and on slicing the liver in different places, irregular depôts of pus were laid open. These were found to be branches of the portal vein in a state of suppuration.

In some the disease appeared to be of long standing, and the coats of the vessels were thickened; in others, it was of more recent date. The larger trunks of the vein near the transverse fissure were filled with firm recent coagula. The gall-bladder contained a nearly colorless watery mucus, and its coats were healthy. At its orifice there was *the cicatrix of an old ulcer, and externally, corresponding to this part, were firm old inflammatory adhesions, highly vascular.* The cystic and the common ducts were greatly distended, so that the little finger could be easily introduced into them, and about an inch from the duodenum a gall-stone, the size of an acorn, was firmly impacted. There was no trace of recent ulceration in any of the ducts examined, although this was carefully looked for. The ducts appeared everywhere healthy, but dilated. The hepatic veins contained no pus, nor was there in the chest or elsewhere any trace of secondary phlebitis.

The liver was generally increased in size, probably weighing between five and six pounds, and the right lobe, as above described, reached to the crest of the ilium.

The spleen was about ten inches in length and uniformly enlarged, flabby, and of a light brownish red color.

The superior mesenteric and the splenic veins were distended by soft recent coagula.

There were old firm adhesions of the pleura on the right side, and some chalky deposits in the lung, but no recent disease of any kind in the chest.

The preceding cases afford strong confirmation of the opinion I have already expressed, that pus-globules brought to the liver by the portal vein usually become all arrested there, and do not pass through, as they often do through the lungs, to cause scattered abscesses in other organs. It is for this reason that suppurative inflammation of a vein that feeds the vena portæ kills less quickly than suppurative inflammation of a vein that returns its blood immediately to the lungs. The blood is filtered, as it were, of pus in passing through the liver, and the local disease is confined to that one organ.

A case very similar to the preceding was published by Dr. Ormerod, in the *Lancet* for May 30, 1846. The inflammation was in this case supposed to result from ulceration of the vermiform appendix, caused by the intrusion of a gall-stone. The trunk of the portal vein was filled with pus, and abscesses were found in the liver, but in no other organ. There were frequently recurring rigors and jaundice. The patient, a man 23 years of age, lived a month after the occurrence of the mischief in the vein.

If, instead of involving the trunk of the portal vein, the inflammation involve only some of its hepatic branches, the patient may recover, and may enjoy tolerable health for years after. This happened, I think, in the person of my late colleague, Mr. Lawson, consulting surgeon of the Seamen's Hospital, who died of dropsy from granular kidney in the spring of 1840.

Mr. Lawson had in early life been much in India, but returned to England ten years before his death, and was soon after appointed resident surgeon to the Seamen's Hospital. He continued in this office several years, and then settled in the city. He occasionally vomited, especially after having eaten or drunk more than usual, and had an occasional fit of gout, but otherwise his health was pretty good till some months before his death. He had a strong impression that he had some disease of the liver, the result of an acute attack he had in India; but few of his medical friends thought so. He was stout and cheerful, had no pain in the side, and his complexion was remarkably clear.

The examination of the body was made by Mr. Busk, in presence of Dr. Bright and myself. The liver had no unnatural adhesions, and there were no marks of inflammation of the capsule, but its surface was deformed by deep linear fissures. On cutting across these fissures, there was found at some points a small stellar cicatrice, of white cartilaginous substance; at other points a small abscess containing white pus. A great number of these abscesses existed, but all were in the lines of the fissures, and all were small; not one was larger than a filbert. The capsule and the peritoneum covering the liver had undergone no change of structure even at the fissures. They were merely drawn in from atrophy of the hepatic substance beneath.

The lungs were not adherent to the pleura costalis, and presented no marks of former inflammation.

The stomach was large, and the pylorus was somewhat contracted by a cartilage-like tissue under the mucous coat—changes which accounted for the vomiting to which Mr. Lawson had been subject.

The vessels of the liver were not traced, and at the time the examination was made the precise seat of the abscesses was not ascertained. The linear fissures on the surface of the liver scarcely, however, leave a doubt that the abscesses were in branches of the portal vein. There had been inflammation of some branches of the vein, a string of small abscesses had formed along them, separated here and there by a plug of lymph, or coagulated blood, the parts of the liver which those branches supplied became atrophied, and, in consequence, the capsule was drawn in, and the surface marked by fissures corresponding to the obliterated branches of the vein. Enough of the liver was left for the purpose of secretion, and the portal blood passed freely through it, so that no serious disorder of health resulted.

Inflammation of a large branch of the portal vein may be caused by an abscess of the liver consequent on phlebitis of some distant part. This happens, however, very rarely; probably on account of the coats of the vein being thick and surrounded by areolar tissue. The only instance of the kind I can cite is one of which notes were sent me by my friend, Dr. James Russel, of Birmingham. The patient, a man of middle age, had his leg amputated on the 18th of March, on account of gangrene occurring after a compound fracture. Three days after the operation he had a rigor, followed by sweating. The rigors recurred, other constitutional symptoms of contamination of the blood by pus came on, he got gradually lower, and died on the 20th of April. Occasional pain at the epigastrium was the only sign that the liver was diseased. An abscess was found in the apex of each lung, and there were three or four abscesses in the liver. A large branch of the portal vein, in contact with one of the abscesses, contained a hollow cylinder of lymph, about two inches in length, filled with pus. The abscess, reaching the coats of the vein, had probably excited inflammation of its lining membrane, just as an abscess reaching the surface of the liver excites inflammation of the peritoneum above it.

Mere *adhesive* inflammation of branches of the portal vein does not prove fatal, like suppurative inflammation ; and on this account, and from the difficulty of distinguishing the different inflammatory diseases of the liver during life, we cannot yet give its clinical history. The patient recovers, and when he dies, perhaps some years after, of another disease, we see merely the ultimate changes to which obliteration of branches of the portal vein leads. These changes are very striking and characteristic. The surface of the liver is marked by deep linear fissures, corresponding to the obliterated branches of the vein, and caused by atrophy of those portions of the liver which the obliterated branches supplied. Rokitansky, who has well described these appearances, states that they are very common in persons who die in the hospitals in Vienna. They are by no means uncommon in this country. During the past year (1844), I have had an opportunity of examining three good specimens of this disease. The first was in a liver, which was sent me by my brother, Dr. William Budd, of Bristol. The person from whom it was obtained was a sailor, who died in St. Peter's Hospital, Bristol, of dropsy from granular disease of the kidney.

He had been a hard drinker, had been in hot climates, and had had remittents—one attack not many months before his death. There was considerable nausea, but no ascites. There had been deep jaundice about a week before death. This had lessened a good deal, but there was still a light yellow stain of the skin.

He died of cerebral disorder, apparently the result of poisoning of the blood by urine and bile.

The liver was much deformed by *deep* linear fissures across its upper and its under surface.

On the upper surface of the right lobe were two spots, nearly the size of a half-crown, covered by a false membrane, a line in thickness, having the toughness and the look of cartilage. From these spots the false membranes shaded away to a thin film, but this did not cover the whole of the convex surface of the right lobe; and on the convex surface of the left lobe, and on the under surface of the liver, there was no false membrane, although the surface was much fissured.

On separating the fissures, and tearing and scraping away the hepatic substance with the handle of the scalpel, solid fibrous twigs were left, which were found to be continuous with branches of the portal vein. The trunk of the portal vein and its first divisions appeared healthy. About the small divisions still pervious the areolar tissue seemed thickened, and the artery and duct were more adherent to the vein than natural. The impervious twigs of the vein, in a section of the liver made across them, looked like small stellar cicatrices, and in many of them could be seen a yellow point, the orifice of a divided gall-duct.

The lobular substance of the liver was of a uniform deep chocolate color, and rather soft, so that it was readily scraped away from the fibrous twigs. The disease was not confined to one part of the liver. One surface was just as much fissured as the other.

The hepatic artery and the hepatic veins appeared healthy.

The gall-bladder and the large ducts were stained with bile, but healthy.

The liver was adherent to the diaphragm and abdominal walls by bands of old tissue at the spots covered by thick false membrane.

The spleen was large and indurated. There were no adhesions, or other traces of peritonitis, anywhere in the abdominal cavity, except on the surface of the liver.

The duodenum was much stained by deep olive bile, and from the opening of the common duct to six or eight inches down, there was deep crimson injection of the mucous coat.

The right lung was universally adherent to the costal pleura; the left lung was quite free.

The heart was immensely hypertrophied. There was no important disease of its valves, but much "atheromatous" deposit in the aorta.

Both kidneys were in a very advanced stage of granular disease.

Another instance of the same disease fell under my notice in King's College Hospital, in a man who died of cancer of the penis. This man, who was a soldier, and had served in the Peninsula, had been at one time a hard drinker. He had neither ascites, jaundice, nor other symptom of diseased liver. The liver, as in the instance just related, was crossed by deep fissures, but there were fewer of them, and there were no marks of inflammation on its capsule. The tissue of the liver seemed healthy, and could be readily scraped away from the obliterated twigs of the portal vein. The spleen was large and firm, and on its capsule, which was everywhere much thickened, there were some cartilaginous-looking plates.

Another specimen, precisely similar, was sent me by Mr. Busk. It was obtained from a sailor, who died of phthisis, much emaciated. There was no mention of hepatic disease in the notes taken of his case. The liver weighed only two pounds one ounce and a half, and, as well as the spleen, adhered to all the surrounding parts by means of old tissue. There were no traces of former peritonitis elsewhere.

It appears, then, that obliteration of branches of the portal vein causes *complete atrophy* of those parts of the liver which the obstructed branches supplied, and consequent diminution of the size of the organ. When an obliterated branch is near the surface, the capsule gets drawn in by the atrophy of the intervening lobular substance, and the surface is marked by a linear fissure. The lobular substance supplied by other branches of the vein may remain uninjured. A portion of the liver is lost, proportionate in amount to the number and size of the obliterated branches of the vein—and the person must suffer all the evils which such a loss entails. The disease, in its effects, is like that form of adhesive inflammation of the substance of the liver which leads to new fibrous tissue in the portal canals of considerable size, and in two of the three instances I have mentioned was attended by marks of disease in the capsule of the liver and in the spleen, such as are usually found in that affection. In these instances it was probably brought on by spirit-drinking. Rokitansky is of opinion that this disease of the liver is in many cases the result of direct communication between the venous system of the liver and that of the body, in consequence of the umbilical vein remaining pervious.

It is probable, from the observations of Mr. Henry Lee, before referred to, that obliteration of branches of the portal vein is sometimes produced, not by inflammation of the vein and the effusion of lymph from its inner surface, but by mere coagulation of the blood within it, caused by the absorption of some noxious matter from the stomach or bowels.

When many branches of the vein are thus obstructed, the impediment to the passage of blood through the liver, as in high degrees of cirrhosis, may cause ascites and slight jaundice, and may lead to great enlargement of the superficial veins of the belly. After a time the enlargement of the superficial veins may form a sufficiently free channel for the blood to the heart, and the ascites may gradually disappear. In the autumn of 1844 I witnessed, in the Seamen's Hospital, a case which I imagine to have been of this kind. The patient, a sailor, was in the hospital eight years before for what was supposed to be some affection of the stomach. The symptoms which led to this inference were soon followed by slight jaundice and by great ascites, for which he was tapped three times in quick succession. The ascites recurred again, but after a time slowly and gradually disappeared of itself. When I saw him he had been long free from ascites or jaundice, but had an enormous bunch of large tortuous veins, which emerged from the belly just above the umbilicus, and ran thence up the chest. He told me that he first noticed these veins four years before, after the ascites had disappeared.

It sometimes, though very rarely, happens that the main trunk of the portal vein becomes completely obstructed in the same way. This usually leads to profuse hemorrhage from the stomach and bowels, the result of the great congestion of their mucous membrane; to great ascites; to deep and persistent jaundice; and to rapid shrinking of the liver. An instance of this, in which, at the end of a month only, the liver was found to be no larger than the two fists of the subject, was published in 1849, by M. Monneret, in a French periodical (*L'Union Médicale*, 1849, No. 13); and several other cases of the same kind are on record. Complete obstruction of the trunk of the portal vein soon destroys life, not, perhaps, so much by stopping the office of the liver, as by preventing the return of blood from the intestinal canal.

Inflammation of a branch of the *hepatic* vein is, as already remarked, occasionally produced by a small abscess in the liver, consequent on phlebitis of some distant part. The abscess touching the thin coat of the vein, sets up inflammation on its inner surface, just as it sets up inflammation of the peritoneum above it when it reaches the surface of the liver. Lymph is effused within the vein at the point where it is touched by the abscess, the canal of the vein becomes closed at that point, and all the branches that feed it, even back to their capillary divisions, become subsequently, and in consequence, choked with fibrin and coagulated blood. If, as more frequently happens, the abscess cause *ulceration* of the coats of the vein before its canal is blocked up, a small quantity of the pus oozes into the vein. The pus coagulates the blood, and thus chokes the vein, and also sets up suppurative inflammation of its inner surface. After death, the vein, backwards from the ulcerated point, is found filled with fibrin and coagulated blood, with here and there a little purulent matter. I have observed these marks of inflammation in a branch of the hepatic vein in two instances in which small abscesses had formed in the liver after amputation. In a portion of liver sent me by Mr. Busk in November, 1843, which was taken from a man who died of phlebitis after amputation of the thigh, several branches of the hepatic vein were inflamed in this way, and obviously from this cause. The liver contained many abscesses of the size of peas, and lined by a distinct, but very thin membrane.

Dr. James Russel, of Birmingham, has sent me notes of a case in which the same changes were observed. The patient died in the Birmingham Hospital, in 1836, eighteen days after amputation of the leg.

A somewhat similar case has been published by M. Lambron, in the *Archives Générales* for June, 1842; but here the abscesses in the liver were most probably caused by a cancerous ulcer of the stomach.

From these instances it is probable that inflammation of one or more branches of the hepatic vein is not uncommon in cases where abscesses form in the liver after injuries of the head or limbs. From want of careful dissection this disease of the vein must be often overlooked.

Inflammation of the hepatic vein from other causes is, I believe, extremely rare. The only instance in which I have seen evidence of it was in a man who died in King's College Hospital in February, 1844. All the hepatic veins seemed thicker and more opaque than natural, and, on examining them closely, I found a thin false membrane on their inner surface, which in the large veins could be readily stripped off. There was a great deal of new fibrous tissue in all the portal canals of considerable size, and some in the small ones also—enough on the whole to render the liver tough, but not distinctly hob-nailed or granular. The liver and the spleen were united to all the adjacent parts by means of old tissue—and there were some adhesions, apparently of the same date, between adjacent coils of intestine. The pericardium adhered to the heart by means of a thick layer of tough fibrous tissue; and both lungs were everywhere adherent to the pleura costalis. The patient was a tailor, fifty-two years of age, and for many years had been in the habit of drinking enormous quantities of gin. It was this probably that caused the adhesive inflammation of which so many traces were found.[1]

[1] There can be little doubt that the adhesive inflammation of which so many traces are found in bodies examined at our hospitals—cirrhosis, obliterated portal veins, thickened capsule of the spleen, puckering of the surface of the kidney from obliterated vessels, stricture of the pylorus, from contracted lymph in the submucous areolar tissue, and, in many cases, adhesions of the pericardium and pleura—are mainly attributable to spirit-drinking. The inflammation which this causes is always *adhesive*.

SECT. V.—*Inflammation of the gall-bladder and gall-ducts—Catarrhal and suppurative inflammation—Croupal, or plastic, inflammation—Ulcerative inflammation—Effect of ulceration of the gall-bladder and gall-ducts—Effect of permanent closure of the cystic and common ducts—Fatty degeneration of the coats of the gall-bladder.*

THE inflammatory diseases of the gall-bladder and gall-ducts, although of frequent occurrence, have been but little studied, and at present we have not materials for anything like a complete history of them. This is to be ascribed, in part, to the ambiguous character of the symptoms of all diseases of the liver; in part, to the small size of the gall-ducts, which causes them to be often overlooked in dissection. It should ever be borne in mind that the ducts, though small, are very important, from being the only outlets for the bile secreted in those portions of the liver to which they lead. Permanent closure of the cystic duct entirely destroys the office of the gall-bladder;—that of the common duct destroys, in the end, the office of the liver itself.

Inflammation of the gall-bladder and gall-ducts probably arises from various causes, each of which determines in great measure the character and course of the inflammation, and its mode of termination—so that we cannot expect a satisfactory account of the different kinds of inflammation until we can arrange them according to the agencies by which they are respectively produced. To attempt such an arrangement at present would be premature. We must be satisfied with what seems the nearest approach to it, viz., an arrangement based on the appearances found after death.

The different forms of inflammation of a mucous membrane, considered with reference to their effects, are,

1st. What may be called *catarrhal* inflammation, which merely increases the quantity and changes the quality of the natural *mucus*, often rendering it viscid, whitish, and opaque. This form of inflammation seems to correspond in degree with the adhesive inflammation of other textures, but it is not *adhesive* in the sense before given to that word, because, by a wise provision, the matter poured out on the free surface of a mucous membrane very rarely becomes organized or permanently adherent to the membrane;

2d. *Suppurative* inflammation, where the matter secreted is purulent;

3d. *Croupal*, or *plastic* inflammation, where the matter effused forms a solid, albuminous layer on the diseased surface, of which, when this is a tube, it becomes a *cast;*

4th. *Ulcerative* inflammation, if, indeed, the process which leads to ulceration can with propriety be classed with those leading to the results before mentioned, and be comprehended with them under the generic term *inflammation.*

All these different forms of inflammation have been observed in the mucous membrane lining the gall-bladder and gall-ducts, but not with equal frequency in its different parts. Inflammation seldom produces changes sufficient to attract notice in the hepatic duct, or in the branches that go to form it. The coats of the gall-bladder, and of the cystic and common ducts, are not unfrequently found ulcerated, or much thickened and otherwise changed in texture; but such changes have been seldom observed, in man, in branches of the hepatic duct. It might have been anticipated that the gall-bladder and the cystic and common ducts would be more liable to inflammation than the branches of the hepatic duct. They are much more liable to be fretted and otherwise injured by gall-stones, which are usually formed in the gall-bladder, and much more liable to irritation from other unhealthy products of secretion. The bile always becomes more concentrated, and, if unhealthy, more irritating, in the gall-bladder, and when unduly detained there, the mixture of bile and mucus undergoes decomposition, and may thus give rise to the formation of matters very hurtful to the mucous membrane.[1] Undue retention, and the consequent decomposition of the contents of the gall-bladder, may

[1] When bile undergoes spontaneous decomposition exposed to the air, oxalic acid is one of the ultimate products, as it is of many other animal substances. Some time ago, Dr. L. S. Beale showed me, in a specimen of ox-bile in an advanced stage of decomposition, a great number of octohedral crystals of oxalate of lime, exactly like the crystals of this substance, which are so commonly found in urine.

result from various conditions—from a mechanical impediment to its escape through the cystic or the common duct; from long fasting; from a disordered state of the nervous system, especially such as exist in low forms of continued fever; and from earthy degeneration of the coats of the gall-bladder itself, which is not an unfrequent condition in persons advanced in life. On these accounts it is, perhaps, best to consider the diseases of the gall-bladder and of the different portions of the ducts separately, as far as this can be done.

Catarrhal inflammation of the gall-ducts is, probably, not uncommon. It is not a fatal disease, and, like catarrhal inflammation of other mucous membranes, may cause no permanent changes, so that it may often have occurred where no traces of it are found. It happens, however, not very unfrequently, that, on squeezing the hepatic ducts, a viscid whitish fluid oozes out, which, on examination through the microscope, is seen to be chiefly made up of the prismatic epithelial cells of the gall-ducts. The symptoms we should expect in catarrhal inflammation of the hepatic ducts are some degree of feverishness, with slight pain in the region of the liver, and, if many of the ducts become closed by thickening of their coats, or be choked by the viscid secretion, slight enlargement of the liver and jaundice.

Many of the cases of simple jaundice coming on in healthy persons, and attended with slight pain and fever, are probably cases of this kind.

In a severer form of inflammation, the matter secreted is purulent, but it has seldom the visible characters of pure pus. The pus is mixed with opaque mucus secreted at the same time, and, it may be, with bile also; and the result is a viscid, greenish, or yellowish fluid, very different in appearance from pure pus.

Inflammation of this degree may likewise subside without leaving permanent traces, and the only evidence of its existence may be an attack of jaundice, attended with more or less pain in the region of the liver, and with some degree of fever.

It happens, however, now and then, in catarrhal or suppurative inflammation of the hepatic ducts, that many of the small ducts become temporarily blocked up at some point, and that the portion behind gets dilated into an irregular pouch, which is filled with a glairy or purulent fluid, more or less tinged with bile. A remarkable instance has been recorded by Cruveilhier (liv. xl. pl. 1), in which, it is reported, there were distributed throughout the liver thousands of small irregular cavities, formed by partial dilatation of the gall-ducts, and containing thick purulent mucus variously tinged with bile. In this instance there were marks of former inflammation about the liver—firm adhesions between the liver and adjacent organs, obliteration of the cystic duct, and narrowing of the duodenal end of the common duct—and the inflammation of the ducts which led to the formation of the sacculated pouches in question was probably the result of permanent obstacle to the free escape of the bile. The hepatic gall-ducts were generally dilated, and in the common duct, above the narrowed portion, was a calculus which did not completely close the canal. The chief symptoms noticed in the ultimate stage of the disease were—jaundice, occasional pain in the region of the liver, a quick pulse, with a sense of general illness, and daily increasing weakness. At length nutrition became very much impaired; there was sloughing at the sacrum, sloughing of the gall-duct, white softening of the brain—and the patient died of exhaustion.

It would seem that sacculated pouches, formed, as in this case, by inflammation of the small hepatic ducts, may, by permanent closure of the duct at the point of obstruction, be converted into small permanent cysts, filled with a glairy fluid, more or less tinged with bile. It is difficult to account in any other way for the cysts of this character that are now and then found in the liver.

Firm, white, nodulous tumors, surrounded by a distinct cyst, and composed of a cheese-like substance, are also now and then found in the liver, and are formed, I believe, in the same way. These cysts are evidently situated in portal canals, and the cheese-like substance of which they consist contains in its middle a small mass of concrete biliary matter, or has solid particles of biliary matter diffused through it which can be seen by means of the microscope. There is usually a false membrane on the surface of the liver at the points where these tumors reach it. In another chapter, a fuller account will be given of these cheesy tubera, which have been generally confounded with cancer. The cheesy matter is very like that of a scrofulous gland, and is probably formed in the same way, by inflammation of the mucous membrane in these portions of the ducts.

These knotty tumors seem, indeed, to differ from the biliary cysts before mentioned only in the consistence of the matter within the cyst—which varies according to the kind and degree of the inflammation by which it is produced.

If a small gall-duct become obstructed in the same way by thick *biliary* matter, or otherwise, the portion behind may, perhaps without inflammation at all, become dilated into a small, irregular, or sacculated cavity, containing mere mucus and bile. Cruveilhier (liv. xii. pl. 4, fig. 3) has given a plate taken from a specimen of this kind. A great number of cysts of various sizes were scattered through the liver, some in its substance, others rising above the surface, completely isolated from the gall-ducts, but containing a deep yellow liquid. Tumors formed in this way never attain a very large size, and are perhaps generally multiple. The large, solitary, encysted tumors, containing a glairy fluid tinged with bile, which are now and then found in the liver, are most of them hydatid cysts (which in man are usually single), in which suppurative inflammation has been set up by the entrance of bile. The greenish glairy fluid is formed by the mixture of bile and pus.

The irregular cysts formed by dilatation of the small gall-ducts, when they contain merely a thin mucous fluid mixed with bile, may contract from absorption of the watery part of their contents, and the cyst may at length close upon a small mass of concrete mucus and bile.

Marks of inflammation and other disease are, as has been already stated, much more common in the gall-bladder and in the cystic and common ducts than in the hepatic ducts.

Inflammation of the mucous membrane may be confined to the lower part of the common duct, or to the gall-bladder; or it may commence in the gall-bladder, and extend down the cystic and common ducts.

The following case, recorded by Andral, is a very instructive example of inflammation of the common duct only; because here, from the disease proving speedily fatal, the source of the symptoms was cleared up by dissection. I have ventured to give the case at length, because a consideration of it may suggest the right interpretation of the symptoms in other cases of the same kind, which usually terminate in recovery.

A shoemaker, thirty-five years of age, was admitted into *La Charité*, the 8th of November, 1821. Six days before, after over-indulgence at table, he was taken with sharp pain at the right of the epigastrium, a little below the edge of the ribs. The next day he remarked that his skin was yellow. On the 9th of November, the seventh day of illness, the conjunctiva and the entire surface of the body had a yellow tint, and there was a dull pain in the right hypochondrium. Below the cartilage of the eleventh rib a pear-shaped tumor was felt, the broad end of which extended a little below the umbilicus, while the narrow end was lost behind the ribs. This tumor, which was supposed to be the gall-bladder distended, was movable under the finger, and not tender.

The tongue was natural. The patient had some thirst; no appetite. The bowels moved seldom; the stools were not colored with bile. The pulse was quick; the skin hot and dry. (Leeches to the anus; whey, with acetate of potash; diet.)

The four following days the tumor grew larger, but no other change took place. On the 13th of November, the eleventh day from his first feeling the pain in the side, the patient was seized, all at once, with a much more severe pain, which, starting from the region of the liver, soon spread over the whole belly.

The pain continued extremely severe, and was much increased by the slightest pressure; the features became pinched, the pulse small and very frequent, and the extremities cold; and the patient died in the afternoon of the next day.

The sac of the peritoneum was filled by a puriform liquid, everywhere yellow, but much more so in the right flank than in other parts. The inner surface of the duodenum was intensely red. The entrance of the common duct was marked by a small round tumor, rising three lines above the surface of the intestine, and pierced at its summit by a capillary orifice, the opening of the duct. The coats of the common duct were much thickened and easily torn, and the canal almost closed.

The hepatic and the cystic ducts and the gall-bladder were dilated. In the hepatic duct, just above its junction with the cystic, was a perforation, having an irregular, roundish outline, and large enough for the passage of a small pea. Around the perforation the texture of the coats of the duct did not seem altered. The tissue of the liver exhibited nothing remarkable. In the stomach were some spots in which the mucous membrane was red. The rest of the alimentary canal, and the other organs, seemed healthy.—(*Clin. Med.*, t. iv. p. 495.)

This case seems to have been an instance of acute inflammation of the duodenum and of the common duct, caused by over-indulgence at table. The symptoms were, pain in the situation of the inflamed duct, soon followed by jaundice and by dilatation of the gall-bladder; loss of appetite, thirst, fever. The disease had lasted eleven days when rupture of the hepatic duct took place, causing peritonitis and rapid collapse.

The inflammation does not seem to have extended above the

common duct. The distended gall-bladder was not painful or tender; and the coats of the hepatic duct about the perforation were not sensibly altered in texture.

The early jaundice and the distension of the gall-bladder were the effect of closure of the common duct by inflammatory swelling of its mucous coat. From the small size of the gall-ducts the passage through them must be completely closed by a very slight thickening of their lining membrane.

Andral gives another case (*Id.*, p. 499), which did not prove fatal, but which, judging from the symptoms, was of the same kind; and two or three similar instances have fallen under my own notice. The symptoms in these cases were pain in the situation of the duct, followed at the end of one or two days by constipation and jaundice, and by distension of the gall-bladder so as to form *a large globular or pear-shaped tumor*, not painful or tender. The symptoms are very like those of obstruction of the common duct by a gall-stone; but the pain occurs less in paroxysms, and vomiting and nausea are, I think, less frequent than when the duct is obstructed by a gall-stone; and the illness usually occurs after over-indulgence at table, or after eating some unwholesome food, sometimes in young men who have had symptoms of gall-stones, and in whom, from their age and mode of life, it is unlikely that gall-stones exist.

In some such cases, especially where active treatment by leeches and blisters has been promptly had recourse to, the inflammation subsides in a few days; the channel of the duct becomes again free; the pent-up bile flows into the bowel, causing griping pain and diarrhœa: and the tumor formed by the distended gall-bladder lessens, and soon completely disappears.

In other cases the inflammation persists, and the jaundice, varying, it may be, in degree, continues for several weeks or months, without much febrile disturbance, but with constant uneasiness in the site of the common gall-duct, and sometimes with occasional severe pain, especially an hour or two after meals, when the food is passing through the duodenum. When the disease is neglected, the inflammation may permanently change the texture of the tube, perhaps permanently narrow its channel; and, by long impeding the passage of the bile, it may give rise to gall-stones, or to destructive inflammation of the mucous membrane of the gall-bladder.

The jaundice and the pain or uneasiness in the side will then persist in varying degrees, and the health will be permanently broken. The illness may be perpetuated in another way still. The inflammation of the ducts, or the absorption of their retained and irritating contents, may lead to enlargement of one of the lymphatic glands that are contiguous to the common duct, and the compression of the duct by the enlarged gland may be a further cause of jaundice. I have met with more than one instance in which jaundice, long continued and ultimately fatal, was ushered in by what was taken for a common bilious attack, and in which, after death, the jaundice was found to be caused by an enlarged lymphatic gland compressing the common duct.

But inflammation may commence in the mucous membrane of the gall-bladder, and for some time may not extend to the ducts. The inflammation is then excited by the irritating nature of the contents of the gall-bladder, and occurs when, from obstruction of the common or the cystic duct, from thickening and induration of the coats of the gall-bladder itself, or from the state of the nervous system, the gall-bladder does not completely empty itself—so that the retained mucus and bile become decomposed, and, when decomposed, irritate the mucous membrane. The inflammation is especially apt to occur when, from a state of fever or any other cause, the secretion of the gall-bladder itself is unhealthy. The chief symptoms of inflammation confined to the gall-bladder are, pain and tenderness in the region of the gall-bladder, vomiting or nausea, and a certain degree of fever. If the inflammation of the gall-bladder be the result of closure of the common duct, these symptoms are of course associated with jaundice. If, from obstruction either of the common or the cystic duct, the bile and the products of inflammation cannot escape, the gall-bladder may become distended so as to form a globular tumor, and, in cases in which the inflammation is suppurative, there are usually recurring rigors.

A very remarkable instance (to which I shall have again to refer) of catarrhal or plastic inflammation, at first confined to the gall-bladder, is related by Dr. Graves in his work on *Clinical Medicine* (p. 463).

The patient, a fine healthy maid-servant, twenty years of age, was attacked with pain in the right hypochondrium, extending into the epigastrium, which was followed at the end of a fortnight by jaundice.

After the skin got yellow the pain in the side diminished; but during the whole time it lasted she had constant vomiting and nausea. The jaundice continued, with tenderness and slight pain in the region of the gall-bladder, and with great irritability of the abdominal muscles, which were thrown into spasm by any attempt to examine the abdomen minutely, but without any other symptoms indicative of especial danger. After the jaundice had lasted about a month she became delirious, and soon after died in a state of coma.

"The liver," Dr. Graves says, "was not by any means enlarged, and a section of it disclosed no excess of blood. It was of a light-brown color, tinged with yellow, as if from a superabundance of the coloring matter of the bile. The gall-bladder was distended, and on being opened was found completely filled by a dark green mass of a tenacious viscid nature, apparently lymph. This substance was of the same pyriform shape as the gall-bladder, and terminated by its narrow extremity at the commencement of the gall-duct. On its removal, the lining membrane of the gall-bladder presented a bright scarlet color and villous appearance, and the natural and beautiful 'honeycomb' arrangement of the mucous membrane was completely effaced. There was no softening or ulceration of the membrane, nor was the color different in any part. It resembled very much the appearance of the mucous membrane in acute laryngitis. The walls of the gall-bladder were much thickened. There was no obstruction of the ductus choledochus, the cystic or hepatic ducts, and their lining membrane was quite free from any unusual vascularity; the duodenum and stomach were stained with the coloring matter of the bile, but in other respects were healthy; no gall-stones or other obstruction; the kidneys were natural."

No morbid appearances were found in the brain.

In this case the disease seems, for the first fortnight, to have been confined to the gall-bladder, and, during that time, the chief symptoms were pain and tenderness in the region of the gall-bladder, with constant nausea and vomiting. Jaundice then came on, and, when it had lasted about a month, the patient became delirious, and soon after died in a state of coma. From the mode of death, and from the circumstance that the liver was not enlarged and that there was no obstruction in the course of the gall-ducts discoverable after death, it is probable that the jaundice and the fatal issue resulted, not from inflammation extending from the gall-bladder to the gall-ducts, but from suppressed or defective secretion of bile.

Suppurative inflammation of the mucous membrane of the gall-bladder, no doubt the result of the undue retention of unhealthy and decomposed secretions, now and then occurs in the course of typhoid fever. M. Louis, in his elaborate work on *Typhoid Fever*, has given three cases (*Obs.* 1, 11, and 28), in which he found a purulent fluid in the gall-bladder mixed with very unhealthy looking reddish bile. In one of these cases (*Obs.* 28), the mucous membrane was a little thickened; but in the others, it presented no other change than slight redness. In not one of them did the gall-ducts exhibit any marks of disease. In the cases related by M. Louis, the inflammation of the gall-bladder gave rise to no symptoms that could be distinguished amidst the general disorder of the fever.

In the following case, which fell under my care in 1849, inflammation of the gall-bladder, occurring during the course of fever, extended to the outer surface of the bladder, and the symptoms were more significant; but here there was an additional cause of disturbance in the presence of numerous gall-stones, one of which had blocked up the cystic duct. The case is further remarkable as affording an instance of gall-stones forming at an unusually early age.

Eliza Smith, a dress-maker, eighteen years of age, was admitted into King's College Hospital on the 17th of March, 1849. She was unmarried, had always lived well, and her health had been habitually good.

Her illness began ten days before with the usual symptoms of typhoid fever—with rigors, followed by noise in the head, pain in the back and limbs, flashes of light before the eyes, loss of appetite, thirst, and great prostration of strength.

On her admission to the hospital, she had the look and the usual symptoms of typhoid fever. The skin was hot, the tongue furred and dry, the pulse 110, and she had great thirst. A few of the maculæ common in typhoid fever existed on the abdomen and back. She appeared restless, but required to be spoken to sharply before she would answer. She had some cough, and on auscultation rhonchus was heard all over the chest, and slight crepitus over the lower part of the left lung behind.

The only symptoms different from those common in typhoid fever were, that the bowels were much confined, and that she lay on her back with her legs drawn up, and complained of pain when the belly was pressed.

She was ordered ʒij of castor oil, and draughts of citrate of ammonia, milk, and beef tea. The castor oil not operating, three grains of calomel, with five of compound extract of colocynth, were afterwards given. This had little effect, and on the 20th, another dose of castor oil was given, which produced several dark and offensive stools.

On the 21st, the tongue was dry and brown; the pulse 120; and the inspirations 30 a minute. She had been delirious during the night. ʒss of aromatic spirits of ammonia, every four hours, was now ordered, instead of the citrate of ammonia, which she had hitherto taken.

On the 23d, ℥vj of wine daily, were ordered in addition; and on the 24th, ℥xij.

For some days, no particular change took place. She was delirious at night, and occasionally passed her water unconsciously. The bowels were confined, but were readily moved by the warm water enema. She always lay with her legs drawn up, and gave signs of pain when the region of the liver was pressed.

On the 26th, she was much in the same state; but when I made pressure on the belly to the right of the epigastrium, she uttered a loud shriek. I now discovered a fulness in that part of the belly, and inferred that there was inflammation of the gall-bladder, or that an abscess existed in the liver.

For several days, there was no further change worth noting. She was generally slightly delirious, took no notice of what was going on around her, and passed her urine and feces under her in bed.

On the 31st, diarrhœa came on, in consequence of which ʒss of tincture of krameria was added to each dose of the medicine.

The diarrhœa ceased in a few days, and did not again recur. The breathing, which had been quick from the beginning, became more oppressed, the respirations being from forty to fifty-six in the minute.

On the 6th of April, she had a distinct shivering fit.

On the 8th, vomiting was noted for the first time; and it recurred on the following days.

She gradually sunk, and died on the 12th.

Up to the time of death, there was constantly some degree of fulness in the site of the gall-bladder, and she always gave signs of pain when this part of the belly was pressed. There was no jaundice.

On examination after death, the gall-bladder was found distended, projecting an inch and a half below the margin of the liver, and united to all the surrounding parts by lymph, which had been recently effused and was readily broken through. There were no marks of peritonitis elsewhere. The gall-bladder contained a puriform matter, and fourteen gall-stones, one of which completely blocked up the cystic duct. The coats of the bladder were much thickened, and flakes of lymph and concrete pus adhered to its inner surface. The gall-stones were of the ordinary kind, consisting of cholesterine, stained by bile, and having a nucleus of inspissated biliary matter. The liver itself presented no unusual appearance.

There was (as is usual in typhoid fever) extensive ulceration of the patches of Peyer and of the solitary glands in the lower part of the small intestine.

The posterior part of the lower lobe of the left lung was in a state of red hepatization ; other parts of the lungs were sound.

No marks of disease were discovered in the brain, or in other organs of the abdomen and chest.

Here, notwithstanding the existence of the fever, it was plain enough from the posture of the patient, and from the constant tenderness and fulness at the right hypochondrium, there was some active inflammatory disease of the gall-bladder or liver. The constipation that existed for some time, the fit of shivering on the 6th of April, and the vomiting that occurred a few days before death, were probably due to this disease.

Suppurative inflammation of the gall-bladder seems especially liable to occur when, by any cause, the cystic duct is permanently closed.

A case in illustration of this fell under my observation in King's College Hospital in 1848. A woman, sixty years of age, was admitted into the hospital on the 23d September, in that year, much emaciated; with jaundice, which had then lasted twelve months, and with other well-marked symptoms of cancer of the liver. The liver was much enlarged, extending an inch below the umbilicus on the right side, and through the wasted walls of the belly it could be felt that the convex surface of the liver was nodulous, and that its lower edge was rounded. At the margin of the liver, near the umbilicus, a firm globular tumor was felt, which was taken to be a distended gall-bladder. The patient remained in the hospital five weeks, during which she had frequent vomiting and much pain in the region of the liver, and then went to her home, where she died on the 7th of December.

The liver was found to contain firm cancerous tumors, of considerable extent, and small masses of cancer were scattered throughout both lungs. The gall-bladder was much distended, and projected beyond the margin of the liver. It contained pus, and many gall-stones; and its mucous membrane, which had quite disappeared in many spots, presented very much the appearance of mucous membrane in the big end of the stomach when corroded by the gastric juice after death. Two gall-stones, moulded upon each other, blocked up the cystic duct. The gall-ducts throughout the liver were dilated. There was much scirrhous matter around the duodenum, through which the common bile duct could not be traced.

Cruveilhier (liv. xxiii. pl. 5) has given a plate of a liver studded with cancerous tumors, in which the cystic duct was obliterated, and the gall-bladder inflamed and full of pus. No notes of the case are given.

A similar instance is recorded by Andral (*Clin. Med.*, iv. 518), in the case of a woman, who died at the age of forty-seven with numerous cancerous tumors in the liver. The gall-bladder was full of pus, and its mucous membrane inflamed. Further on, other instances will be related and referred to which serve to illustrate the same fact.

Suppurative inflammation of the gall-bladder seldom proves fatal of itself, except when, from closure of the cystic or the common duct, there is no outlet for the matter; or when from previous disease of its coats the gall-bladder cannot empty itself *completely*, so that some irritating matter is constantly contained in it; or when from any other cause the inflammatory process leads to *ulceration*. Under other circumstances the inflammation subsides after a time, and the general health is restored. In some instances of recovery no traces of the disease remain; in others, in which the inflammation was more protracted, or in which it involved the outer coats of the bladder, some visible changes of structure are left. I have twice found the gall-bladder and cystic duct contracted, and their coats thickened, in young persons who died of other diseases, and in whom there were no gall-stones, nor any trace of inflammation of the common or hepatic ducts, or of the capsule or substance of the liver. I refrain from giving any details of these cases, as no particulars were noted that can serve to mark even the date of disease of the gall-bladder.

Occasionally the coats of the common duct, as well as those of the gall-bladder and cystic duct, are found thickened and indurated, without gall-stones or trace of inflammation in other tissues of the liver. It is probable that in most cases of this kind inflammation is set up first in the gall-bladder by long retention of irritating bile, and afterwards in the ducts by the passage of this together with irritating secretions from the bladder.

In persons dead of granular liver, with ascites, it is not very uncommon to find the gall-bladder and cystic duct much contracted, and their coats thickened and indurated. The canal of the duct is much narrowed, and now and then completely closed, so that the duct is transformed into a fibrous cord. When this is the case, the gall-bladder contains yellowish mucus, or is moulded on a gall-stone, formed of mucus and the yellow matter of the bile. In some cases the gall-bladder and cystic duct become inflamed, secondarily, like the capsule of the liver (*Clin. Med.*, iv. obs. 51 and 52); and the inflammation is seated in the outer coats. From the presence of other disease of the liver, it is difficult to determine in what degree the symptoms depend on disease of the gall-bladder and gall-duct.

Sometimes the coats of the common duct, as well as those of the cystic, are thickened and indurated, and the canal much contracted. When this happens, the hepatic duct and its branches are found dilated and filled with thick yellow bile; the tissue of the liver is greenish or olive (*Clin. Med.*, iv. obs. 49, 50); and there is a deeper jaundice than belongs to mere cirrhosis.

Another and much more common cause of inflammation of the gall-bladder, and of the cystic and common ducts, at least among the rich, is the mechanical irritation of gall-stones. But this gives rise to ulceration, rather than to the diffuse catarrhal or suppurative inflammation we have hitherto chiefly considered.

Croupal or *plastic* inflammation of the mucous membrane of the gall-bladder and gall-ducts is very rare. Rokitansky says he has observed it in the ducts within the liver, in what has been called the secondary fever of cholera, and as a sequel of ordinary typhoid fever. It produces within the gall-ducts membranous tubes, in which the bile forms tree-like concretions; and this, again, by blocking up the passage, causes distension of the capillary ducts behind.

Ulceration of the Gall-bladder and Gall-ducts.

Ulceration of the gall-bladder has been more commonly remarked than the forms of inflammation yet considered, and occurs in various circumstances.

It has been noticed by more than one observer among the morbid appearances of remittent fever.

Sir G. Blane, in his account of the Walcheren fever, states that the mucous membrane of the gall-bladder was frequently found inflamed and ulcerated; the ulcers having in such cases the conical or tubercular form sometimes seen in dysentery. The gall-bladder was generally distended with bile, which, in those persons who died early, was of a deep green or dark brown, but in more protracted cases had the consistence and the color of tar. This tar-like fluid did not taste bitter like bile, and when mixed with water did not impart any yellowness to it, while it was often so acrid as to excoriate the lip. (Williams' *Morbid Poisons*, vol. ii. p. 470.)

Mr. Boyle, speaking of the Sierra-Leone fever, says there were in almost all cases traces of inflammation in the pyloric extremity of the stomach, extending thence along the duodenum to the entrance of the gall-duct, about which, for the space of a Spanish dollar, the inflammation seemed to have attained the greatest height. The duct was ordinarily choked by dark-colored, viscid bile. The gall-bladder was probably not examined. The other abdominal viscera are stated to have been congested, but otherwise healthy. (*Id.*, p. 478.)

In the yellow fever at Barcelona, in 1821, there were usually traces of inflammation of the stomach, small intestine, and duodenum, not unfrequently extending to the gall-bladder. (*Id.*, p. 473.)

The acrid quality of the bile in the Walcheren fever, and the circumstance that in Dr. Boyle's dissections the strongest marks of inflammation in the intestinal canal were about the entrance of the common duct into the duodenum, render it probable that the inflammation of the gall-bladder and duodenum, in remittent fever, is caused by unhealthy or decomposed and irritating bile. As in typhoid fever, the symptoms of inflammation of the gall-bladder are not distinguishable in the midst of the general disorder that constitutes the fever and the symptoms of inflammation of other parts that likewise occur in its course.

In this country, ulceration of the gall-bladder is produced, perhaps not unfrequently, by the irritation of gall-stones.

Ulcerations of the gall-bladder and gall-stones are often found together, but it must not be inferred, in all such cases, that the ulcers were produced by the gall-stones. Both the ulcers and the gall-stones may have originated from unhealthy or decomposed bile.

When there is only one ulcer in the bladder and a large or hard gall-stone is found resting upon it, it is perhaps safe to infer that the mechanical irritation of the stone was the cause of the ulcer. Gall-stones too large to pass through the cystic duct, not unfrequently cause ulceration of the lower or depending part of the gall-bladder; lymph is poured out on the peritoneal coat below the ulcer; the gall-bladder becomes united by this means to the duodenum or colon; the ulcer eats likewise through the coats of the intestine at this point; and the gall-stone escapes into the intestinal canal. The processes of ulceration and adhesion take place very slowly, and are seldom attended by alarming symptoms. Often, indeed, the first clear intimation that such an event has happened is the discharge of a large gall-stone from the bowel.

In other cases we find many small round ulcers in the gall-bladder, and perhaps in the common duct, and small gall-stones in the bladder not resting on the ulcers. When it is considered that most human gall-stones are so light as to float in bile—since they almost float in water, which is of much lower specific gravity—and that, consequently, they can exert no pressure on the coats of the gall-bladder from their *weight*, when there is bile enough in the bladder to keep them afloat;—it seems most reasonable to infer both ulcers and gall-stones in these cases to an unhealthy state of the bile.

Extensive ulceration of the gall-bladder sometimes occurs without gall-stones, when from any condition the passage of bile into the duodenum is stopped, so that bile and mucus are long retained, and undergo decomposition in the gall-bladder. An instance of this occurred in the following case, which fell under my care in King's College Hospital, in the autumn of 1856, and which is further interesting as showing the effects of obliteration of both the pancreatic duct and the common gall-duct, uncomplicated at first with other disease. I was out of town when the patient was admitted into the hospital, so that the account of his condition then, and for three weeks afterwards, is derived from the hospital case-book:—

Michael Donaghan, a working tailor, forty years of age, was admitted into King's College Hospital on the 6th of September, 1856. He stated that he had been rather a hard drinker—generally drinking to excess at the end of each week, from Saturday till Monday—and that he had of late had a good deal of anxiety and suffered from lowness of spirits, but that his health was good until seven weeks before his admission into the hospital, when jaundice came on, together with a dull pain in the hepatic region, but without any severe pain or spasm. The jaundice persisted. The dull pain in the hepatic region also continued, but in less degree than at first. His appetite remained tolerably good, but he had, he said, great thirst, and drank large quantities of water to appease it. The bowels were generally costive; the motions constantly pale, and the urine dark-colored, as is usual in jaundice. From the commencement of his illness he had gradually lost flesh and strength.

On his admission to the hospital he was deeply jaundiced, and complained of a dull pain about the ensiform cartilage. He complained also of a sense of fulness in the stomach, and of nausea, but had no vomiting. The tongue was somewhat dry, but clean, and he was very thirsty. The appetite was tolerably good. His spirits were much depressed, his sleep was interrupted by troubled dreams, and he had occasional headache. The pulse was counted 64, the inspirations 18, in a minute. No distinct enlargement of the liver seems to have been made out. The urine, which was deeply stained with bile, contained no albumen.

He was ordered five grains of blue pill, night and morning, and a drachm of sulphate of magnesia, with ten minims of dilute sulphuric acid, three times a day.

From this time there was no appreciable change in his condition till the 16th of September. He complained constantly of a dull pain across the stomach, of great thirst, and of a sense of nausea—but did not vomit. In the daytime he was observed to be generally somewhat drowsy.

On the 16th of September, at 4 P. M., he had a severe rigor. The following day he was much in the same state as before. The pulse was 80 in the minute, and it was noticed that the urine had a greasy film of phosphates on the surface. The former medicines were then left off, and he was ordered ten minims of dilute nitro-muriatic acid, with infusion of quassia, three times a day.

From this time he went on much as before till the 24th of October. His appetite was tolerably good, his bowels moved regularly, and he complained chiefly of pain across the epigastrium. The urine, which continued to be deeply stained with bile, constantly presented a greasy film on its surface. Nothing more was remarked in the discharges from the bowels than the continued absence of bile. The skin was perspiring.

The dose of the dilute nitro-muriatic acid was increased to twenty minims three times a day, but the greasy film on the surface of the urine still continued to appear.

In the evening of the 24th of October he had another rigor, followed by heat of skin and sweating, and afterwards for two or three successive nights he had a similar aguish attack. It was ascertained that he had never previously had ague.

On the 27th it was noted that the liver extended a little below the false ribs, but that no unevenness of its surface could be detected. In the right iliac fossa a globular tumor was felt, extending three or four inches below the edge of the liver, but traceable to it, and somewhat tender to the touch—which tumor, from its form and position, and from the evident stoppage to the flow of bile, was inferred to be the gall-bladder distended. The skin was frequently perspiring, but Donaghan complained of great general chilliness, and could not bear to be a moment uncovered.

He was now ordered, instead of his former medicines, ℨss of aromatic spirits of ammonia, every four hours, and four ounces of wine daily; and from this time no rigors occurred for several days. The appetite was still tolerably good, and the bowels were disposed to be costive.

It was subsequently noted that on the 3d of November he had a shivering fit, which began at 11 A. M. and lasted an hour, and another at 7 P. M., lasting fifteen minutes; that he had another shivering fit in the evening of the 5th, beginning at 8 P. M., and lasting about two hours; and another in the morning of the 6th, beginning at 8 A. M., and lasting three-quarters of an hour.

The tumor in the right iliac fossa remained of the same size, and the urine was constantly covered with a greasy film of phosphates. He continued to lose flesh. The pulse was latterly more frequent than at first, having been counted 80 and 84 in the intervals of the aguish attacks. In consequence of these irregular aguish attacks, it was inferred that suppuration had occurred in the liver.

In the morning of the 8th of November a considerable quantity of blood, about a pint it was said, was ejected from the mouth, part of it in clots. On the 10th it was found that there was some ascites, slight œdema of both feet, and œdema of the right side of the belly and right thigh, on which he had been lying; and that the superficial veins of the belly were enlarged. No fresh shiverings had occurred since the morning of the 6th.

In the morning of the 13th, he was in a drowsy state, and answered questions incoherently; and in the afternoon of that day he died.

Since the 28th of September he had constantly had the milk diet of the hospital, with an extra daily allowance of a slice of meat, and half a pound of potatoes.

The body was examined twenty-three hours after death.

It was *extremely* emaciated. The abdominal parietes were very thin, and contained hardly any fat. On opening the abdomen, about three pints of serous fluid, tinged with bile, escaped.

The tumor on the right side of the belly was found to be the gall-bladder greatly distended, reaching four inches below the edge of the liver. There was no inflammation of the peritoneum either of the gall-bladder or liver, or elsewhere, and there were no unnatural adhesions of the liver. The common gall-duct was *obliterated* by inflammatory thickening about it just as it enters the coats of the duodenum, and above this was dilated to the size of a large thumb. The larger hepatic ducts were also greatly dilated, but there was very little dilatation of the cystic duct. The gall-bladder contained thirteen ounces of a dirty chocolate-colored fluid, which, under the microscope, exhibited pus-globules, detached epithelium, and small plates of cholesterine. In that portion of it which was undermost in the recumbent posture of the body, the mucous membrane was almost entirely destroyed by ulceration in a space equal to half its extent; and around this space were many round or oval detached sloughing ulcers, varying in size from the diameter of a pea to that of a florin. The liver itself was of a mottled dark olive color, and rather more friable than natural, and exhibited under the microscope cells charged with biliary coloring matter, but containing very little oil. The pancreatic duct was involved in the same condensed tissue as the gall-duct, and was likewise obliterated just before it enters the duodenum; and the duct behind this was dilated and filled with a yellowish, puriform fluid. The head of the pancreas for an inch in length seemed to be converted for the most part into fatty tissue by the wasting of the gland-structure and the formation of fat. Behind this portion the gland was a good deal atrophied about the dilated ducts.

On examining the duodenum, an ulcer was found partially cicatrized about an inch and a half in length, and half an inch broad, commencing immediately above the papilla which marks the entrance of the gall and pancreatic ducts, and extending lengthwise up the intestine. In the stomach, also, an oval ulcer was found, about the size of a florin, situated on the posterior surface, very near the lesser curvature, and within an inch of the cardiac orifice. This ulcer, which had entirely destroyed the mucous membrane, appeared to be recent, as there was no thickening or induration at its margin. No other disease was found in the body.

In this instance the pancreatic duct and the common gall-duct were involved in a small mass of condensed tissue—apparently the result of inflammatory effusion—and were in consequence permanently closed, just at their point of entrance into the duodenum.

The ultimate effect was the same as if, without violence or other injury, a ligature had been there placed on the ducts.

The obstruction of the gall-duct caused, as it necessarily does, persisting jaundice and dilatation of the hepatic ducts; and also caused, after a time, great dilatation of the gall-bladder and sloughing ulceration of its mucous membrane. The effects of obliteration of the pancreatic duct may have been equally important, as regards the general condition of the patient; but they were less striking, and during life less distinctive. The conjoint obliteration of the two ducts caused, directly and by its after-effects, continuous wasting—so that, although the diet was sufficient for the maintenance of health, and the appetite continued tolerably good, and there was neither diarrhœa nor vomiting, the patient died, about four months after the occurrence of jaundice, in a state of *extreme* emaciation.

It is difficult to fix the time when inflammation of the gall-bladder set in, but it no doubt existed on the 16th of October, nearly a month before death, when the first distinct rigor occurred.

Ulceration of the gall-bladder is sometimes caused by irritating bile, independently of fever or gall-stones, and when there is no stoppage of the common or the cystic duct. A very remarkable instance of this kind, recorded by Dance, will be related further on.

Ulceration of the gall-bladder seems especially liable to occur in persons in whom the gall-bladder has suffered from former disease. The following case, which fell under my care in 1837, affords an instance of this, and further shows that an ulcer in the gall-bladder, like an ulcer in the stomach or duodenum, may cause profuse vomiting of blood:—

John Sibston, æt. 18, a collier, was admitted into the Seamen's Hospital, the 21st of September, 1837, on account of vomiting of blood, which had come on that morning. He stated that he was quite well previously.

During the 21st, he suffered great pain at the epigastrium, vomited blood several times, and had several loose stools. Eighteen leeches were applied to the epigastrium, and he was ordered dilute sulphuric acid, ♏vij every four hours.

On the 22d, he did not vomit. He was bled from the arm to ℥viij, and xij leeches were applied to the epigastrium.

On the 23d, the first time I saw him, the skin was hotter than natural; the pulse 100. There was still tenderness, and some tension, at the epigastrium. The tongue had a yellowish paste on its middle, but was red at the edges; he was thirsty, and had no appetite; had vomited once that morning, but no blood; had slept tolerably. The blood drawn the day before was not buffed or cupped. He was put on fever diet; and the sulphuric acid was continued.

On the 25th, the epigastrium was still tender, and the skin hot; but the pulse was 90; there was less thirst; and the coat on the tongue was white. No vomiting had occurred since the morning of the 23d. The bowels were rather confined. The sulphuric acid was left off, and common effervescing draughts were given instead.

26th. Tenderness at the epigastrium had ceased; no vomiting; bowels confined; some appetite; no thirst; has slept well. A dose of salts and senna was given, and the effervescing draughts were continued.

28th. No vomiting; bowels rather confined; appetite good; sleeps well. Beef-tea, Oij.

On the 4th of October he was put on meat diet.

He continued on this diet, walking about the wards, seemingly in full convalescence (his appetite good, bowels regular, sleep sound), until the evening of the 10th of October, when he was taken with malignant cholera. He soon fell into a state of collapse, and died early in the morning of the 12th.

At that time cholera prevailed in the Seamen's Hospital. Twenty-one of the patients fell ill of it in the course of three weeks.

The body was examined ten hours after death.

The cardiac extremity of the stomach was united to the under surface of the left lobe of the liver by a false membrane, in which were some chalky bodies, the size of small peas. The pyloric end of the stomach and the colon were firmly united to the gall-bladder, whose coats were much thickened.

The gall-bladder contained some pus, and its mucous membrane was extensively ulcerated. On the surface in contact with the liver, there was an ulcer as large as a shilling, and several smaller ones. On the opposite surface, there were some very small circular ulcers, scarcely larger than a pin's head. The ulcers had eaten through the mucous coat. There were no gall-stones, and the tissue of the liver appeared to be healthy.

The mucous membrane of the stomach in its splenic extremity was soft and thin, and red from the injection of small vessels, visible to the naked eye. The rest of the intestinal canal presented only the appearances usual in persons dead of cholera. The mesenteric glands were enlarged. In the transverse meso-colon were many bodies, about the size of a hazel-nut, composed of matter resembling soft cheese or glazier's putty, in a very distinct capsule. The spleen was firmer than usual, but of the usual size.

The left lung was united to the pleura costalis by old tissue; the right lung was free. Both lungs were healthy.

The heart and the kidneys were sound. There were yellow fibrous clots in the right auricle and ventricle, but none in the left chambers of the heart.

In this case inflammation of the gall-bladder seems to have come on in the midst of apparent health. The symptoms, at first, were vomiting of blood, which recurred several times, severe pain, with tenderness and some tension, at the epigastrium, some fever, with loss of appetite, thirst, and a foul tongue. These symptoms passed off in a few days, and the patient seemed convalescent, when he fell ill of malignant cholera, of which he soon died. The case shows that there may be extensive ulceration of the gall-bladder without any special symptoms to denote it. For a fortnight before the attack of cholera, there was no pain or tenderness at the epigastrium, and no vomiting, although there can be little doubt that the ulcers of the gall-bladder then existed.

Andral has published a case (*Clin. Med.*, t. iv. p. 500) in which ulceration of the gall-bladder, or sloughing of it from defective nutrition, occurred in a man 64 years of age, in whom the coats of the cystic and common ducts had been much thickened, and their channel much narrowed by former inflammation. Perforation of the gall-bladder took place, and the patient died speedily of the resulting peritonitis.

Cruveilhier (liv. xxix.), has published another case, in which suppurative inflammation and ulceration occurred in a gall-bladder previously diseased; but here there was an additional cause for disease of the gall-bladder in the cystic duct being closed by a gall-stone. The patient was a strong woman, 34 years of age, and death resulted from peritoneal inflammation, caused by the perforation of the gall-bladder.

I am indebted to Mr. Bowman for notes of a case observed by himself in which sloughing ulceration of the mucous membrane of the gall-bladder occurred during typhoid fever, in a housemaid, 16 years of age. The coats of the gall-bladder were somewhat indurated and thickened, and the cystic duct has been obliterated by previous disease. As in the cases recorded by Louis, already alluded to, in which suppurative inflammation of the gall-bladder occurred during typhoid fever, there were no symptoms by which the disease of the gall-bladder could be detected amidst the general disorder.

Thickening and other changes of texture in the coats of the gall-bladder, and narrowing of the cystic or the common duct, dispose to ulceration of the gall-bladder, just as paraplegia, or stricture of the urethra, or enlarged prostate, disposes to inflammation of the urinary bladder, by preventing the bladder from *completely* emptying itself, so that its contents undergo decomposition, and thus become irritating to the mucous membrane.

An ulcer in the gall-bladder, however it may have originated, is very difficult to heal while the cystic duct remains open, because the bile with which the ulcer is then constantly bathed is very irritating to a raw surface. An ulcer in the stomach or in the urinary bladder is in the same way constantly fretted by irritating fluids, and is consequently very difficult to heal.

Ulceration of the gall-bladder and gall-ducts may have various results.

1st. An ulcer, commencing in the mucous membrane of the gall-bladder, or of the common duct, may eat through its different coats until the peritoneal coat is laid bare. The bile brought in contact with this coat causes it to slough, and the contents of the gall-bladder are poured suddenly into the cavity of the peritoneum. When this happens, diffuse suppurative inflammation of the peritoneum is set up, which destroys life in a few hours; quicker, perhaps, in most cases, than the peritonitis that follows rupture of the bowel.

If, however, the cystic duct has been long closed, and the gall-bladder contain no bile, its contents may escape into the cavity of the peritoneum by *oozing*. When the mucous coat is eaten through, the matter may filter between it and the other coats, and may escape by a rent of the peritoneal coat, at a point that does not correspond to the ulcer of the mucous coat. The matter escaping drop by drop causes inflammation of the serous membrane, which is limited to the vicinity of the gall-bladder by adhesions of coagulable lymph, so as to form a circumscribed abscess in the cavity of the peritoneum. I have before referred to a case recorded by Cruveilhier, in which this happened.

When the gall-bladder contains bile this never occurs, because when the bile reaches the peritoneum it causes it to slough, and the contents of the bladder are discharged at once.

2d. When an ulcer of the gall-bladder or gall-ducts is caused by a gall-stone, adhesive inflammation of the serous membrane is usually set up before perforation takes place; the gall-bladder or gall-duct becomes united to some adjacent part, generally the duodenum or the colon; the coats of the intestine are eaten through after those of the bladder or duct; and the gall-stone passes into the intestinal canal.

Inflammation of the gall-bladder from gall-stones is less extensive, is attended with less severe symptoms, and is less dangerous in its results, than inflammation from other causes. The processes of ulceration and adhesion are slow, and give rise to no violent symptoms.

I have met with no instance of ulceration of the gall-bladder extending in this way through the coats of the bowel, except when produced by a gall-stone.

3d. Ulceration of the gall-bladder or gall-ducts, like ulceration of other mucous surfaces that return their blood to the portal vein, may lead to scattered abscesses in the substance of the liver. In the chapter on suppurative inflammation of the liver, several cases are referred to in which abscesses in the substance of the liver seemed to have their origin in ulceration of the gall-bladder or gall-ducts. The abscesses in such cases are probably the immediate consequence of suppurative inflammation of a small vein in the vicinity of the ulcer, or of the absorption of the ichorous matter of the ulcer.

In the large ducts, which lie close on the large branches of the portal vein, an ulcer may eat into a branch of the vein, and set up suppurative inflammation within it; and the consequences will, if possible, be worse than those of ordinary suppurative inflammation of the portal vein, because bile, as well as pus, will be mixed with the portal blood. The dreadful effects of this are fully exhibited in the following case, published by Dance (*Archives Générales*, t. xix. p. 40, 1828), in which an ulcer in the common duct ate into the portal vein:—

A hairdresser, aged twenty-five, of lymphatic temperament, was taken, without known cause, in the beginning of October, 1828, with lassitude, loss of appetite, thirst, and pain at the epigastrium. Some leeches applied there produced only slight relief. The 12th of October he was brought to the *Hôtel Dieu*, with these symptoms, but the pain at the epigastrium had increased, and the tongue was then red and dry, yet the pulse was but little quicker, the skin little hotter, than natural. Twenty leeches were applied to the anus;—little amendment. The next day fifteen leeches were applied to the epigastrium;—considerable abatement of pain.

During five days he continued to mend, the tongue became nearly natural. Later, at two different times, the severe symptoms recurred, probably from errors of diet. The first time they were calmed by leeches to the epigastrium; the second, they subsided without treatment.

At the end of October the patient seemed convalescent, but he still suffered at the epigastrium, and there was something in his condition altogether that we could not explain. At this time pain in the right hypochondrium, at first obscure, then more distinct, accompanied by bilious vomiting, and by purging; moderate fever, tongue natural. (Twenty leeches to the anus; bath.) Abatement of pain, continuance of vomiting and purging; the skin gradually acquired the tint of decided jaundice.

The patient continued nearly in this state till the 12th of November; then rigors, recurring at irregular intervals, followed by frequency of pulse, heat, and dryness of skin.

Two days later acute deep-seated pain about the right shoulder came on suddenly, swelling and tenderness of the soft parts about the joint, movements of the arm very painful. (Poultices; v. s. ℥viij.) The blood not buffed.

Eight days had elapsed from the appearance of this new train of symptoms, when, all at once, the middle of the forehead became the seat of severe pain, soon followed by swelling and tension, without change of color in the skin. At the end of two days the same phenomena at the left temple. The swelling extends, by degrees, to the face and to the entire head, which acquires an enormous size.

In the midst of these varied and serious disorders the pulse is small, not very frequent, compressible; the heat of the skin moderate; the vomiting, purging, and jaundice continue; the pains in the belly have ceased.

The swellings at the middle of the forehead and at the left temple go on increasing; bullæ filled with bloody serum appear here and there, and, bursting, leave small spots where the skin seems mortified. These spots extending, run together and form a single one, on the forehead and on the temple, as large as a crown-piece, the surface of which is riddled with small openings, from which small drops of pus can be pressed.

Some days before death the tongue becomes red and dry, then black; the lips and teeth become covered with sordes; the skin of the nose acquires a brownish tint. Petechiæ and small nodulous swellings appear on the skin, and in the subcutaneous areolar tissue of the limbs and of the trunk; the patient falls into a state of prostration and quiet delirium, and dies at 3 P. M., on the 2d of December.

Sectio cadaveris eighteen hours after death.

Limbs not rigid. The surface of the skin sprinkled with petechiæ. By the side of the petechial spots are blackish, lenticular pustules, some containing a sanious fluid, others a white homogeneous pus. These last extended into the subcutaneous areolar tissue, which was there infiltrated with pus. This eruption was thicker on the legs than on the arms; in front of the trunk than behind.

Head and face enormously swelled. Nose covered with a blackish crust, involving the skin, which here appeared gangrenous. On the middle of the forehead, on the left temple, and behind the left ear, soft, grayish, fetid sloughs, under which the areolar tissue is infiltered with pus. The skin of the forehead and of the anterior left half of the skull was transformed into a substance resembling bacon-rind, an inch thick, in the midst of which could be distinguished many veins filled with pus. These veins went to form the temporal veins, which, in the midst and on the surface of the temporal muscle, in the zygomatic and pterygoid fossæ, formed an immense plexus, of which all the branches were filled with pus, and bounded above by the black and softened fibres of the aforesaid muscle, below by dense yellowish areolar tissue. The left parotid, quadrupled in size, exhibited, when cut across, a granular surface, from which pus flowed, by a thousand different points, in small round drops, that came solely from the orifices of the numerous veins in the substance of the gland, many of whose branches were traced, all filled with pus. These branches terminated in the external jugular vein, which was inflamed as low as the middle of the neck, and offered on the outside an unnatural volume and hardness; on the inside, a reddish, roughened surface, covered with thick false membranes, and, lower down, with clots of blood mixed with pus.

On the right side of the head, and under the scalp, abundant infiltration of yellowish lymph, of the appearance of gelatine; the temporal muscle pale and soft; the parotid and external jugular veins healthy; the anterior branch of the temporal vein and all its divisions contain pus, collected into masses by small whitish bands, interrupted here and there by small clots of blood. The deltoid muscle on the right side blackish, softened, traversed by a considerable number of veins containing thick yellow pus. Muscles in other parts of the body brownish, and easily torn. The right shoulder and elbow joints contained shreds of false membrane, and a small quantity of puriform synovia. The other joints healthy.

Brain.—Sinuses of the dura mater distended with black grumous blood, without change of their coats. The cerebral substance pale, and as if œdematous. The ventricles distended by colorless serum. The membranes healthy.

Chest.—Heart of the usual size, color, and consistence, containing a small quantity of black fluid blood, presenting no trace of inflammation in its cavities or in the coats of the vessels that terminate in it.

Pleura not inflamed, and free from adhesions.

The lungs sprinkled with millions of small solid masses ("engorgemens"), of various forms and sizes, more numerous in the right lung than in the left, and in greatest number near the pleura, under which they formed prominences visible to the eye. Some of these solid masses had a blackish tint, others were whitish and granular, and broken down into a puriform matter by slight pressure. None of them were converted into abscesses. The pulmonary tissue around them was healthy, or slightly engorged with bloody serum. It was ascertained, by a careful dissection, that these masses were formed, in great part, of a mass of pulmonary veins, filled with pus in their smallest ramifications. The veins of the lung contained pus in no other points.

Abdomen.—The liver of a dark brown color, likewise containing many purulent masses ("noyaux"), most of them visible on the surface of the organ, but without projecting above it. These masses appeared to be formed of veins filled with pus, or, at least, to be the termination of them. We ascertained their continuation with the radicals of the vena portæ. Many branches of this vein and its trunk were full of a pulpy and puriform matter, of a yellowish color, like that of bile, mixed with liquid blood and with black or colorless clots, free or adherent. The inner membrane of these vessels was covered by a thick layer of pus, and had below this a rough and granular aspect; but, in the greatest part of its extent, it retained its natural polish, and was only whiter and more opaque than usual. Matter of the same kind was contained in the mesenteric veins which come from the small intestine, in those which come from the pancreas, and in the splenic vein. The coats of these vessels offered the same changes as those of the former vessels.

All these veins, before reaching the trunk of the portal vein, traversed a considerable mass (d'engorgement), formed, in front of the vertebral column, and in the whole length of the mesentery, by a collection of large red glands, suppurating at the centre, and surrounded by dense areolar tissue infiltered with pus.

The gall-bladder, filled with turbid serous bile, presented, towards its base, four small, round, blackish ulcers, extending through the mucous membrane. The common duct was destroyed in its entire length, and converted into an oblong winding cavity, containing membranous shreds detached from its coats, and stained with bile. Behind, this canal offered several deep ulcers, which extended through all its coats, and also through those of some large veins adjacent. One of these ulcers opened into the superior mesenteric vein by an orifice a line in breadth, presenting a projecting and greenish edge in the inner surface of the vein. The others might easily admit a moderate-sized probe.

The mucous membrane of the stomach and of the intestines everywhere in its natural state, of good consistence, remarkably white, only coated by thick, grayish mucus. About the entrance of the common gall-duct into the duodenum, for the space of a half-crown, the mucous membrane was of a slate color, softened, and presented four or five small deep ulcers.

The spleen was of a black-brown, and softened, but contained no pus.

Kidneys firm, pale, healthy.

Bladder healthy, filled with urine.

In the history of this case, the different stages of the disease are marked out with tolerable distinctness. During the month of October, it seems to have been confined to the mucous membrane of the gall-bladder and gall-ducts, and the symptoms were pain—which was twice relieved by leeches to the epigastrium—lassitude, loss of appetite, and thirst, without much fever. At the end of October, during apparent convalescence, inflammation seems to have been set up outside the common duct by the ulcers eating through it, and fresh symptoms occurred—return of pain in the right hypochondrium, bilious vomiting, purging, increased fever, jaundice. On the 12th of November, one of the ulcers had probably eaten into a branch of the portal vein; rigors recurring at irregular intervals, frequent pulse, and hot dry skin—the phenomena then noted—being constant symptoms in suppurative inflammation of a large vein.

In the cases of suppurative inflammation of the trunk of the portal vein before related, the local mischief was confined to the liver. The pus globules seemed all to be stopped there. In this case, at the end of two days, the patient was seized suddenly with pain and swelling about the right shoulder; at the end of eight days, with pain and swelling at the middle of the forehead; at the end of ten days, with pain and swelling of the left temple. Later still, petechiæ appeared on the skin, and gangrenous pustules on the limbs and trunk, and the patient died in a low typhoid state on the 2d of December. After death, shreds of lymph and purulent synovia were found in the right shoulder and elbow joints, and small circumscribed masses in different stages towards suppuration, in the lungs and liver.

The effects resembled those of suppurative phlebitis occurring after injury of the head or limbs, but the inflammation set up in so many distant points was more gangrenous than that consequent on ordinary phlebitis.

The dissection rendered it clear that the disease of the parts remote from the liver resulted from contamination of the blood with bile and pus, and that the morbid changes in those parts began in inflammation of the minute veins.

The circumstance that there were no gall-stones, and that ulcers were found in the duodenum, *immediately around the opening of the common duct*, as well as in the gall-bladder and in the duct, scarcely leaves a doubt that the ulcers, from which all the subsequent mischief resulted, were caused by irritating bile. It is worthy of remark, that there were no ulcers in the large intestines, or anywhere in the intestinal canal, except immediately about the opening of the common duct. It would seem that the bile, mixed with the food, and diluted, if we may so speak, with the pancreatic juice and the secretions of the bowel itself, became less irritating as it moved downwards.

The case confirms in a striking manner the opinion advanced in a former chapter on the relation between abscesses of the liver and dysentery.

It shows, too, how serious may be the consequence of faulty states of the bile, which in themselves may be transient, and of which at present nothing is known.

Another occasional effect of the diseases we have been considering is permanent closure of the cystic or of the common duct. This may, indeed, arise from various causes besides inflammation. Permanent closure of the *cystic* duct is not unfrequently caused by a gall-stone. The stone forms in the gall-bladder, and grows too large to pass through the duct. It is carried with the bile, in which it floats, into the mouth of the duct, and gets firmly lodged there. Circumscribed inflammation of the duct about the gall-stone is then set up, by which the duct is in general permanently closed beyond the stone, in the direction of the hepatic ducts. Sometimes the channel of the duct is thus obliterated on the other side also, so that the stone is inclosed in the cyst. Now and then the *common* duct is closed in the same way, but much less frequently, because the common duct is larger and straighter than the cystic duct, so that when a gall-stone has passed through the cystic duct, it in most cases passes through the common duct. The common duct is also liable to be closed by cancerous and other tumors, especially by cancerous or other enlargement of the lymphatic glands that lie upon it, and by malignant disease of the head of the pancreas. Further on a case will be related in which the duct, near its duodenal end, was completely obstructed, so as to cause persisting and fatal jaundice,-by a wart-like body, the size of a small bean, growing from the lining membrane of the duct. A few instances have been recorded in which the common duct was permanently closed by some foreign body getting into it from the duodenum.

The effects of mere closure of the ducts are just the same, whatever be its cause, and it is as well, therefore, to speak of them once for all.

Closure of the *cystic* duct destroys the office of the gall-bladder, and leads to various changes in it, which depend chiefly on the length of time the duct has been closed, and on the previous condition of the gall-bladder.

When the cystic duct is closed by adhesive inflammation of the capsule of the liver, and the mucous membrane of the gall-bladder is healthy, the bile in the gall-bladder soon gets absorbed, and its place occupied by a glairy fluid, of the consistence of mucus or synovia, and not at all tinged, or but very slightly tinged, with bile. After a time, this fluid is secreted in less abundance, and the gall-bladder contracts and shrivels—in some cases almost to the size of an almond.

When the coats of the gall-bladder were previously diseased and secreting cholesterine, which is generally the case when the cystic duct is closed by a gall-stone, the gall-bladder, after the closure of the duct, contains a viscid mucus, sparkling with scales of cholesterine, or is moulded on calculi almost entirely composed of that substance.

If, at the time of the closure, the gall-bladder contained unhealthy mucus or bile, this may undergo decomposition and set up, as we have already seen, suppurative inflammation of the mucous membrane, so that the gall-bladder may become filled with pus.

It would seem from the cases before related that closure of the cystic duct impairs the nutrition of the gall-bladder, and in this way also renders it more liable to inflammation and sloughing than in its natural state.

The effects of closure of the cystic duct on digestion and the general health are much less serious than might have been expected, and sometimes are of very little import. I have lately met with a striking instance of this in a man, 64 years of age, who died in King's College Hospital of extensive softening of the brain, and of inflammation of the urinary bladder which was consequent on the cerebral disorder. I did not expect to find anything amiss in the liver. The man's complexion was remarkably clear, and in the notes of his case, which were taken with much care, there was no mention of any disorder of digestion. The gall-bladder was filled by a mass of small stones, which choked the mouth of the duct, and completely prevented the entrance of bile. (See plate 2, fig. 3.) From subsequent inquiry among his friends, I learnt that he had never had jaundice, and never complained of disordered digestion.

Another instance of the same kind fell under my observation in King's College Hospital, in 1851. The gall-bladder was contracted upon an oval gall-stone, and seemed to have been long obliterated, in a woman who died of phthisis, and in whom no disease of the liver was suspected.

My friend, Dr. Scott Alison, some time ago sent me a gall-bladder, in which the orifice of the cystic duct was closed, and apparently had been closed long before death, by a gall-stone, the size of a hazel-nut. The bladder was filled with viscid mucus, sparkling with scales of cholesterine, and its coats were diseased. It was taken from a lady who died, at the age of 79, of acute bronchitis, of eight days' date, and who, before this illness, had been particularly healthy. She was of very temperate habits, and had never had jaundice or other symptoms to lead to the inference that the liver was diseased.

It has been stated that closure of the cystic duct, by causing the bile to flow continuously into the duodenum, increases the appetite in a remarkable degree (*Dict. de Méd.*, t. v. p. 241)—but this effect was not noticed in the cases just mentioned, nor in many others to which I could refer.

Closure of the *common* duct has far more serious effects.

The most immediate of these are deep jaundice, dilatation of the gall-bladder and hepatic ducts, and retention of bile in the lobular substance of the liver, which acquires in consequence a deep olive color. By the retention of bile the liver at first grows larger; but when the duct has been closed for some months it ceases to enlarge further, and subsequently, from atrophy of the lobular substance and from absorption of the retained bile, it may shrink again, and in the end, notwithstanding the dilatation of the gall-ducts, may become even smaller than in health.

When the liver is enlarged from the mere retention of bile, its edge is not rounded as in the fatty or scrofulous enlargement, but remains sharp and thin; and if the patient be much wasted, the sharp thin edge can sometimes be distinctly felt through the walls of the belly.

If the closure of the common duct occur suddenly, the gall-bladder, or one of the ducts behind the obstruction, may be distended so rapidly as to burst. Several cases of this kind are recorded.

When the obstruction occurs gradually, the bladder and ducts are distended more slowly, and when the duct has been long completely closed, are sometimes found of enormous size. Abercrombie (*Diseases of Stomach, &c.*, 2d edition, p. 364) cites from Boismont, a case in which the hepatic gall-ducts were so distended in this way, and the lobular substance of the liver was so wasted, that the liver had the appearance of a large undulating cyst. The closure of the common duct was caused by a membranous band which passed over it.

The ultimate effect of closure of the common duct on the *lobular substance* of the liver is very remarkable. The cells which go to form this substance, and which secrete the bile, are destroyed; the capillary vessels of the lobules, which minister to secretion, become atrophied; the liver, in consequence, no longer presents an appearance of lobules; and the office of the lobular substance can no longer in any degree be performed.

The destruction of the proper cells of the liver was first noticed by Dr. Thomas Williams, in a paper "on the Pathology of Cells," published in *Guy's Hospital Reports*, for October, 1843. Dr. Williams remarked it in a man who died in Guy's Hospital of malignant disease of the duodenal end of the pancreas, which so pressed upon the common duct that the bile could have passed into the duodenum only in very small quantity and very slowly. The gall-bladder and gall-ducts were extremely distended, and the whole organ was considerably enlarged. "The liver had lost its fragile, solid character, and had become soft, flabby, and not capable of being easily broken down by pressure. On the application of the microscope for the purpose of examining the ultimate structure, the extraordinary fact was developed, that scarcely a *single* nucleated glandular cell in a perfect state could be found. Different portions of the organ were carefully and repeatedly prepared, in order to remove every possibility of mistake or misobservation; the conclusions were uniformly the same, that the true parenchymal cells of the organ were certainly *not present*. These preparations were also seen and examined by several excellent observers about the hospital. In each portion of the organ mounted for inspection nothing more than minute *free* fatty particles, and equally free, floating amorphous, granular matter, could be discovered: it was very seldom that a *whole* nucleated cell could be seen. The following cut may serve to convey a conception of the microscopic characters of these objects."

Fig. 12.

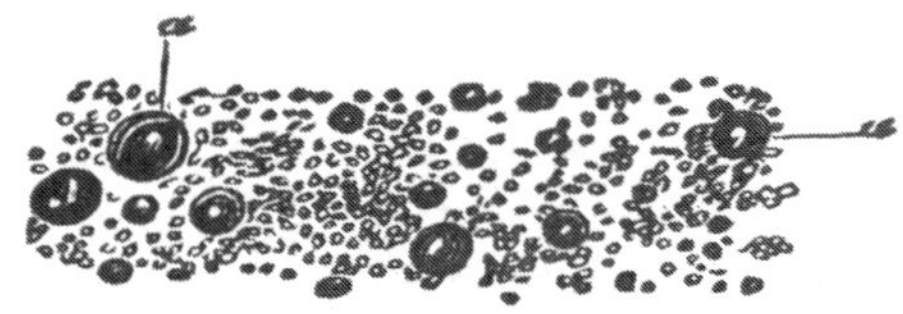

a, *a*, fat particles, free.

In the spring of 1844 I met with a case in which, from long closure of the common duct, the cells of the liver were perhaps even more completely destroyed than in the case related by Dr. Williams. I shall give the case in detail, because from there being no disease elsewhere to render the result ambiguous, it shows, clearer than any of the experiments made on animals, the effect of closure of the common duct.

CASE.—Ann Diprose, aged sixty-three, a sempstress, was admitted into King's College Hospital on the 18th of May, 1843. She was born in London, and had passed her life in it; of temperate habits, never taking spirits; married; had had six children, and five miscarriages; the catamenia appeared at the age of seventeen, were regular, except when interrupted by pregnancy and suckling, and ceased at the age of thirty-eight. Enjoyed good health till about fifteen years ago, when, after a fire which destroyed much of her husband's property, she was seized with violent pains, extending from the feet to the thighs, which continued for some time. A year after this the muscles on the right side of the face were spasmodically contracted for six weeks. About eleven years ago she fell down suddenly in the street, with loss of sensation and motion, from which she perfectly recovered in six weeks. She had no further illness till five years ago, when she suffered from pain and swelling in the right iliac region, attended with constipation. The pain gradually became very severe. It yielded to leeches, blisters, and low diet, after continuing from three weeks to a month. She perfectly recovered from this attack, and her health was good till her present illness, which began seven months ago, after great fatigue and anxiety in attending her mother, who was then, in her 91st year, operated on successfully for strangulated hernia.

At this time her face and body became *gradually* of a deep yellow color, which, with some diminution for one interval of three weeks, has continued ever since. The jaundice came on without pain, but with some degree of nausea, and was followed, at the end of two months, by vomiting, which has recurred at intervals up to the present time.

The appetite, at times, has been quite gone ; at other times ravenous. She has always found herself worse, and the jaundice deeper, after anxiety or fatigue.

Four months ago was salivated, without relief. Has wasted much since her illness.

On her admission to the hospital, the conjunctivæ and the whole surface of the body were of a greenish color. She was thin, but not emaciated. There was much itching of the skin ; surface cold ; frequent shivers. Pulse, 88 ; regular. Respiration, 22. Nothing discovered amiss in the heart or lungs by auscultation and percussion.

The tongue was clean ; the appetite very variable, and sometimes voracious ; occasional nausea, but no vomiting for the last week ; bowels confined ; evacuations clay-colored and fetid. Great tenderness over the whole belly, but no pain. There was dulness on percussion over the epigastrium, and for some distance below the right false ribs, which was ascribed to enlargement of the liver. No ascites. The abdominal muscles irritable.

The urine was of dark color ; s. g. 1015 : nitric acid produced at first a deep green, and when added in excess, a purple color.

Some headache and depression of spirits. Sleep good, but easily disturbed. She was ordered ♏xx of dilute nitric acid, three times a day ; and compound colocynth pills, when necessary, to keep the bowels open.

She remained in the hospital till the 8th of June, and during this time the symptoms underwent no material change. There was no fever ; the skin was cool ; the tongue moist, pallid, and indented ; and she was seldom thirsty ; the pulse ranged from 86 to 90 ; the s. g. of the urine from 1015—1020. She complained often of tenderness at the epigastrium, and at times of a gnawing pain there, which was relieved by taking food. Had frequent nausea, especially when the stomach was empty, but only vomited once—and then in the morning, in consequence, as she thought, of having taken the night before a draught containing the fourth of a grain of muriate of morphia.

A few days after she left the hospital she was much troubled by her husband returning to her ill—and from that time she became much weaker, and did not afterwards leave her bed, except for a short time in the evenings. She continued to take the nitric acid, which she thought did her good. There was great tenderness over the epigastrium and right hypochondrium, with *rigidity of the abdominal muscles;* she was unable to lie on the right side, and generally preferred the supine posture. She was very nervous—the least noise, or even sewing or reading, producing a "fluttering of the chest;"—and her sleep was more disturbed than it had been previously. She often became hot and feverish about night-fall, and continued so during the night. Complained at times of pain in the ankles and wrists, but these joints were not red or swollen. She had no vomiting. Her appetite was at times voracious; and she had a craving for oysters and small shell-fish, which, even in large quantities, never disagreed with her. She had an aversion to meat, and porter, and milk,—which she said disordered her.

One evening, after imprudently eating gooseberry tart, she was seized with violent pain and spasm under the right false ribs, which exhausted her very much, but did not cause vomiting.

On the 27th of June the nitric acid was exchanged for sulphate of quinine and dilute sulphuric acid; and this, again, was soon exchanged for nitro-muriatic acid, which she continued to take, with short interruptions, till the end of December.

During this time she grew weaker and thinner, and was harassed by occasional hectic at night. In other respects, her symptoms underwent little change. Her appetite was almost constantly craving, and she still had great desire for mussels and oysters. There was no vomiting. Her bowels habitually required purgative medicines; but in the middle of December she had diarrhœa, which lasted for a week, during which she felt better. She always complained of pain and tenderness of the belly, and often of itching of the skin. Slept badly by night, and was drowsy by day. The pulse ranged from 88 to 100; the respiration from 20 to 24. She had frequent cough, but did not expectorate. The urine was ever high-colored, fetid, stained linen yellow, and, on the addition of nitric acid, became first of a beautiful green, and then of a purple color. It was sometimes clear, at other times turbid, but never deposited a sediment approaching to pink.

A little before Christmas she suffered much from thirst, and effervescent draughts were given to allay it. She relished them very much, and continued to take them till her death, which happened on the 10th of March.

In the beginning of February she lost one of her sons, who died rather suddenly, from disease of the heart. From this time her appetite began to fail, and the last few weeks of her life she ate very little. She complained of nausea, and now and then vomited. Often had shivers, followed by burning heat of skin. Complained greatly of pain and soreness of the belly; and at times of pain of the head of a throbbing character. About a week before her death vomiting of blood came on, and recurred two or three times. The last week her mind wandered a little at night; but, with this exception, she continued rational up to her death, which seemed to result from exhaustion.

The urine was examined for the last time on the 21st of February. It had the same characters as previously, and its s. g. was 1012.

Two or three times morphia and conium were given to procure sleep, but these medicines disordered her, and increased her sufferings.

The body was examined twenty-two hours after death.

It was much emaciated, and of a greenish-yellow color.

The belly was large. The cavity of the peritoneum contained three or four pints of a serous fluid, and the intestines were much distended with gas.

The colon was closely united to the gall-bladder by false membranes of old date; but its canal was not contracted at this point.

The duodenum also adhered firmly to the gall-bladder for a very small space, about an inch and half below the pylorus. The canal of the intestine was a little curved by this adhesion, but not sensibly contracted.

There were a few threads of false membrane uniting contiguous loops of intestine.

The mucous membrane of the stomach and intestines presented no sensible change of structure. The duodenum contained a whitish pulpy matter; the large intestine firm white fecal matter, and much gas.

The liver was *smaller* than natural, and looked flattened. It was of a deep olive, finely mottled with yellow. Its surface presented no traces of peritonitis, except about the gall-bladder, and was readily thrown into fine wrinkles. The hepatic gall-ducts were enormously dilated, every section of the liver presenting some of the size of goose-quills. The tissue of the liver was flabby, but not easily broken down by the finger. The cut surface was of a deep olive, finely sprinkled with yellow—having somewhat the appearance of fine grained granite—but the lobules could not be distinguished in it.

When some of the tissue from any part of the liver was examined under the microscope, nothing was seen but numerous oil globules, and irregular particles of yellow and orange biliary matter, which was in many places agglomerated into roundish masses. *No distinct cells were visible.* The matter taken from the yellow points appeared to differ from the matter of the olive portions only in containing more oil globules and less biliary matter.

The tissue of the liver was in the same state throughout.

The gall-bladder and the cystic duct were enlarged, the latter to the size of the little finger. Their coats were much thickened. The outer coat had a dead-white color, and was of the firmness of cartilage, but presented no calcareous plates. Both were stuffed with small irregular tetrahedral calculi, the interstices of which were filled by a light yellow fluid, of the consistence of thin cream, which, under the microscope, presented nothing but a mass of very minute crystals of cholesterine (some of which were stained yellow), with here and there a particle of biliary matter.

The thickened coats of the gall-bladder and cystic duct exhibited under the microscope oil globules and plates of cholesterine.

The common duct was completely closed just below the point where the cystic duct enters it. Between this point and its opening into the duodenum *it was very narrow, just admitting a small probe.* Its coats not at all thickened or diseased, and not stained with bile. Immediately above the entrance of the cystic duct, the hepatic ducts were dilated to the size of a man's thumb. Their coats were stained of a deep olive, but were not thickened. Some of the dilated ducts contained a little dark green fluid.

The gall-bladder was not quite closed to the hepatic ducts. Some of the contents of those ducts might soak into the gall-bladder through the impacted mass of calculi.

The hepatic artery appeared to be of its natural size. The portal vein was healthy, and did not seem compressed by the gall-bladder and cystic duct.

In the loose areolar tissue, near the entrance of the portal canal, were some lymphatic glands of a dark olive color.

The thoracic duct was small; in the posterior mediastinum not larger than the quill of a hen.

The spleen had thick white spots of false membrane on its capsule, but was firm, and not enlarged.

The kidneys were healthy.

The heart healthy. Its ventricles, which were contracted, contained only very small fragments of fibrin.

The lungs were sound, but were united to the pleura costalis on each side by a few threadlike bands. There were no false membranes uniting the lower lobe of the right lung to the diaphragm.

There was some serous fluid in each pleural cavity.

In the case just related, closure of the common duct was evidently the chief, if not the sole, cause of the woman's sufferings during more than the last year of her life. The gall-bladder and the cystic duct were indeed stuffed with small gall-stones, but there were no marks of recent inflammation about them, and there was no disease elsewhere by which the symptoms could have been produced. It is difficult to fix the precise time when the duct became completely closed. From the circumstance that the jaundice came on *gradually and without pain*, the inference can scarcely be avoided that the occlusion took place gradually, for the sudden closure of the common duct by a gall-stone usually gives rise to a train of more urgent symptoms—to vomiting and paroxysms of severe pain, soon followed by deep jaundice. It is not improbable that in this case the first occurrence of vomiting, about two months after the onset of the disease, and about fifteen months before death, marked the completion of the process.

Among the many points of interest which the case presents, we may notice first, the effect which this long closure of the common duct had on the liver itself. Great dilatation of the gall-ducts and a dark green color of the liver are results which might have been predicted; but results far more curious and interesting are, the shrinking and flattening of the liver, the absence of distinct lobules in its substance, and the complete disappearance of the nucleated cells by which the bile is secreted. The substance of the liver was made up of vessels and areolar tissue connecting them with the free oil-globules and solid particles of yellow and orange biliary matter that were left when the watery and more soluble parts of the retained bile were absorbed. The objects seen when some of the tissue from any part of the liver was examined under the microscope were just the same as in the case related by Dr. Williams, and confirm in almost every respect Dr. Williams's account.

Destruction of the proper cells of the liver seems to occasion atrophy of the capillary vessels subservient to their secretion, and the two circumstances combined explain the shrinking of the liver in this case, and the absence of any appearance of lobules.

Other points worthy of notice in the history of the case, and which were among the effects of closure of the common duct, are:—

1st.—The constipation, and the relief derived from purgatives, and once from diarrhœa, that occurred without purgative medicine. Much of the pain and tenderness of the belly complained of was probably owing to distension of the intestine by feces and gas, and to irritation of its mucous membrane by the contact of matters chemically different from those natural to it.

2d.—The ravenous appetite that so long existed, which probably depended, as in diabetes, on imperfect digestion. I have known the same thing happen where the common duct was closed by the pressure of a cancerous tumor.

3d.—The desire that existed for shell-fish, especially oysters and mussels, which, in quantity to satisfy a craving appetite, never caused disorder.

4th.—The fetid urine; which was at times turbid with pale lithates, but never had a *pinkish sediment.* The absence of a pink sediment may help to distinguish such cases from cases in which the common duct is closed by the pressure of a cancerous tumor, and in which a sediment of this tint is often observed in the urine.

5th.—But perhaps the most striking circumstance of all was that although for a long time before death the liver must have ceased to separate bile from the blood, there were no symptoms of cerebral poisoning, and the mind remained clear to the last. This circumstance will appear still more remarkable if we compare this case with other cases in which suppressed secretion of bile is attended with delirium, or with stupor and convulsions, soon ending in fatal coma. Dr. Alison, in a paper published in the *Edinburgh Medical and Surgical Journal*, for 1835, has collected many cases of this latter kind, and, from a review of them, he concludes that it is jaundice from *suppressed secretion*, and not from obstructed gall-ducts, that is peculiarly, if not exclusively, liable to be followed by delirium, coma, and speedy death. He explains this by supposing that "the retention in the blood of matter destined to excretion is much more generally hurtful to the living body than the *re-absorption* into the blood of matters which have been excreted at their appropriate organs, but not thrown out of the body, in consequence of obstruction at their outlets." The fact is, I believe, correct, but Dr. Alison's explanation is not satisfactory, since, in this case, for a long time before death, there could have been no bile *secreted*, and yet there was no disorder of the brain.

6th.—The case further shows that life may continue for fifteen months after bile has ceased to flow into the intestinal canal; and thus proves that all the staminal principles of the food may be digested and absorbed without its aid. The absence of bile in the intestine, or destruction of the secreting element of the liver, proves fatal, however, in the end, by impairing nutrition, and causing slow but progressive wasting. The time requisite to wear out life must depend on the age and previous strength of the patient, his powers of digestion and assimilation, the nature and quantity of the food taken, and the various other circumstances that influence nutrition. It will, of course, be shortened by the injudicious employment of lowering measures. In Mrs. Diprose, the cells in the lobules of the liver had probably disappeared, and the organ ceased altogether to secrete bile some months before death.

In the summer of 1851, a very remarkable case of complete closure of the common duct by a gall-stone fell under my observation at King's College Hospital. The patient, a poor woman, became deeply jaundiced from this cause, when four months gone in pregnancy; yet, in spite of the deep and persisting jaundice, she brought forth, at the proper time, a living child, and suckled it up to the time of her death, which happened three months after the birth of the child, and between eight and nine months after the occurrence of the jaundice. She often came to see me, as an out-patient; but, from an unwillingness to leave her young children, constantly refused to come into the hospital. The following notes of the case were partly entered in my hospital case-book by Mr. Jordan, who was physician's assistant at the hospital when the poor woman first applied there, and partly procured for me by Dr. Henry Salter, who held the same office at the time of her death.

CASE.—Margaret Beglin, aged twenty-nine, married, and the mother of five children, is a native of Ireland, but has lived in London the last sixteen years. Her husband has secondary syphilis; she has miscarried once (six years ago) at the third month. She has always been of temperate habits, and was living in comparative comfort until the last two years, when, from her husband's illness (epilepsy from syphilitic cranial periostitis), she became poor, and has since suffered much privation. She is now living in a wretched place in Clement's Lane.

She was a stout, hearty girl, when she came to London, and had good health until her marriage at the age of nineteen.

Three years ago, she went to Dublin, and during her stay there caught a severe cold, which confined her to bed for three weeks. She recovered from this illness, but remained very weak, and could not get proper nourishment, and in about two months after had an attack of jaundice. There was then very severe pain in the right side, extending to the right shoulder, and swelling of the belly came on, which has continued ever since. The bowels were always loose and the stools white. She has never been "regular" from that date. though she had always previously been so.

The jaundice continued for about four months, at the end of which time she recovered her health, but the belly remained large. She came to England, and remained free from jaundice for nine months. Eight months ago jaundice recurred, and has continued ever since. At its recurrence, there was pain in the chest, and in the right side and right shoulder, and slight cough. Ever since, the bowels have been loose, as before, and the stools white.

About three months ago, she had a child at full term. The jaundice, therefore, came on in the fourth month of pregnancy. The child was "yellow as a guinea" when born, but acquired the natural color in two or three days. This child she is now suckling. Her milk has been, and is, perfectly white. After her confinement, she had severe flooding for five days.

At present (August 12, 1851), she is attending the hospital as an outpatient, deeply jaundiced. She lives badly, and is very weak, and suffers a good deal from giddiness and headache, but is yet able to walk about well, and suckles her baby. She complains of itching of the skin, which has existed from the commencement of the jaundice, and of pains in "the small of the back," and in different parts of the limbs, along the thigh and in the hip, which are not worse at night. She likewise complains of almost constant pain in the region of the liver, and of occasional severe pain in the right shoulder. At times, she has had pain, amounting to agony, stretching from the navel to the chest; and, during these paroxysms, has vomited a sour watery fluid. She has cough, and spits dark-colored catarrhal mucus, and catarrhal sounds are heard on the chest.

The diarrhœa, which has existed ever since the occurrence of the jaundice, has been much checked by infusion of logwood and chalk mixture, which have been given her at the hospital; but the bowels are still moved two or three times a day, and the stools are loose. Her skin is generally damp and perspiring; and her expression cheerful. She sleeps badly, but her appetite is very good. She has a sense of distension of the stomach after meals, but no pain. Feels occasionally sick and faint, but does not vomit. Has piles, and has lost a small quantity of blood from them. Has lately had many fits of shivering, and sweats much at night. Never had ague, and the spleen is not enlarged. Since her confinement, her legs and feet have swollen a little. The pulse 98, the inspirations 20, in a minute.

The belly is protuberant, like that of a woman eight months advanced in pregnancy, and the liver is much enlarged. The lower edge of the liver can be traced, stretching from the left hypochondrium, in a curved line, to a spot about half an inch below the umbilicus, and thence down into the right iliac region, a great part of which it occupies. To judge from percussion, it does not encroach much on the lungs. Its outer surface seems quite smooth to the touch; and its lower edge, which can be grasped between the fingers for some distance near the umbilicus, is felt to be *sharp*. The liver does not appear to be adherent to the abdominal parietes, since, by pressure, it can be shifted from its position and moved up. There is but little pain on pressure over the liver, the greatest being in the right iliac region. The superficial veins of the belly are not enlarged, and there does not seem to be any fluid in the peritoneal sac. There is no rigidity of the recti or other abdominal muscles.

Half a drachm of aromatic spirits of ammonia was ordered to be taken in an astringent mixture three times a day; and she was urged, in vain, to wean the baby, and to come into the hospital.

From this time she was not seen by any of the medical officers of the hospital until her death, which happened on Sunday, the 24th of August. The following statement of her condition during this interval was obtained from her husband:—

She first appeared to get worse about a week before her death. The pain in the right side then became much more severe, shooting down to the bottom of the belly, and being much aggravated by any movement, so that she was hardly able to walk, and suffered great pain in getting in and out of bed; and a difficulty in passing her water, which existed for some weeks before her death, increased, so that at times she would sit on the urinal in great agony for a quarter of an hour, and pass none. Towards the close of her life, the diarrhœa, which had existed for some months, likewise increased greatly. During the last week her appetite failed, and she was in a state of extreme weakness, hardly able to move about, and occasionally for a minute or two losing her sight.

On the evening of the 21st, when her husband came home, he found her very ill, sitting by the fire. She said she had been very ill all day, and had been passing from the bowels "black lumps" mixed with blood. The pain in the side was worse, and pain in the head, which subsequently became very severe, also came on. She continued to past "black lumps" from the bowels up to the time of her death, and was very faint and thirsty, but was quite sensible to the last, except during a short fit, in which she lost her speech, and fell out of bed insensible. After the fit she was sick, and threw up a dark brown matter like coffee. She seemed to suffer most from pain in the head, and at last did not complain of pain in the side or belly—the pain in the head appearing by its severity to obscure all the other pains.

On the evening of the 23d she looked and spoke somewhat better, ate a biscuit, and then slept for two or three hours. The rest of the night she complained of pain in the head, and was tossing about, seeming very faint. At six A. M., on the 24th, she became insensible, and, at seven, died very quietly. Two or three hours before her death she suckled her child.

On the morning of the 27th the body was examined by Mr. Jordan and Dr. Salter.

On opening the belly, a small amount of fluid was found in the cavity of the peritoneum, but no more than was probably cadaveric. The intestines, large and small, were blown out with gas. The intestinal canal throughout was stained of a dark purple, and on cutting into it the cause of this was revealed, the whole of the intestines being filled with blood; the entire alimentary canal was taken out and washed; but, though stained with blood, as before stated, no ulcer or abrasion of the mucous membrane was detected.

The liver was about three times the natural size, very flat, and not thickened, and its lower edge was very sharp. It looked fatty, and its texture was mottled and uneven. On examining the gall-duct, the secret of the disease was explained. A gall-stone, as large as a walnut, was found firmly impacted in the common duct, about two inches from its duodenal end. The duct was hard, like a cord, below the obstruction towards the duodenum, and very much dilated above. Its coats were much thickened, and all its ramifications in the liver were enormously dilated, so as to look like sinuses as large as the branches of the portal vein. The cystic duct and the gall-bladder were atrophied and quite shrivelled up. No ulcer could be found anywhere in the ducts, and the mucous membrane, even where the gall-stone was impacted, was perfectly unbroken. On examination under the microscope, the liver was found to contain a great deal of oil, in globules of various sizes, but no cells belonging to the lobular substance were seen.

The kidneys were large, soft, and congested, and looked fatty.

The brain and other organs were not examined.

In this case, as in the preceding, closure of the common duct by a gall-stone was the primary cause of illness; and the effects of this were, in the main, the same—deep and persisting jaundice; very slow, but progressive, wasting; destruction of the cells in the lobular substance of the liver; after a time, more or less fever, of the character of hectic; and, finally, hemorrhage from the intestinal canal, and death from exhaustion—the mind remaining clear almost to the last.

This case differs, however, from the preceding in the existence of almost constant diarrhœa; and in the circumstance, that the liver, instead of being smaller than natural, as it was in the preceding case, was much enlarged by the dilatation of the ducts and the accumulation of oil and biliary matter within it.

It will be seen that in both cases the portion of the common duct, between the obstructing gall-stone and the duodenum, was found very much contracted after death. In the first case it only just admitted a small probe; and in the second it was like a hard cord. When the common duct is thus completely closed by a gall-stone, contraction and atrophy of the lower end of the duct necessarily take place; and as it renders the future passage of the stone along the duct impossible, the prognosis in such cases is very unfavorable when the closure of the duct has existed for some months. The course of the bile can then be restored only by the gall-stone working its way, *by ulceration*, into the intestinal canal.

The case last related shows quite as clearly as the one before it, that all the staminal principles of the food can for a considerable time be digested without the presence of bile in the alimentary canal; for the poor woman, although her health was doubtless impaired by the former attack of jaundice, which had left the liver enlarged, and although she lived badly and suffered many hardships, and lost much blood after her confinement, lived between eight and nine months after bile had ceased to flow into the duodenum, and during this time not only supported herself, but brought to maturity and suckled an infant.

I have since met with another instance quite as conclusive in showing that fatty matters at least—to the digestion of which bile is supposed especially to contribute—may, under certain circumstances, continue to be sufficiently absorbed for a long time after bile has ceased to flow into the intestinal canal. A gentleman, about fifty years of age, fell under my care in the beginning of November, 1854, on account of jaundice, which came on towards the end of June preceding, in consequence, as he supposed, of a bilious attack. A short time before I saw him he had undergone an operation for fistula, and there was still, and for several months afterwards, a considerable discharge of pus from the rectum. At the epigastrium a large tumor was felt, which turned out to be the omentum thickened and contracted, and the liver, as a *post mortem* examination showed, was in a state of cirrhosis. Notwithstanding these conditions and continued complete obstruction of the common gall-duct, he lived till the end of March, 1856,—or for more than twenty months after the occurrence of jaundice. A short time before death, ascites came on—the result of the cirrhosis—on account of which he was tapped twice. The strength slowly declined, but at the time of death the body was still tolerably fat. The obstruction of the gall-duct was caused by the pressure of a tumor, the size of a walnut, which proved to be an enlarged lymphatic gland.

It is worthy of notice that, in two of the cases just related, hemorrhage took place from the intestinal canal a short time before death. Since these cases fell under my observation I have met with several other instances of long-continued and ultimately fatal juandice from obstruction of the common gall-duct, in which the same thing happened; and have no doubt that permanent closure of the duct, after it has existed a long time, has, in some way or other, an especial tendency to cause hemorrhage from the bowel.

The intestinal hemorrhage in these cases occurred without hemorrhage elsewhere, and cannot therefore be attributed solely to a general disposition to hemorrhage, which is not unfrequently seen in cases of jaundice. The question then arises, On what other condition did the hemorrhage depend? If it has resulted from pressure on the trunk of the portal vein by the gall-stones, or by a tumor, obstructing the common duct—or from mechanical impediment to the passage of blood through the liver, caused by wasting of the capillary vessels in the lobular substance, consequent on the destruction of the cells—there would, probably, as in cases of cirrhosis, have been a greater degree of ascites. A *sudden* impediment to the passage of the blood through the liver may cause great congestion of the mucous membrane of the intestinal canal, and hemorrhage from it, without ascites; but an abiding impediment, as is seen in cases of cirrhosis, and in those cases of cancer of the liver in which the trunk or a large branch of the portal vein is compressed by a cancerous tumor, causes ascites rather than hemorrhage, and usually leads to a high degree of ascites before any hemorrhage takes place.

As no ulceration of the intestine had been observed in these cases, my impression at one time was that the hemorrhage resulted from a state of *congestion* of the mucous membrane, and that this congestion of the secreting membrane of the stomach or intestines was caused in some way or other, not by *mechanical* impediment to the passage of the blood through the liver, but by cessation of the process of secretion in it.

In the summer of 1855 a case fell under my observation, in King's College Hospital, which in some degree shook my belief in the truth of this explanation. The patient, a man fifty-three years of age, became rather suddenly affected with jaundice in the month of January. The jaundice continued, and he died on the 6th of July following. A short time before death he vomited a large quantity of blood. On examination of the body, the jaundice was found to be caused by a wart-like growth of the mucous membrane of the common duct, which completely blocked up the duct, about half an inch from its duodenal end. In the duodenum there was a large ragged ulcer. There was no ulceration elsewhere in the intestines, and no disease worthy of note was discovered in other parts of the body. In the autumn of the present year (1856) I met with another instance (the case of Donaghan, before related, p. 212), in which, after jaundice from obstruction of the duct had existed many months, vomiting of blood occurred. In this instance, both the pancreatic duct and the common gall-duct were obliterated just at their point of entrance into the duodenum by being involved in a small mass of indurated tissue—apparently the result of inflammatory infusion. In the duodenum an ulcer was found partially cicatrized, an inch and a half long and half an inch broad, commencing immediately above the papilla, which marks the entrance of the gall-duct, and extending lengthwise up the intestine. In the stomach there was another ulcer, about the size of a florin, that had the appearance of having been recently formed.

In these instances the ulcers were certainly the most probable source of the hemorrhage; and the coincidence of the ulcers with long-continued obstruction of the duct raises the suspicion that the ulcers may have been caused by the obstruction, and that in some of the other cases of long-continued obstruction of the duct, in which intestinal hemorrhage occurred, an ulcer may have existed in the duodenum and have escaped notice. It is possible, however, that both explanations may be in part true—that permanent stoppage of the common gall-duct may lead, after a time, to congestion of the mucous membrane of the duodenum, and subsequently to ulceration, and that hemorrhage may occur in either stage of disease A careful examination of the duodenum and stomach in a few more cases of long-continued jaundice from obstruction of the duct will settle the point.

Simple closure of the common gall-duct, when it occurs in a person previously well nourished and placed in favorable circumstances, sometimes causes very slight constitutional disorder, and no great loss of strength, for several months. The patient, in some instances, would hardly consider himself ill, if he were not jaundiced, and I have more than once known a man in whom deep jaundice from this cause had lasted six or seven months, still able to walk several miles without fatigue. After a time, however, digestion becomes a good deal disordered; slight fever, of the character of hectic, sets in; the loss of flesh and strength, though still very gradual, becomes greater than before; and at length—usually after the lapse of from twelve to twenty months from the occurrence of the jaundice—the patient dies from exhaustion, which, as we have just seen, is sometimes hastened by hemorrhage from the intestinal canal. A short time before death, slight dropsical effusion now and then occurs—the result, probably, of the joint influence of an impoverished state of the blood and of feeble propulsive power in the heart.

In cases of this kind the deepest possible jaundice may exist for many months—the skin may be of a brownish green, instead of yellow, from the accumulation of biliary pigment and the action of the air upon it—and no disorder of intellect whatever, may occur. The patient gradually loses flesh and strength, and having become very thin and anemic, at length dies—simply from exhaustion. These facts are sufficient to justify the inference that in cases of jaundice which prove rapidly fatal from delirium and coma—and many such cases will be related in the next chapter—the fatal cerebral disorder is owing, not to the mere suppressed secretion of bile, but to some peculiar noxious matter developed in the system.

When permanent closure of the duct occurs in a person in a faulty state of nutrition, or in one who has insufficient means of support, the hectic fever sets in earlier, the wasting is more rapid, and the strength may be exhausted in seven or eight months.

In some instances, as we have seen, the retention of the mucus and bile causes suppurative inflammation of the gall-bladder, and death is still further hastened by the severe constitutional disorder which this occasions.

It sometimes happens that, after complete closure of the common duct has existed many months, and while no bile flows through it into the intestine, the jaundice of the skin becomes very much less deep, and the urine very much less deeply stained with bile. I have, indeed, more than once known the jaundice gradually diminish and almost entirely disappear after the lapse of twelve months, to the great satisfaction of the patient, although the color of the intestinal discharges, and an examination of the body after death, showed that the closure of the duct was still complete. These facts strongly support the opinion that the coloring matters of the bile are formed primarily, at least for the most part, within the liver—as the resinous acids of the bile appear to be—through the agency of the cells in its lobular substance.

In other cases of the same kind, the jaundice, perhaps from retention of the biliary matter in the skin, remains deep to the last.

The question may here be asked—in what degree does the progressive anemia, and the gradual loss of flesh and strength ending in death, in cases of simple closure of the common gall-duct, result from the want of bile in the intestinal canal; and in what degree from the unhealthy condition of the blood and from the impairment of digestion caused, more directly, by the total destruction of the cells in the lobular substance of the liver? Destruction of the hepatic cells leads to an unhealthy condition of the blood, not only by preventing the elimination of those effete matters which contribute to form the bile, but also by preventing those reparative changes which the blood naturally undergoes in its passage through the liver; and the suppressed secretion of bile, which is a consequence of destruction of the hepatic cells, directly impairs digestion by lessening, or vitiating, the secretions of the stomach and other parts of the intestinal canal. The opinion was advanced by Dr. Prout, that the principal digestive organs, taken together, form a kind of galvanic apparatus, of which the mucous membrane of the stomach and intestinal canal generally may be considered the acid or positive pole, the hepatic system, the alkaline or negative pole. There is much in favor of this opinion, but whether the relation between the stomach and the liver be *electrical* or not, there can be no doubt that there is an intimate relation between them, and that cessation or derangement of secretion in one of those organs affects more or less the secretion of the other.

If we consider that for many months from the commencement of illness, in cases of this kind, the strength is often tolerably maintained, and the signs of disordered digestion are slight, that the strength usually declines more rapidly, and the disorder of digestion becomes greater as time wears on, it seems most probable that the defective regeneration of the blood and the gradual wasting of flesh are owing much less to the mere absence of bile in the intestinal canal than to the other conditions just mentioned.

This inference is confirmed by the result of an experiment performed by M. Blondlot, in which he succeeded in tying the common gall-duct in a pointer bitch, between three and four years old, and afterwards establishing a biliary fistula from the gall-bladder, so as to allow the bile to escape from the gall-bladder through the side.

After the operation, the stools had no tinge of bile, but the bitch had an excellent appetite, and her health was so good that she littered every year, and occasionally hunted with eagerness. The bile continued to flow from the fistula with its habitual characters, but in a manner in some degree intermittent. When the animal was fasting no more than a few drops escaped, while some minutes after taking food it issued in abundance, and continued to do so during the whole time of digestion. This state of things continued for five years, after which the animal wasted for some time, and then died without the occurrence of any remarkable incident.

On examination after death, the common gall-duct was found perfectly obliterated, so that all the bile secreted by the liver must have passed out of the body through the fistula. The gall-bladder, although adherent to the abdominal walls, and having a fistulous opening through them, had preserved its natural form and dimensions. The cystic duct was very much dilated. The liver itself was contracted and hard, and had the appearance of a liver affected with cirrhosis.[1]

In three of the cases related above, the patients lived at least fifteen months after the closure of the duct. Other cases have occurred in which, judging from the duration of complete jaundice or the state of the liver after death, life must have continued much longer after this had happened.

Some months ago my attention was called by Mr. Busk to a patient in the Seamen's Hospital, who had then been jaundiced for four years, and, as I imagined, from closure of the common duct. During this time but little bile seems to have passed into the bowel. The feces were reported to have been always pale; and the year before I saw him he had taken strong emetics, which produced free

[1] Comptes Rendus de l'Académie des Sciences, 23 Juin, 1851.

vomiting, but, as he stated, nothing *bilious* was brought up. He was still tolerably stout and muscular. In the case related by Boismont, already alluded to, where, from extreme dilatation of the gall-ducts and wasting of the lobular substance, the liver had the appearance of a large cyst, the cells in the lobular substance must, for the most part, have disappeared, and the action of this portion of the liver could have been performed but to very small extent, long before death.

These cases might lead us to expect (what indeed happens) that persons who, from obliteration of branches of the portal vein, or from the changes so frequently produced by long residence in tropical or malarious climates, have very little liver left,—to use a common expression, but which, if we consider the liver as a mere agent of secretion, is strictly correct — might often, by careful management, enjoy tolerable comfort for many years.

Complete atrophy of the cells in the lobular substance of the liver, from permanent closure of the common gall-duct, is not a singular fact in pathology. When the ureter is *completely* stopped, as it sometimes is by a calculus formed in the pelvis of the kidney, the secreting structure of the kidney wastes, and at length entirely disappears, so that the organ is reduced to a cyst, which may not be larger than a small apple.[1] Wasting of the gland-structure of the pancreas results from stoppage of the pancreatic duct—and probably the same thing happens for other excreting glands. In the liver, for complete disappearance of the cells in the lobular substance after closure of the duct a variable time is required. In the case of Donaghan, before related (p. 212), where death occurred from closure of the pancreatic duct and the common gall-duct, between six and seven months after the gall-duct was completely and permanently stopped, every particle of the liver that was examined under the microscope contained a great number of perfect cells, highly charged with biliary matter. Atrophy of the liver-cells takes place the more slowly, when the common gall-duct is stopped, because the products of their secretion are still taken up and carried out of the liver by the capillary vessels of the lobular network and by the numerous lymphatics which are spread over the hepatic ducts, and consequently the cells can, to some extent, continue in

[1] Two preparations, which exemplify this fact, are preserved in King's College Museum—one of them placed there by myself.

the performance of their appointed function—which, doubtless, prevents their decay. In glands where the secreted products are not carried off with the same facility by the bloodvessels and lymphatics, closure of the excreting duct probably causes a much earlier atrophy of the gland-structure.

Another circumstance worthy of notice in the first of the cases of closure of the common duct related above, is the state of the coats of the gall-bladder, which were thickened and opaque, and, when examined under the microscope, exhibited numerous oil globules and transparent scales of cholesterine. This disease of the gall-bladder is analogous to the "atheromatous" disease of arteries, which Mr. Gulliver has lately designated "fatty degeneration of arteries," from having discovered that the atheromatous matter is chiefly composed of fat, in the form of oil-globules and scales of cholesterine. This disease of the gall-bladder may therefore be termed, with equal propriety, *fatty degeneration of the gall-bladder*—an expression which has the merit of involving no theory as to the cause of the disease, but merely announcing the fact. In the gall-bladder, as in the arteries, phosphate of lime is often deposited with the fatty matter, and sometimes in such quantities as to form large bony plates, which on the inside of the gall-bladder are usually bare, or merely covered by a soft pulpy matter, which may be readily scraped away. Sometimes the earthy matter is in such quantity that the gall-bladder is almost converted into a bony cyst.

In some cases the entire gall-bladder has undergone this change; in other cases, merely a part of it. In a gall-bladder sent me by Dr. Alison (of which I have already spoken), which was taken from a lady who died at the age of 79, much of the under and free surface was rigid from calcareous plates, which on the inside were covered only by a soft pulpy mass, composed of fatty matters and mucus. About the neck of the gall-bladder, and on the side of it attached to the liver, the coats were not at all thickened, and seemed healthy. The diseased part was limited by a well-defined line, readily seen on the inside of the bladder. The mouth of the cystic duct was blocked up by a calculus, composed almost entirely of cholesterine, and the bladder was filled with a viscid matter of a dirty yellowish-green and sparkling with small scales of cholesterine.

This disease of the gall-bladder, according to my own observation, is much more common, as gall-stones are, in women than in men. It occurs especially in the decline of life, like the atheromatous disease of arteries, and seldom exists in the highest degree under the age of 50. Sedentary habits, and modes of life conducive to fatty degeneration of other tissues, doubtless favor its production; but some local condition directly affecting the nutrition of the coats of the bladder—such as inflammation, or prolonged irritation by unhealthy bile or gall-stones—seems generally to have contributed to bring it on. It does not always co-exist with atheromatous disease of the arteries, as it probably would do if it depended entirely on general or constitutional causes. I have met with it in the highest degree when there was little disease of the arteries; and have met with atheromatous disease of the arteries in the highest degree in persons advanced in life, in whom the coats of the gall-bladder were sound. The disease is very important, because it is not uncommon in the decline of life, and may have very serious results. It is always attended with an abundant secretion of cholesterine in the gall-bladder, which frequently leads to the formation of gall-stones, and thus to all the evils which gall-stones occasion. After a time, it causes sloughing of the lining membrane of the bladder, and by rendering the coats of the bladder rigid, prevents it from ever being completely emptied. The bile and the unhealthy secretions of the bladder being retained there, undergo decomposition, and set up persisting inflammation of its inner surface. If the cystic duct should become blocked up by a gall-stone, or otherwise, which not unfrequently happens, the gall-bladder is converted into an abscess, with rigid and uncontractile walls, which almost necessarily causes great and protracted suffering, and may destroy life in various ways.

The cases that have been related in this chapter exhibit the chief forms of inflammation of the gall-bladder and gall ducts. We may gather from them, that when *catarrhal* or *suppurative* inflammation is confined to the gall-bladder, or to the gall-bladder and cystic duct, the chief symptoms are, pain and tenderness in the site of the gall-bladder, vomiting or nausea, and a certain degree of fever. When from the first the inflammation is not severe, or when its first flush has passed by, these symptoms may be very slight, and excite little attention, or be even entirely disregarded. When, again, inflammation of the gall-bladder occurs during typhoid fever or in the midst of other severe constitutional disorder in which sensation is blunted, pain is little complained of, and the other symptoms lose almost all their significance. *Ulceration* of the gall-bladder, when it involves only a small part of the organ, may exist without fever or other constitutional disturbance, and with only occasional pain, and may be almost unheeded, till, by sloughing of the peritoneal coat, the contents of the bladder are poured into the cavity of the peritoneum. The symptoms that precede this accident are not such as to impress us with a notion of danger, and we require fuller knowledge than we now have of the circumstances in which ulceration of the gall-bladder occurs, to make us alive to their true meaning. When inflammation involves the hepatic ducts or still more the common duct, and, by causing thickening of their mucous membrane or secretion of viscid mucus, prevents the passage of bile, in addition to the symptoms mentioned above—that is, more or less pain and tenderness, which we may expect to be more diffused than when the gall-bladder alone is diseased; vomiting, perhaps, or nausea; and more or less fever—there will be jaundice. The jaundice, attended by slight pain in the region of the liver and by slight fever, that occurs in young and previously healthy persons, depends, perhaps generally, on an inflamed state of the gall-ducts, which, from their small size, must be readily closed by swelling of their mucous membrane or by a viscid secretion from it.

When inflammation involves the lower end of the common duct only, and is of such a nature as to close it, the symptoms are very peculiar—pain confined to a small spot in the situation of the common duct, early jaundice, and early distension of the gall-bladder, so as to form a large, movable, pear-shaped tumor, which, at first, is not painful or tender.

In the *treatment* of inflammation of the gall-bladder and gall-ducts, a most important principle is the early employment of local depletion. Leeches, as was seen distinctly enough in some of the cases that have been related, relieve the pain and tenderness, and no doubt mitigate the inflammation, and, in consequence, lessen the danger of perforation and of permanent closure of the ducts. The value of this practice has been more or less vaguely recognized in *jaundice*, but its importance in the class of cases we have been considering has not perhaps been sufficiently inculcated. It should always be borne in mind, that, here, a disease attended with but little pain and fever, and, at first, with no alarming symptoms, and indeed trivial in itself, may, *from its situation*, prove mortal. The precept to be drawn from this truth may be made general. In all cases where *canals* form an essential part of vital organs, mechanical considerations come to be paramount, and give an importance to diseases which in themselves are trivial. In stricture of the pylorus from thickening and induration of the submucous areolar tissue, and in the endocarditis of acute rheumatism, this truth is strikingly exemplified. In such cases our object must be, not so much to relieve the present symptoms, which are often slight, as to prevent those changes of structure which, slowly it may be, but inevitably, and with much suffering, destroy life. How valuable, then, is that insight which enables us to perceive the danger before it is revealed to other eyes, and when alone we can effectually guard against it! This insight we can derive only from knowledge of the circumstances under which these forms of disease occur; knowledge, which gives meaning to symptoms otherwise vague, and perhaps so slight as to be scarcely regarded.

Blisters have the same kind of efficacy as leeches. Like these they often greatly relieve the pain and tenderness, and, therefore, we may infer, tend also to prevent permanent changes of structure. The proper time for blistering is when the pain and fever have abated under leeches and other measures, and it is no longer deemed advisable to take away blood.

Another important principle in the treatment of these diseases is the strict enforcement of a simple diet. In certain cases the free use of diluents may have some peculiar advantages. By filling the stomach, they help to empty the gall-bladder by the pressure they exert upon it, and, after absorption, they pass out of the circulation again, in part, by the liver, and thus dilute the bile.

In cases in which the ducts are still pervious, signal benefit often results from the judicious use of mercury, which probably acts beneficially in two ways—first, by increasing the quantity and promoting the flow of bile; and secondly, by causing changes in its quality, which render it less irritating. These are the objects to be kept in view in its administration, and they are best attained, not by the more powerful and constitutional action of the drug—which should be studiously avoided—but by small doses of its milder preparations, repeated as need may be. It is to the striking influence in increasing the secretion of bile, which mercury, used in this way, sometimes has, that this medicine owes the high reputation it has long had as a remedy in liver diseases.

Soda, like mercury, is much in use in the treatment of such cases, and there is reason to believe that it deserves the esteem in which it is generally held. Soda, which is a natural constituent of bile and readily excreted by the liver, not only, when given in appropriate doses, increases the secretion of bile, but probably renders the matter secreted by the inflamed gall-ducts less viscid, and has the same sort of efficacy in these cases as in catarrhal diseases of the lungs, in which this and other alkalies have been long used as expectorants.

The muriate of ammonia is another medicine which is often of service in inflammatory diseases of the gall-bladder and gall-ducts. It has a less special action on the liver than the salts of soda, but a more general action on other secreting organs; and does good, not only by increasing the flow of bile, but also by the indirect relief it gives to the liver by exciting the action of the kidneys and skin.

As most diseases of the biliary passages may be traced to a faulty condition of the bile, so it may be stated, as a general principle, that, as far as medicines are concerned, the best remedies for them are to be found among those agents which modify the qualities of that fluid. Among these, taraxacum holds an important rank. Its powers in increasing the secretion and modifying the qualities of the bile are very variously estimated, but reasons have already been given for believing that its efficacy, like that of cholagogue medicines generally, is more likely to be under than overrated. That it should continue to be held in such high esteem by so many accurate observers is a strong testimony in its favor; and as it has the further advantage of being perfectly safe and harmless, there is every motive for giving it an extensive trial in the treatment of these forms of disease.

In cases of long-continued jaundice from obstruction of the common gall-duct, the treatment should be regulated by the opinion formed of the cause of obstruction. In many such cases all active treatment is obviously injurious. When, for example, the common duct is obliterated, or when it is closed by the pressure of a cancerous tumor, or by a calculus irremovably impacted in it, mercury and other lowering measures must do positive mischief, and the rule of treatment should be that of avoiding all active interference. In such cases there is little more to be done than to regulate the diet; to endeavor to control, by the appropriate remedies, whatever disorder there may be of the stomach and bowels; to keep up the action of the kidneys and skin; and to obviate all avoidable causes of exhaustion. In other cases, where the closure of the duct is caused by the pressure of an enlarged gland, or by inflammatory effusion and thickening about the duct (and several such cases have been referred to in this chapter), benefit may result from mercury, cautiously administered, even when the jaundice has lasted many months. The great question is—How can the actual cause of obstruction be ascertained? When for a long time the jaundice has been *complete*—that is, when the discharges from the bowels have exhibited no trace of bile—this circumstance is, of itself, almost proof that the jaundice results from mechanical obstruction of the common duct; and the cause of the obstruction must be inferred from the symptoms attending the onset of the jaundice, from the history of the illness, and from the age and general condition of the patient. It must now and then happen that with all the information that can be derived from these different sources the precise cause of obstruction will be a matter of doubt. In that case it may be right to give the patient the chance afforded by the more active treatment, and in the endeavor to do good we must run the risk of doing harm. This is but one of the countless questions which continually call up the remark, that, in diseases of the liver, beyond all others, diagnosis is the very foundation of treatment, and that to render our diagnosis more sure, should, for the present, be the chief object of our researches. This end will be best attained by more perfect knowledge of the healthy action of the liver, and by a more accurate study of the circumstances under which its various diseases arise.

CHAPTER III.

DISEASES WHICH RESULT FROM FAULTY NUTRITION OF THE LIVER, OR FAULTY SECRETION.

SECT. I.—*Softening of the liver—Destruction of the hepatic cells—Suppressed secretion of bile—Fatal jaundice.*

HAVING considered the inflammatory diseases of the liver, we may pass on to a class of diseases quite as important, but at present less understood—diseases in which, without any process to which the term inflammation can be rightly employed, the secreting power, or the nutrition of the hepatic cells, is seriously disordered. These diseases may be divided into two principal groups. One of these groups is characterized by suspension of the secretion of bile; the distinctive peculiarity of the other is, that the hepatic cells separate from the blood some abnormal matter, which, instead of passing freely out of the liver in the bile, is retained there, adding to the size of the liver, and more or less changing its appearance and texture.

To understand how changes in the appearance and texture of the liver are produced in this way, we must again refer for a moment to the intimate structure of the organ.

We have seen that the lobules of the liver are spaces mapped out by the ultimate twigs of the portal vein, which are hairy, as it were, with capillaries springing from them on every side and forming a close and continuous network; and that the interstices of these capillaries are filled with nucleated cells. It is in these cells that the vital chemistry of secretion goes on. It is seen by the microscope, that in different livers the cells vary in size; that in some they are almost transparent, in others opaque, and apparently more solid; that in some they contain but a few very small oil-globules, while in others they are distended almost to bursting with globules of oil; that in some they are colorless or nearly so, and in others yellow with bile; that in some specimens, again, as in cases before related, they are broken down and destroyed. It is probable, too, that in some cases the cells are only slowly reproduced; so that at length the number of active cells in the lobular substance is much diminished.

These differences in the condition of the cells cause, of course, corresponding differences in the size, color, and texture of the liver—differences which were noticed long before that knowledge of the intimate structure of the organ was obtained by which we are now enabled to explain them.

When the cells are small, or few in number, and the spaces between the capillaries in the lobules are not distended with the products of secretion, the lobules are small and indistinct, and the liver is small and flattened, and its lower edge is thin. When, on the contrary, the cells or their interstices are distended with oil, or with any other product of secretion, as in the fatty and the scrofulous liver, the lobules are larger than natural, and the liver is large and thick, and its lower edge is blunted.

The most remarkable and most serious change is where the cells are completely broken down and destroyed. It has been seen that this may result from long retention of the secreted bile from closure of the common gall-duct. In consequence of this, the hepatic gall-ducts become enormously dilated, and the whole liver acquires a deep olive color. Its tissue is then flabby, but not readily broken down by the finger, and *presents no appearance of lobules.* Every part of the liver is affected alike, and exhibits under the microscope, in the place of the secreting cells of the lobular substance, nothing but free oil-globules and irregular particles of solid biliary matter. The liver contains but little blood, and partly from this, but chiefly from loss of the cells, it may be smaller than in health, and its surface wrinkled, notwithstanding the biliary matter accumulated in it.

But destruction of the hepatic cells may take place rapidly, without any obstruction of the gall-ducts, and instead of being consequent on protracted jaundice, the impaired nutrition of the cells may be the cause of jaundice that proves rapidly fatal from disorder of the functions of the brain.

It has been long known that cases of jaundice now and then occur which prove fatal in this way; and that in such cases it frequently happens that no obstruction can be found in the gall-ducts—which are pale and empty of bile—and no effusions characteristic of inflammation in any part of the liver. In some such cases, no change of structure has been remarked in the liver, and the disease has been described as fatal jaundice from suppressed secretion. In other cases, the liver has been found unusually small, much softened, and changed in color, and the disease has been spoken of as *softening* of the liver, or *simple softening*, or *black softening*, according to the color of the liver in the individual case.

The two following cases, published by Dr. Alison, in the *Edinburgh Medical and Surgical Journal* for 1835, are examples of this terrible form of disease.

CASE 1.—Pêter Schread, aged about twenty-five, a German sailor, was admitted into the clinical ward the 26th of February, 1826, in a state of complete delirium, with tendency to violence, but alternating with drowsiness. His skin and the *tunica conjunctiva* of the eyes were of a bright yellow color; he had no tenderness of abdomen; his pulse was 60, of irregular frequency; tongue moist; extremities rather cold; he had occasional *singultus;* he passed a copious bilious stool, and also urine in bed, soon after his admission.

His companion reported that he had a severe attack of flux in Java, in the summer previous; that he had been in good health at Antwerp from September till December, but that since the 1st of January, when he arrived at Leith, he had complained often of pain and heat in the abdomen, chiefly towards the right side, with thirst and chilliness; that eight days before admission, he had become jaundiced, and two days before admission, had become delirious.

His head was shaved, bathed, and blistered, and he had one dose of calomel, and several of tartar emetic (the only medicines that could be got down), which produced copious bilious stools, all passed in bed; but the delirium passed into complete coma, with dilated pupils and stertor; his pulse rose to 120, and became feeble; some purplish spots appeared on the skin, and he died on the evening of the 28th—ten days after the appearance of jaundice.

The following account of the dissection was drawn up by Dr. C. Henry, of Manchester, then one of the clinical clerks in the infirmary:—

"The skin and subjacent cellular tissue were universally of a bright yellow color. This tinge extended also to the pericranium, and to both surfaces of the *dura mater*, which was rather more vascular than natural. The other membranes of the brain were dry and glistening. The bloody points were somewhat more numerous than usual. There was very slight distension of the left lateral ventricle, the contained serum not exceeding half a drachm. That found in the right was still less considerable, and there was hardly any at the base of the brain, which appeared somewhat vascular. The consistency of the cerebral structure was perfectly healthy. The surfaces and central points of the cartilages of the ribs were tinged with bile, as were the peritoneum and pleura.

"The liver, when incised, appeared of a light yellow color; it was smaller than natural, its structure dense and resisting compression, but in mass it was remarkably loose[1] and flexible. The calibre of the cystic duct seemed to be in part obliterated, but the hepatic and common biliary ducts were quite pervious. Their mucous membrane was unnaturally white. The gall-bladder contained a greenish, viscous, semi-fluid matter.

"The spleen was somewhat firmer than natural. The pancreas was healthy. The contents of the intestinal canal were tinged, though slightly, by a greenish bile—those of the lower part of the ileum less than of the larger intestines. There was no vascularity of their lining membrane, but that of the great intestines appeared somewhat thicker than usual. The mucous coat of the bladder had acquired a deep yellow tinge, and contained urine of similar appearance."

Here the patient seems to have been ailing for several weeks, often complaining of pain and heat in the abdomen, with thirst and chilliness, before he became jaundiced. When the jaundice had existed six days, delirium came on, and life ended in a state of complete coma four days afterwards, that is, ten days from the first appearance of jaundice.

On examination after death, it was evident that the jaundice resulted from suppressed secretion, and not from an impediment to the passage of the bile through the ducts; for the liver was of a light yellow color, and smaller than natural, and the hepatic and common ducts were found to be quite pervious, and their lining membrane was unnaturally white.

The man was under medical observation only two days before death, and after the occurrence of delirium, so that no full report of the illness was made. It was noted, however, that after his admission to the hospital, he was in a state of depression, the pulse being 60, of irregular frequency, and the extremities rather cold; that he had no tenderness of the abdomen; that he had occasional *singultus;* that he had copious *bilious* stools, which were passed in bed; and that before death some purpuric spots appeared on the skin.

CASE 2.—Agnes Anderson, aged thirty-five, was admitted into the clinical ward on the 10th of December, 1830, with symptoms of jaundice (of a fortnight's standing), and occasional pain across the epigastrium, but little constitutional disturbance. She had recently suffered much mental distress, having been abandoned by a man with whom she had co-

---

[1] In Dr. Alison's paper, it is printed "large and flexible," which, considering what goes before, does not make sense. "Large" is probably a misprint for "loose."

habited, and was in a state of agitation, and, being apprehensive of catching fever, she suddenly left the house the same day. After this, as we subsequently learned, the pain at the epigastrium increased; on the 14th, she was observed to stagger in walking, and became drowsy and occasionally incoherent, without complaining of headache. On the 17th, she was re-admitted, deeply jaundiced and perfectly comatose; her pulse was 118, soft; the surface rather cold; the respiration somewhat stertorous, but of natural frequency; the pupils somewhat dilated; the teeth firmly closed, and inclosing the apex of the tongue, which was bleeding. There was no rigidity of other muscles; she had occasional fits of hurried breathing, with partial spasm, during which the pupils became quite immovable. Her bladder was much distended, and five pounds of deep yellow-colored urine were drawn off by the catheter.

Blistering and enemata were tried without any effect. The breathing became more rapid and heaving, and the pulse feebler, and she died twenty-four hours after admission—three weeks after the first appearance of jaundice.

The following report of the appearances on dissection was drawn up by Dr. J. Reid, then clinical clerk:—

"The skin had assumed a deeper tinge of yellow since death. Upon removing the skull-cap, the dura mater was observed to have also a yellowish tinge. The veins upon the surface of the brain were somewhat tinged. There was no effusion under the arachnoid, or at the base of the brain; but a small quantity of yellowish serum was contained in the ventricles. Upon cutting the brain in thin longitudinal slices, every part of it appeared quite healthy, and nothing presented itself about which there was the slightest doubt, except the appearance of the choroid plexus, which was of a dark red color, and a vein distended with blood was seen running along each of its portions situate in the lateral ventricle. Along with the red points which usually appear upon the cut surface of the brain, a little yellowish serum exuded.

"The liver was small, soft, and of a peculiar brownish-yellow color. The gall-bladder *was collapsed,* and *contained a small quantity of bile.* All the bile-ducts were of the usual color, at no point more dilated than another, perfectly pervious throughout, and almost completely empty of bile. It was doubtful whether the mucous membrane of the duodenum was very slightly thickened or not; but there was *certainly no decided change upon it.*"

In this case, a woman, thirty-five years of age, after much mental distress, became affected with jaundice. The jaundice was attended with occasional pain at the epigastrium, but with little constitutional disturbance. After it had lasted eighteen days she was observed to stagger in walking, and became drowsy and incoherent. The drowsiness was followed by clenching of the jaws, and other occasional partial spasms, and she died in a state of coma, three days after the occurrence of cerebral disorder, and three weeks after the first appearance of jaundice. On examination of the body it was clear, as in the former case, that the jaundice resulted from suppressed secretion; the liver was small, soft, and of a peculiar brownish-yellow color; and the gall-ducts were perfectly pervious throughout, and almost completely empty of bile. Here, also, the patient was under continuous medical observation only for a short time, and the account of the illness is very imperfect. It was noted, however, that after her admission to the hospital, five pounds of deep yellow-colored urine were drawn off by the catheter, so that, while the secretion of bile was suppressed, the state of coma seems to have had on the kidneys the effect of increasing secretion—an effect which Bernard has shown it usually has on all secreting organs.

Most medical men who have been some years in practice have probably witnessed this form of disease. More than one instance of it fell under my own notice, when I was not sufficiently alive to their interest, and my notes of them are very imperfect. I shall not, therefore, relate them, but cite instead the two following cases, which were published by Dr. Bright, in an excellent paper on jaundice, in the first volume of *Guy's Hospital Reports*, and which are counterparts of the cases already quoted from Dr. Alison.

CASE 3.—Keatrina Pfifrein, aged eighteen, was admitted into the clinical ward January 11, 1832, laboring under icterus. She was an assistant to a German broom-maker, and was unable to speak any English. The skin was of a brilliant yellow; and the cheeks, which were flushed, were of the color of a very ripe apricot; she appeared exhausted; and though she answered questions pretty readily, we were cautioned by a woman who brought her that her replies were incorrect. Pulse 120, very small and weak; feet and body very cold. We learned, that when she came to London, about a fortnight ago, she had been already unwell about a fortnight; and her skin had a decidedly yellow tinge, which had daily increased, attended by an inactivity amounting almost to torpor; so that, when removed from her bed, and placed by the fire, which was all she could bear of late, she sat constantly in a kind of doze. We were told that her bowels had been relaxed, without much abdominal pain; and she had not suffered from sickness. She had complained but little of headache; tongue moist, and slightly furred; the papillæ prominent.

She was ordered a moderate dose of hyd. c. cretâ, three times a day, and light nourishment and warmth; and should it not prove, as had been stated, that her bowels were relaxed, she was to take some colocynth pills at night.

Jan. 12th.—She was sick yesterday evening, vomiting a good deal; she lay in a perfectly torpid state the whole night, apparently suffering no pain; but towards the morning became delirious, so that it was with difficulty she could be restrained in her bed. At the time of the visit she was very restless, and seemed to suffer pain; but was unable to answer any questions; indeed, except that she swallowed what was given to her, she seemed scarcely conscious; and it was quite uncertain whether pressure on the abdomen gave her any pain. The pupils were dilated; the bowels had not been opened, although she had taken two compound colocynth pills; pulse 106, thrilling, and compressible; tongue moist and clean.

She was ordered two grains of calomel every two hours, and the ammonia julep every four hours, besides wine, if she became more depressed. Her head was shaved, and a blister applied over the liver; mustard poultices to the feet; and camphor mixture was to be given freely, in case the delirium should return; injections were to be repeated till the bowels acted freely.

During the night, the purging injections, with colocynth and castor oil, were administered three times; she lay completely comatose the whole night; the pulse sometimes at 140, and extremely weak, when not raised by stimulants.

No dejection having been passed at ten o'clock in the morning, another colocynth injection was administered, which produced copious, rather dark, unhealthy, feculent motions, mixed with some sanguinolent fluid; and there was likewise an appearance like pus. The blister discharged very abundantly; the urine was passed involuntarily, and in considerable quantity; mouth and lips covered with sordes; pulse 120, weak.

A blister to the crown of the head; the calomel to be repeated.

She continued to sink during the day, and died at ten o'clock in the evening.

Sectio cadaveris.—The whole external surface of a deep yellow color; the adipose matter was also yellow, as were the cartilages of the ribs.

The lungs were healthy, but the posterier portions gorged with blood, probably the result of her having been lying for two days on the back. The pleura of the left lung of a slight yellow tinge; the heart healthy.

The whole of the abdominal viscera, when first exposed to view, were remarkably tinged with bile; the stomach of a vivid yellow; the intestines looked green; the liver was unusually small, and, for the most part, of a brightish yellow color, with portions marked with purple or deep brown; and, in parts, a finely spotted appearance was yielded by the acini. On cutting into the liver, the same yellow color, with fine dark spots, pervaded it. The gall-bladder was very small aud collapsed, and contained less than a teaspoonful of thick ropy mucus, of a bright green color. The cystic duct appeared to be quite contracted; so that neither could a fine probe, nor the point of a scissors, be carried along more than two-thirds of its length upwards; nor could the tenacious mucus of the gall-bladder be forced down it. However, there was no appearance of thickening, or of morbid deposit, either within or around the duct, which, when laid open with the scalpel, presented the corrugated valvular appearance peculiar to that part of the duct. The lower part of the cystic duct, as well as the whole of the hepatic duct and the common duct, quite into the duodenum, were pervious, and not at all thickened or diminished from the natural calibre. There was no trace of bile in either of the ducts; and following the hepatic ducts quite into the substance of the liver, no bile was detected; but, on squeezing the liver, the small secondary and tertiary subdivisions of the ducts were seen filled with thick tenacious mucus, of an exceedingly faint lemon-yellow color.

The mucous membrane of the alimentary canal was perfectly healthy, but the contents were very unnatural; in some parts of the ileum and jejunum, there was yellow mucus; in others, an olive-green mucous excrement; and in the colon, a drab-colored and gray mass, characteristic of that which usually composes the feces of jaundiced patients.

The spleen soft; pancreas healthy. Kidneys tinged throughout with bile. Bladder somewhat distended, rising to view above the pubis, and containing, probably, a pint of clear yellow urine.

The thoracic duct quite empty. The arteries deeply tinged with bile.

The dura mater was of a brilliant yellow color; the arachnoid not vascular, and quite untinged with bile; there was no unnatural effusion of serum beneath it, but the small quantity which collected in a few of the sulci was very slightly tinged with yellow, as were the few drops which collected in the base of the skull, when the brain was removed. When slices of the brain were taken horizontally, a moderate number of cut vessels were seen; many of the small points of blood gave a stain of beautifully yellow bile around them; and some points gave out the yellow serum without any blood appearing. The ventricles contained an unusually small quantity of serum, and that was not tinged with bile. The quantity of serum throughout the whole brain was decidedly deficient. There was no structural lesion nor irregularity in the brain.

Here, as in the two former cases, the patient was under medical observation only a short time before death, and the account of the illness is, in consequence, very meagre; but the body was carefully examined, and the state of the liver is fully described.

The poor broom girl had been jaundiced from two to four weeks, when she was brought to the hospital in a state of much exhaustion, and with the mind wandering. It was stated that, for the fortnight preceding, she had been in a state of inactivity, almost amounting to torpor; that the bowels had been relaxed, without much abdominal pain; and that she had not suffered from sickness.

She vomited a good deal the evening of the day on which she was brought to the hospital, and the next morning was violently delirious. The delirium passed into coma, in which she died the evening of the following day.

The bowels were confined, after her admission to the hospital, but the day on which she died, copious feculent stools, mixed with some sanguinolent fluid, were brought away by purgative injections. As in the preceding case, the action of the kidneys was probably increased during the state of coma, for, on the morning of death, urine was passed in considerable quantity, and at the time of death, the urinary bladder was somewhat distended.

The liver was found to be unusually small, as in the former cases, and, for the most part, of a brightish yellow color, with portions marked with purple or deep brown. The hepatic and the common gall-ducts were pervious throughout, and quite empty of bile. It was clear, from these facts, that the jaundice resulted, not from a mechanical obstruction in the gall-ducts, but from defective action of the secreting apparatus of the liver. No change in the texture of the kidneys was noticed.

CASE 4.—Sarah ——, aged 28, was admitted into Guy's Hospital, as a surgeon's patient, on the 6th of August. She was a married woman, and had borne two or three children; but had latterly been separated from her husband, and was said to be much addicted to drinking. As she had sores of a very suspicious character, she was ordered to take sarsaparilla three times a day, with five grains of the compound ipecacuanha powder, and of the Plummer's pill, every night, which she continued for a considerable time. On the 13th of November, I was requested to take charge of her, as she was apparently very ill; had been complaining of abdominal pain for the last week; and during the last two days had become jaundiced. I found the bowels rather confined; urine tinged with bile; pulse moderate, but quick; slight tenderness at the pit of the stomach.

(Fourteen ounces of blood were ordered to be drawn by cupping from the region of the liver; the belly to be fomented: five grains of mercury with chalk to be taken immediately, and ℥ss of castor oil four hours after, and to be repeated until the bowels should be relaxed.)

14th.—There is still some tenderness on pressure at the pit of the stomach, and accelerated pulse.

(Fifteen leeches to the pit of stomach; the mercury with chalk, and the castor oil to be repeated.)

The yellowness increased; the stools continued of a pale clay color; the tenderness of the upper part of the abdomen continued.

It is unnecessary to give a detail of all the daily symptoms. Cupping, mercurial purges, and blue pill, with fomentations, were continued; and during ten days no very remarkable change occurred.

24th.—Slight tenderness over the whole abdomen; color very intense; pulse 96, small, and rather sharp; respiration, 27; bowels confined; thirst; occasional sickness; and occasional pains in the abdomen, much relieved by the fomentation.

28th.—She generally prefers the sitting posture in bed. Lips dry; tongue moist and red; some sluggishness in her mode of speech, and a plaintive tone; pulse, 88; no sickness; six or seven loose dejections.

(Twelve leeches to the pit of the stomach; a linseed poultice to the belly.)

29th.—One copious lumpy white stool. Pulse, 96; slight tenderness of pit of stomach; respiration tranquil; tongue moist, but more red at the edges.

December 1st.—Her pupils are rather dilated; her mode of utterance is dull and indistinct; complains of loss of power in the left hand; the right is already disabled by disease.

2d.—Is lying on her right side, drowsy, with her legs drawn up, moving her left hand with a kind of jactitation, often raising it to her head; she is capable of being so far roused as to put out her tongue when pressed to do so. Tongue moist, and red at the edges; the pupils are dilated.

(A blister to the crown of the head; a cathartic enema.)

3d.—Yesterday evening she was screaming loudly, with her tongue protruded between her teeth. To-day she is in a state of perfect coma, with the eyes turned up. She is incapable of being roused, and has taken no nourishment or medicine since yesterday.

She died the following day.

Sectio cadaveris.—The color of the whole body of the brightest yellow which jaundice yields. Not less than an inch of adipose matter over the whole abdomen. On removing the calvaria, the dura mater was found tinged of a brilliant yellow color, and very vascular; raising this, the surface of the brain showed the vessels loaded with blood; and beneath the arachnoid, in the convolutions, lay a small quantity of serum, probably not more than natural, of a decidedly yellow color. As the brain was sliced away, numerous points of fluid blood appeared; and from many of them the serum which issued with the blood was of a bright gamboge yellow, presenting points of that color mingled with red points. The whole of the vessels and the sinuses of the brain were unusually loaded with blood; the ventricles unnaturally dry; scarcely could a drop of serum be discovered. The heart healthy. The pulmonary and other vessels deeply tinged with bile. The peritoneum, also, was peculiarly dry. The omentum was beautifully spread over the viscera. The colon, when the omentum was turned back, was seen contracted and very yellow; while the portion of the omentum, closely attached, was spotted with ecchymosis, and loaded with fat.

The liver weighed only two pounds five ounces. It was soft or flaccid to the touch; quite free from any mark of peritoneal inflammation. Its external appearance was mottled dark-red liver-color, with yellow stone-color. The acini were pretty distinctly to be traced throughout—red at their centres, and yellow in their circumferences; and in most parts the yellow bore a large proportion to the whole. The gall-bladder was contracted; and contained about half a drachm of mucus, very slightly tinged with green. The ducts were all pervious and healthy, and were not even stained with bile. Pancreas, quite healthy. Spleen, large. Kidneys remarkably lobulated, and tinged throughout with bile, particularly the membrane lining the pelvis. Ovaries, externally very yellow. Uterus, also yellow, with some ecchymosis in its fundus.

This case is more complete than the three preceding cases, as the patient was under observation long before the occurrence of jaundice, and during its entire course. The jaundice was preceded for some days by abdominal pain; and throughout its course there was some tenderness at the pit of the stomach, with occasional pains in the belly. The pulse was quicker than natural; the bowels were generally confined, and the stools of a pale clay color; and it is once mentioned that there was occasional vomiting. When the jaundice had lasted twenty days cerebral disorder came on, and the woman died three days afterwards, in a state of complete coma.

The gall-ducts were pervious and healthy, as in the former cases, and not even stained by bile.

The liver was small, weighing only two pounds five ounces, and soft or flaccid to the touch, and quite free from peritoneal inflammation. It was of a mottled red and yellow color, and the lobules were pretty distinctly to be traced throughout.

I had been for some time looking out for an instance of this form of disease, wishing to examine the liver minutely, when an opportunity of doing so was afforded me by Mr. Busk, who at once observed that in the portions of the liver that were most diseased the cells were completely destroyed.

The following notes of the patient's illness were kindly furnished me by Mr. Clapp, then assistant surgeon of the Seamen's Hospital:—

CASE 5 —Abdul, a lascar, aged 50—60, was admitted into the Seamen's Hospital, the 16th of January, 1844, jaundiced, and with constant hiccough, which was stated to have lasted three days.

He was in a state of half stupor, and but little concerning his feelings could be elicited from him. He appeared, however, to have some pain in the region of the liver, but there was no tumor in that situation. A few hours after his admission, Mr. Clapp observed his pupils to be much contracted, and, from his look, suspected that he had taken opium; and on searching his clothes and bed, a small tin box containing opium was found. No cough or other symptom of pulmonary disease was observed; and the hiccough continued the only prominent symptom to the time of his death, which happened on the 18th.

The body was examined on the 20th, about forty hours after death.

The rigidity of the muscles was nearly gone. The surface was deeply jaundiced. No hardness or fulness in any part of the abdomen.

The *head* was carefully examined, but no morbid appearance noticed, except the yellow tint of jaundice.

Chest.—The right lung adhered slightly to the diaphragm, in a small space at the centre of its base, and the greater part of its lower lobe was in a state of red hepatization. The other lobes of this lung were congested, and infiltrated with red frothy fluid. The small bronchial tubes were filled with a thin mucus fluid, brownish, and also tinged with bile. The left lung was nowhere adherent to the pleura costalis. Its lower lobe was of a dark purple, from extreme congestion, but was not solid. The upper lobe slightly congested, but not otherwise altered. There was no fluid in either pleural cavity. There was a large, irregular, superficial ulcer on the back of the larynx, just below the base of the arytenoid cartilages, and the mucous membrane over the cartilages was slightly raised by effusion into the areolar tissue beneath it. The ulcer was surrounded by a narrow vascular zone. The mucous membrane of the trachea and bronchi was injected, and the surface covered with thin brown mucus.

Heart, large and fat. Valves perfect. Muscular substance colored in parts by bile. Left cavities empty. Small fibrinous clots, colored with bile, in the right cavities. Blood, grumous and clotted.

Œsophagus, pale, and healthy throughout.

Stomach.—Mucous membrane grayish and "mammillated;" everywhere of natural thickness and firmness. Duodenum perfectly natural, as was also the small intestine, to within a few feet of the lower end of the ileum, below which it exhibited a few vascular patches, and some serous fluid was infiltrated in the submucous tissue.

The ileo-cæcal valve at first sight appeared to be slightly ulcerated; but on looking closer, this appearance was found to be caused by the edges of the folds of the mucous membrane being of a dark purple from congestion, and having shreds of lymph on the surface.

Large intestine.—Mucous membrane having the edge of the rugæ of a deep red, and with small shreds of lymph on their surface; but everywhere else of natural color, thickness, and consistence.

There was no bile in any part of the intestinal canal, nor did the mucous membrane appear jaundiced in any part. A large quantity of fecal matter, of a pale clay color, was found in the large intestine.

The kidneys were jaundiced, but otherwise perfectly natural. Bladder empty.

Spleen, large, firm, rather pale.

Pancreas, healthy.

The liver was rather large, and weighed four pounds four ounces. The whole gland, except a very small portion of the extreme right, was remarkably soft, flabby, and easily torn. This condition was most marked in the lobulus Spigelii and adjacent parts. There was no disease in the gall-bladder or gall-ducts, which were carefully examined, nor any obstruction at the duodenal orifice of the common duct. The bile could be very readily made to flow into the intestine. The gall-bladder contained about an ounce of thick bile, sparkling with distinct scales of cholesterine, but otherwise of natural appearance.

On examination by the microscope, Mr. Busk found that in the firm portion the proper cells of the liver contained a good deal of bile, but were otherwise quite natural; while in the softened portion there were *hardly any cells to be found.* Nothing was seen but a confused mass of amorphous particles and oil-globules.

Here, as in the former cases, the jaundice resulted from defective secretion, for the large gall-ducts were pervious and healthy. The illness seems to have been of short duration; and this circumstance will probably serve to explain the fact, that the liver, instead of being small, as in the former cases, was rather large. A great portion of the liver was remarkably soft and easily torn, and in this portion hardly any hepatic cells could be found, while in the firmer portion the cells presented nearly their natural appearance.

The objects seen when these two portions of the liver were examined under the microscope are represented in the annexed woodcut, which was made from a drawing by Mr. Busk.

Fig. 13.

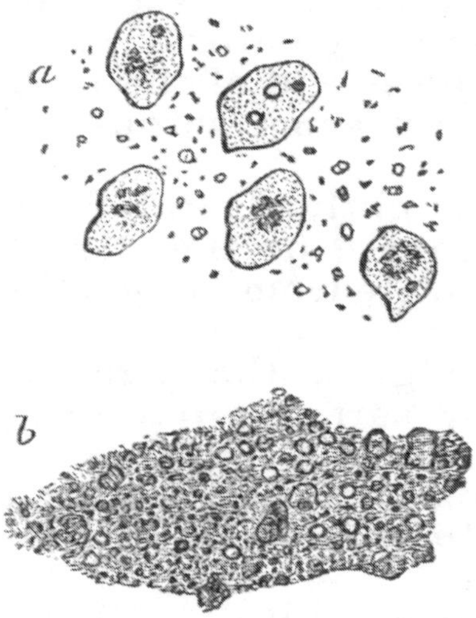

(*a*) Represents cells from the firm portion of the liver. The dark spots within them are particles of biliary matter, which was in greater quantity than usual. Some cells contain small oil-globules, marked by the clear rings. Between the cells are seen small free oil-globules and particles of granular matter.

(*b*) The appearance presented by a particle from the softened portion of the liver, showing an irregular aggregation of oil-globules, particles of solid biliary matter, and amorphous granular matter.

Mr. Busk sent me the liver to examine, and I was enabled to satisfy myself that the description of the microscopic appearances which he sent with it, and which is given above, was perfectly accurate. All I observed besides was, that the firm portion was hardly so firm as is natural, and was of a mottled yellowish, nutmeg appearance, the lobules being distinct to the eye. The soft portion was of a uniform dirty color—a compound of yellowish-brown and red—and presented no appearance of lobules. It had no smell of gangrene.

It may, perhaps, be supposed, from the time after death at which the body was examined, that these changes resulted from common putrefaction, but it was clearly not so. The secreting cells of the liver do not break up quickly after death. In ordinary cases they present no such appearances as are described above, even when the decomposition of the body is much further advanced; and in the solid part of this liver, which was kept, and several times examined by Mr. Busk and myself, the cells were distinctly visible two days afterwards. Destruction of the cells was doubtless the result of disease, and took place, or at least commenced, during life. The existence of jaundice, which could not be accounted for by any impediment to the passage of the bile through the ducts, is sufficient proof that in great part of the liver the secreting cells did not adequately perform their office.

In this case the cells were broken down, just as they were in the case of Mrs. Diprose, related in the preceding chapter (p. 227), in which this change was a remote effect of closure of the common gall-duct; but the condition of the liver in the two cases was in many respects different.

1st. The liver was here *readily torn or broken down by the finger;* while that of Mrs. Diprose, though feeling equally flabby, was not.

2d. The softened portion of the liver was brown or reddish-brown, and not much colored with bile; while in Mrs. Diprose the liver was throughout of a deep olive, mottled with yellow, solely from the presence of bile.

3d. The liver seemed to contain more fluid, certainly contained more blood, than that of Mrs. Diprose; and under the microscope it exhibited more amorphous granular matter, and less solid biliary matter and oil.

4th. In the one case a small portion of the liver remained tolerably healthy, and continued to secrete bile of natural color and appearance; in the other, the secreting cells of every part of the liver were disorganized.

There are still greater differences in the symptoms, and in the state of other organs, in the two cases. The case of obstructed gall-duct was very lingering; the patient died much emaciated, and all organs besides the liver were sound. Here, the disease proved fatal very quickly; and besides this change in the liver, there was hepatization of the right lung, and a large ulcer in the larynx, and the folds of the mucous membrane of the large intestine were purple, or of a deep-red, and covered with lymph.

No cause could be assigned for this terrible disease, and but little is known of its real pathology. The symptoms and the marks of inflammation in various parts of the body are sufficient evidence that there was a poisoned or unhealthy state of the blood; but it is impossible to say in what degree this resulted from defective action of the liver and the rapid disorganization of a part of its substance, and in what degree from the noxious influence, whatever it might be, by which this defective action of the liver and change in its texture were brought about. Up to this time such cases have been considered cases of jaundice, depending, not on obstructed gall-ducts, but on suppressed secretion of bile; and the changes in the liver have been overlooked, or their outward and obvious characters only have been noticed.

It would appear that the disease is not necessarily fatal. It happened that, on the 21st of January, four days after the admission of Abdul, another lascar was brought into the Seamen's Hospital from the same ship, who was also jaundiced and semi-comatose, passing blood in considerable quantity from the bowels, and with very evident tenderness in the right hypochondrium, but without hiccough or vomiting. His disease was considered to be the same as that of Abdul, and the same issue was expected; but in a few days he got very much better, and soon recovered sufficiently to leave the hospital. Numbers of other lascars from the same ship were brought into the hospital, and several of them were observed to be more or less jaundiced, so that it is not improbable that these also had the same disease in a less degree. All these men lived in the same way, and were subjected to the same influences of diet and locality.

Since my attention was called to the facts related above, I have examined the livers of three persons, who died in a state of jaundice from suppressed secretion.

The first was that of a sailor, aged twenty-four, who died in the Seamen's Hospital, on the 10th of December, 1844. The particulars I learned respecting the patient were these:—

Case 6.—He arrived in the port of London in the middle of October, and when he had been ashore about a fortnight he was taken ill with pain in the right side of the belly, and headache. A week afterwards he became jaundiced, and began to vomit. On the 16th of November he was brought to the hospital in deep jaundice. From that time there was tenderness in the region of the liver, and occasional vomiting. The stools were generally clay-colored, but for a few days were stained with bile. After the jaundice had lasted about a month, violent delirium came on, soon followed by death.

The liver was rather small, and of a pale yellowish color, but was not softened. The lobules were indistinct. The secreting cells, which contained fine granular matter, and a few very small oil-globules, were smaller than usual.

The gall-bladder and gall-ducts were pervious, and empty of bile.

The next fatal case of this kind to which my attention was called occurred about a year afterwards. On the 28th of November, 1845, I went to the Seamen's Hospital, at the request of Mr. Busk, to see a lad who had been jaundiced for some time, and who was then in a state of delirium. The lad died the next day, and on the 30th the liver was sent to me for examination. The following particulars of the illness were recorded :—

CASE 7.—George Chambers, aged seventeen, was admitted into the Seamen's Hospital, under Mr. Busk, on the 17th of November, 1845, with several ash-colored non-indurated sores on the glans penis and prepuce, and also with deep jaundice, which commenced without apparent cause three weeks before.

He belonged to one of the Scotch steamers, but had lately been living at Greenwich, and was reported to have been leading a dissolute life.

The black-wash was applied to the sores, and he was ordered ʒss of acetate of potash three times a day.

The following notes were afterwards taken :—

Nov. 18th.—No better; in fact, the color of the skin is darker. Urine very high colored. Stools perfectly white, and very fetid; has never had any pain or uneasy feeling in the abdomen, except from wind; sleeps badly, but does not dream. Nausea, anorexia, thirst; bowels relaxed (two or three stools daily). No fulness or tenderness in the region of the liver; no pain in the shoulder; no pain in the region of the kidneys; tongue clean, clammy.

℞. Ammoniæ sesquicarb. gr. v; sodæ bicarb. gr. x; aquæ carui ℥j; sextis horis sumendus. Empl. lyttæ regioni hepatis. Milk diet.

19th.—No change; color of the skin, if anything, more intense. Urine less highly colored. Two stools, without bile. Has vomited several times.

℞. Hydrarg. chlorid. gr. x, statim.

20th.—Color of the skin rather higher; urine much lighter; feels less bloated with wind. Has had one copious stool.

℞. Repet. hydrarg. chlorid. gr. x.

21st.—Has passed a large quantity of feculent matter, of a pale clay color.

℞. Ext. colocynth. co. gr. x.

22d.—Much the same, except that he vomits more frequently. One stool of the same pale color; urine of a bright yellow. No pain.

℞. Hydrarg. chlorid. gr. v; ext. colocynth co. gr. viij; statim. Magnes. sulphat., sodæ bicarb., āā ℈j; tinct. card. co. ʒss; aquæ ℥ij, 6tis horis, cum acid. tartaric gr. xviij.

23d.—No change. One clay-colored solid motion; frequent vomiting, which always occurs after taking food. Matters vomited contain no bile. Urine not high colored, though still bilious. Pulse 60—soft, irregular both in frequency and in force.

24th.—No stool, though he has continued the sulphate of magnesia in effervescence, every six hours. The vomiting is less frequent; there is a yellowish tinge from bile in the matters vomited. He is very dull this morning, and not altogether rational. Lies with his eyes closed, and frequently grinds his teeth. No headache; pupils natural; pulse 60, regular, soft.

℞. Hydrarg. chlorid. statim; enema terebinth. statim.

25th.—More comatose. Yesterday morning was very noisy for a short time. Is now roused with great difficulty, and then will not speak, but throws himself about in a sullen way, trying to hide his face in the bed.

26th.—No bile in the motions, of which he has had two, one immediately after the enema, and one since. Pulse 54; pupils natural.

℞. Hydrarg. chlorid. gr. ij, 4tis horis. Empl. lyttæ nuchæ.

On the 28th, when I saw him, he was confined in a strait waistcoat, in a state of raving delirium, and constantly grinding his teeth. There was no enlargement of the liver, and no expression of pain was elicited by pressing on the belly. The feces were slightly tinged with bile.

He gradually became more and more insensible, and died in a state of coma at 3 P. M., on the 29th.

The body was opened the next day, twenty-two hours after death, and the liver and omentum were immediately sent to me.

The liver was small, weighing only 2 lbs. 2½ oz., extremely flabby, and great part of it (all the right lobe towards the diaphragm) was of a uniform yellowish-brown, and so much softened that, when the capsule was removed, it tore with the greatest readiness in any direction, and broke down under slight pressure into a soft, pulpy mass, like a soft spleen. The rest of the liver (the left lobe, and the right lobe near its lower edge) had more of the purple tint of venous blood, and was firmer, so that it resisted slight pressure; but even these parts were much softer than natural.

The softened yellow portion projected slightly above the level of the darker and firmer portion, and the lobules were visible in it through the transparent capsule of the gland. When the capsule was divided, the subjacent substance projected through the incision. The darker and firmer portions seemed to be much wasted, especially the left lobe, which was very thin, and no lobules could be distinguished in them. The hepatic substance looked very much like compressed lung.

When a particle of the softest part, prepared with the greatest care to avoid disintegration, was examined under the microscope, a confused granular mass was seen, in which were scattered numerous liver-cells, of the natural size, filled with a brown granular matter. Here and there were seen cells containing oil, but not much more than natural.

In a particle taken from the firmer part, the cells were very few in number, and much smaller than natural, and did not contain so much of the brown matter.

Here, the two parts of the liver so distinguished by difference of color and consistence doubtless presented different stages, or different degrees, of the same morbid processes. The circumstance that in the dark-colored part, which was much thinner than natural, the lobules could not be distinguished and the cells were very few and small, led to the inference that this part had undergone atrophy through the destruction or diminished fertility of its cells.

The capsule of the liver could be readily stripped off, and presented no marks of inflammation or other disease.

The gall-bladder was empty, its inner surface being only just moistened with olive-colored bile. The gall-ducts were not dilated, and their inner surface, like that of the gall-bladder, was tinged with bile. Some of the bile taken from them exhibited under the microscope only the prismatic cells of the ducts.

The omentum presented a curious appearance from being sprinkled with numerous clots of blood, each of the size of a split pea, or rather smaller, which were all situated in the course of the vessels.

The spleen was small, and adherent to contiguous organs. Its capsule was thickened by an irregular deposit of false membrane of old date, and its substance was soft, affording a creamy purple fluid on the slightest pressure.

There was no fluid in the peritoneum, and the stomach and intestines were healthy throughout.

The kidneys were large, soft, and easily torn. The capsule readily detached, but bringing up here and there portions of the cortical substance. The surface and the cortical substance throughout were of a pale yellow; the tubular portions of a deep purple. Examined microscopically, the cortical substance afforded, on the slightest pressure between the glasses, a large quantity of opaque fluid, which was composed of cells, more or less perfect, filled with granular matter; fragmentary remains of cells; a large proportion of irregular amorphous particles of various sizes; a great abundance of oil-globules; and some particles of yellow biliary matter. Besides these objects, there was occasionally seen a more adherent mass, composed of the above constituents, evidently moulded in a uriniferous tube.

There were no marks of recent disease in the lungs.

The pericardium contained several ounces of a deep brownish-red serum, but exhibited no traces of inflammation.

The head was not examined.

The body, twenty-two hours after death, showed that *decomposition was already considerably advanced. The surface of the belly was green, and the course of the superficial veins was marked by purple lines.*

In this case, a lad, seventeen years of age, who had been leading a dissolute life, became jaundiced. The jaundice had continued three weeks before he came under observation, and, it would seem, before he was compelled to lay up. At the end of that time it was attended with much depression and with considerable gastric and intestinal disorder; but there was no tenderness in the region of the liver, nor pain of any kind. The matters discharged from the stomach and bowels were seldom tinged with bile. At the end of another week, without any other striking change having occurred, delirium came on, and he died five days afterwards in a state of coma.

On examination after death great part of the liver was of a yellowish-brown color, and much softened, presenting disintegrated cells, but not entirely disorganized, and still showing the lobular structure. The rest of the liver, which was firmer, and of the dark color of venous blood, seemed already to have undergone atrophy from destruction of the cells. The lobules could not be distinguished in it, and when a particle from it was placed under the microscope, only a few small hepatic cells could be seen.

The cortical substance of the kidneys was large, soft, and friable; and was clearly the seat of a morbid process analogous to that which had so changed the texture of the liver.

Hemorrhage from the stomach or bowels, which occurred in some of the preceding cases, was not noticed; but the omentum was thickly sprinkled with ecchymosed spots.

Other circumstances worthy of note are, the early decomposition of the body, and the entire absence of any marks of recent inflammation in the liver.

In 1848, the following case, which is of the same kind, fell under my observation in King's College Hospital:—

CASE 8.—John Granfield, aged twenty-two, was admitted into King's College Hospital on the 13th of March, 1848, jaundiced, and in a state of raving delirium.

The following particulars respecting him were learned from his father: He was bred up at Portsmouth, but had lived the last four years in Lambeth; was single; very temperate in his habits; and, with exception of an attack of typhus fever, three years before, his general health had been good. He was a house-painter by trade, but had been for some time out of work, and had been living badly in consequence.

Three weeks before his admission to the hospital, while in the act of stretching himself, he was struck rather violently at the pit of the stomach, and from that time had pain there, which he felt especially on coughing, and some degree of tenderness.

The pain, however, was not severe enough to prevent him from living as before. Four days after the blow, he made a very hearty supper, which was followed by much sickness and faintness. The next day, February 29th, he went to live as a waiter in a public house, at the back of Exeter Hall; still so ailing that he applied to a medical man, who told him he had had a surfeit, and gave him some aperient medicine. After this, some red blotches (urticaria?) appeared on the skin, but they soon went away.

On the 2d of March, slight yellowness of the skin was noticed, which became deeper day after day. From this time his bowels were much relaxed, and he often complained of faintness and nausea, and sometimes vomited, especially after a full meal. Notwithstanding these ailments, his spirits were good, and he continued to work hard.

On the 12th of March, the day before his admission to the hospital, he felt so ill that he was obliged to give up his work. His manner was then noticed to be strange, and soon afterwards active delirium came on.

When brought into the hospital, he was raving violently, but became more tranquil on being placed in bed. I saw him soon afterwards, and he was then totally unable to answer questions; his skin was of a rich yellow; his features were pinched; and his mouth was clenched. The belly was drawn in, and the liver was clearly not enlarged. There was no unnatural heat of skin, and the pulse was very feeble. The body was in a state of good muscular nutrition.

He was ordered to take ʒss of aromatic spirits of ammonia every four hours, and ℥xij of wine daily, and a turpentine enema was directed to be given immediately.

Before the enema was administered, he had one stool, which was loose and yellow. During the night and following morning, he had four stools more, which were clay-colored.

During the 14th, he was very quiet, but never rational. He took, with apparent satisfaction, wine and beef-tea, when they were presented to him. The pupils were of the natural size.

He was reported to have slept well the following night.

At five A. M., on the 15th, he was fed, and then slept again till eight. When he awoke at the latter hour, it was evident that a change for the worse had taken place. He was weaker and more comatose; his breathing was quicker, and mucus, which he was unable to spit up, collected in the bronchial tubes. He soon passed into a state of complete coma, and died at half-past eleven A. M.

When seen by the clinical clerk at eleven A. M., he was lying on his back quite insensible, and with the pupils much dilated. His breathing was laborious, the inspirations forty a minute. The pulse was ninety; the sounds of the heart were very feeble; the belly was still drawn in.

The liver was smaller than natural, and weighed twenty-three ounces. It was flaccid, so that its surface could be readily thrown into wrinkles, and its color was a reddish-brown, mixed with yellow.

Some patches in the upper part of the right lobe were reduced almost to a pulp, so that irregular cavities were formed when they were gently pressed by the finger. Other portions of the liver were not remarkably soft.

In the softened portions, scarcely any entire hepatic cells could be found, all that appeared under the microscope being irregular granular matter, apparently consisting of disintegrated cells.

In the rest of the liver, the cells were entire, and contained a variable quantity of oil and of biliary coloring matter. Most of them were pale, and contained less oil than usual. The gall-bladder was flaccid, and contained a very small quantity of dark-green bile, which presented under the microscope no visible objects. The gall-ducts were very small, and but slightly tinged with bile.

There were no marks of inflammation on the capsule of the liver, or anywhere in its substance.

The spleen was small and tolerably firm, and its surface was wrinkled.

The stomach in the big end had been slightly acted on by the gastric juice after death, but, in other respects, was sound and had its natural appearance.

The intestines contained nothing more than fecal matter, tinged with bile, and their inner surface was quite sound.

The kidneys presented to the naked eye their natural appearance, but the tubules were stained with bile, and contained an excess of epithelium, which rendered them opaque.

The lungs were healthy, except in the lower and posterior part, which was, in each, gorged with dark blood, and unnaturally friable, though it still crepitated under the finger. There were no marks of recent inflammation of the pleura.

The brain, when sliced, presented many bloody points, but had everywhere its natural consistence.

No other marks of disease were discovered in the body.

Small fibrinous coagula were found in the cavities of the heart.

Here a young man of very temperate habits, and seemingly of sound constitution, but who had been for some time out of work, and, in consequence, had been living badly, and been probably depressed in mind, receives, while in the act of stretching himself, a rather violent blow on the pit of the stomach. From this time he complains of pain and tenderness at the pit of the stomach, but the pain is not severe enough to make him change his mode of life. At the end of four days, after a hearty supper, he becomes very sick and faint. The next day, still ailing, he goes to a new situation—that of waiter at a public-house. Two days afterwards (March 2) jaundice comes on, which grows gradually deeper. From this time his bowels were relaxed, and he felt occasionally sick and faint; but he continued to work hard for ten days longer, till the 12th of March, when violent delirium came on. The delirium passed into a state of coma, and he died on the 15th, just a fortnight after the occurrence of jaundice.

On the examination after death portions of the liver were found disorganized in the way described above; and it was clear that the jaundice resulted, not from an impediment to the flow of bile into the duodenum, but from defective secretion.

In 1847, Dr. Handfield Jones presented to the Pathological Society the liver of a girl who died in St. George's Hospital, and the following interesting report of the case was published in the *Medical Gazette* for December 31 of that year:—

Case 9.—The patient, a girl, aged 18, was admitted into St. George's Hospital on the 17th of November, 1847.

She complained of amenorrhœa, slight cough, and palpitation, and was weak and cachectic.

When eight years old she had a rheumatic attack, with pain in the chest, and ever since had been subject to palpitation and dyspnœa.

At the apex of the right lung some degree of dulness was noticed on percussion; and here, also, the breathing was coarse, the expiratory sound prolonged, and there was increased vocal resonance. The heart's action was increased, there was extended dulness in the cardiac region, the sounds were audible over the whole chest, and there was a loud murmur accompanying the first at the apex.

The tongue was clean and moist, and the bowels were open.

During four days she remained in much the same state. On the 24th, vomiting occurred, and continued incessantly in spite of various remedies. At this time the urine was examined (not microscopically), and found apparently healthy; the cough increased; the sputa became muco-purulent, and afterwards somewhat rusty; the action of the heart very turbulent.

On the 29th jaundice made its appearance, the stools also being white; diarrhœa succeeded, and the vomiting continued till the 4th of December, when it subsided, and she expressed herself as feeling better; but the jaundice did not diminish, the features became collapsed, and she sank on the 6th of December, a slight attack of erysipelas having occurred on the face a day or two before death.

Post-mortem examination.—The mucous membrane of the fauces, and of the upper part of the pharynx and larynx was red, covered with tenacious mucus, and with a thin layer of lymph in some parts.

The lungs were very much congested throughout; in some parts there almost appeared to be extravasation of blood, forming numerous dark but small patches, the lower lobe of the left lung being incompletely hepatized. A portion of one of the lungs, where it was least congested, was examined by the microscope, which showed a very great increase in the epithelium lining the air cells; multitudes of pale granular cells being found in this situation, together with a few exudation corpuscles, instead of the mere nuclei or feebly developed cells which should normally exist. A moderate quantity of serum, with some flakes of lymph floating in it, existed in the pericardium. The heart was large, its cavities distended with coagula; the left ventricle much dilated, its walls slightly thickened, its cavities occupied by *a large firm fibrinous coagulum;* small fibrinous fringes on the aortic valves, the mitral valve thickened, and the orifice of the aortic valves somewhat narrowed.

The liver was of a deep yellow color; on making a section, the interlobular veins were seen highly congested, the lobules themselves not at all; the gall-bladder was full of bile, the ducts quite pervious. On examining these sections under the microscope, it was immediately seen that the secreting structure was seriously affected. On the margins of the lobules cells still existed, and their nuclei were distinctly visible, though they were gorged with bile of a deep yellow tint; in by far, however, the greatest extent of the lobules no cells could be discerned; a densely aggregated group of oil-globules formed a zone concentric to the marginal one, where the bile-laden cells still retained their forms; within this there was nothing but coarse granular and amorphous matter, with a few groups of oil-globules. The relative size of this interior part, where the degeneration was most complete, varied in different lobules, but in some it occupied nearly one-half of the whole extent.

The spleen was unusually firm, many of its nuclei developing fibres from the opposite extremities.

The kidneys were very firm, not congested, but perhaps rather pale; microscopic examination showed the tubuli of the left kidney tolerably healthy, but the granular matter of the epithelium perhaps rather coarse. On cutting into the right kidney, there was seen a large patch of yellow color, extending throughout the cortical substance, and which was accurately bounded and separated from the surrounding healthy part by a broad line of deep red color, which was happily compared by Dr. Nairne to the boundary line of gangrene which had ceased to spread. The discoloration of the tissue extended to the surface of the organ; the corresponding part of the capsule was similarly discolored, and also evidently thickened. On viewing these sections of the altered portion, it was very apparent that the secreting tubuli were principally affected, in some specimens being completely destroyed; numerous coarsely granular cells, the remains of their epithelium, being alone visible. In the majority of instances, however, the tubes still remained, but were so bloated and opaque as to be evidently unfit for the discharge of their functions—resembling in many respects the diseased tubes which are found in a kidney which has suffered consecutively to scarlatina. On close examination, several of these tubes were still seen to be invested by a basement membrane, in the interior of which were dense masses of large, coarse epithelial cells, which completely filled the cavity and obstructed the passage. The matrix was unaffected; in particular the capsules of the Malpighian tufts were beautifully seen; no trace of any fibrinous or other deposits could be found in the portions examined by Dr. Jones and Mr. Simon, though Dr. Bence Jones had found a considerable quantity of free oily matter in a specimen from this same kidney. The Malpighian tufts themselves separated with great readiness from their capsules; their capillaries had quite lost their natural aspect, and appeared of an indistinct fibrous or granular texture.

In this case, a girl, aged seventeen, with valvular disease of the heart, most probably the effect of an attack of rheumatism, which she had nine years before, was brought into the hospital on the 17th of November, weak and cachectic, and complaining of amenorrhœa, slight cough, and palpitation. No particular change in her condition was noticed till the 21st, when she was taken with vomiting, which continued incessantly in spite of various remedies. The sputa now became muco-purulent, and afterwards somewhat rusty.

On the 29th jaundice came on, succeeded by diarrhœa. The vomiting continued till the 4th of December, when it subsided, and she expressed herself as feeling better. The jaundice, however, did not diminish; erysipelas appeared on the face; and she died on the 6th, fifteen days after the occurrence of vomiting, seven days after the occurrence of jaundice. No mention is made of delirium or other cerebral disorder.

On examination after death marks of recent inflammation, which was probably erysipelatous, were found in the fauces and in the upper part of the larynx, and also in the pericardium.

The lower lobe of the left lung was completely hepatized, and the lungs were very much congested throughout.

The liver had undergone the same morbid process as in the preceding cases; but, from the shorter duration of the malady, the disorganization of the cells was complete only in the central portions of the lobules.

The kidneys exhibited, in different degrees, changes in the secreting tubules like those found in kidneys that have suffered from scarlatina; and in the right was a large patch of yellow, which extended through the cortical substance, and which was separated from the surrounding part by a broad, deep red line. In this yellow portion the tubes were blocked up, and the circulation had evidently ceased some time before death.

I have twice found a similar pale spot in the cortical substance of the kidney, separated from the rest of the organ by a red line, where death had resulted from acute dropsy, consequent on cold and fatigue.

The disease of the kidney doubtless came on after the occurrence of the gastric disorder, which was followed by the jaundice; for, on the 21st of November, when the vomiting occurred, the urine was submitted to the ordinary examination, and considered to be healthy. The most probable supposition is, that it was consecutive to the jaundice, and that it was caused by the elimination of some noxious matter through the kidneys.

In the month of July, 1850, one of my brothers sent me the following brief account of a case of fatal jaundice from suppressed secretion, in which the additional fact was observed, that the bile in the gall-bladder, and the liver itself, had an acid reaction:—

Case 10.—A few days ago I was called to a case of jaundice, the particulars of which may have some interest for you. The subject of it was a married lady, thirty-seven years of age, delicate, but sound. On Monday, July 1, she was quite well; on Tuesday, ailing; on Wednesday, jaundiced, but not ill enough to keep her bed. On Thursday and Friday she kept her bed, and was frequently very sick, but was sprightly and cheerful, and without a single alarming symptom. Little or no fever, or, indeed, general disorder of any kind. In the course of Friday evening she bacame worse, chiefly in the way of sickness. All the early part of the night she was harassed by almost incessant vomiting. At five in the morning she became *suddenly* incoherent, knowing no one, and making continual efforts to get out of bed. At eight o'clock she was quite *unconscious*. It was about half-past eight that I first saw her. She was then lying in a state of profound stupor; her surface very yellow, her lips and nose livid, her extremities cold, her pulse scarcely to be felt. The pupils were much dilated, and the right was sensibly larger than the left. The mouth was drawn to the left side. To say the truth, she was already moribund. She never recovered consciousness, and died at a quarter before nine the same evening—that is to say, in less than fourteen hours after the supervention of the first head-symptoms. For some time before her death her breath had a peculiar and sickening smell.

I made the *post-mortem* examination thirty-six hours after death, and although, from circumstances, it was not so complete as could be desired, the particulars are worthy of notice. In the first place, the liver presented no single mark of inflammation. It was not swelled, but, of the two, rather small than large. The capsule smooth, and peeling readily; its edges sharp. In mass the organ was flaccid, but its substance was pretty firm and not readily broken up. It presented but one color, and that color was *red.* It did not contain much blood. There was about a drachm of chocolate-colored bile in the gall-bladder. The ducts were empty, and all pervious. Blue litmus-paper placed in contact with the liver was immediately *changed to a bright red*, and the bile in the gall-bladder appeared also, by the same test, to be *intensely acid.* The stomach contained about three pints of black fluid, identical in appearance and character with that which is known as "the black vomit." This fluid had been poured out when there was no longer power to eject it. In the small intestine there was mucus, abundantly stained with green bile; and I may here add that, during life, the stools were never entirely devoid of bile. There were three other circumstances especially worthy of remark: rapid tendency to putrefaction; a fluid state of the blood; and an immense number of large ecchymoses. With the exception of a very small fibrinous clot in the left ventricle, the blood was everywhere fluid. Hundreds of ecchymoses, varying in size from that of a split pea to large blotches as broad as a shilling, were scattered over the mesentery. Similar extravasations had occurred in the fat of the abdominal parietes, as also in the anterior mediastinum. There was a great number under the parietal pleura on both sides, and the whole surface of the heart was variegated by them, It was probable that something of the same kind had occurred in the brain. but unfortunately the head was not allowed to be opened. The marks of rapidly progressing putrefaction were everywhere conspicuous. The blood in the right ventricle was frothy from evolution of gas; the mesentery, near the upper part of the duodenum, was emphysematous, and the whole of the mucous membrane of the small intestine was blown up, and partially separated from the coats beneath by a similar change. The kidneys and spleen were sound; the lungs much gorged in their posterior or undermost half, but not diseased. I had no time to make a microscopic examination of the liver until the next morning. There was not then a single cell to be seen, but decomposition had gone on so rapidly, that no inference could be drawn from the fact.

There can be no doubt that in this case, as in the former cases, the jaundice resulted from defective secretion; and as there appears to have been no moral influence at work that could have arrested the action of the liver, we can hardly avoid the inference that it was caused by some special poison introduced from without, or engendered in the body by faulty digestion or assimilation. The disorder of the brain occurred, as in Case 5, only a few days after the occurrence of jaundice, and proved more speedily fatal than in any of the preceding cases. On the Thursday and Friday this lady was ill enough to keep her bed, but was sprightly and cheerful, without a single alarming symptom. Early on the Saturday morning she became suddenly incoherent, and the same evening she died in a state of coma.

The strongly acid reaction of the bile in the gall-bladder and of the juices of the liver is a remarkable fact, and probably will turn out to be very important when the true explanation of this terrible disease is discovered.

The instances that have been related serve to show the remarkable changes which the lobular substance of the liver undergoes in fatal cases of jaundice from defective secretion.

When death occurs early, the liver is softer than natural, and of a dirty yellowish, or yellowish-brown color, but is nearly of its former size, and the lobules are distinctly visible. The secreting cells are entire, but contain fine granular matter, and are consequently more opaque than natural.

From the beginning the liver ceases almost entirely to secrete bile, and before long the secreting cells break down, or are not reproduced; and, in consequence, the lobules, which owe much of their bulk to the cells and the products of secretion, waste, and the liver shrinks rapidly. At the end of some weeks the liver is much diminished in size and weight, and the lobules are very indistinct. Different parts of the liver may present different stages of the disease. In one part the lobular substance may be slightly raised above the general level of the surface, and soft, and of a dirty yellow, or yellowish-brown, and the lobules may be distinct. In another part the substance may be firmer, but more wasted, and its color may be more owing to the blood in the vessels. In this part the lobules are very indistinct, and the secreting cells are few and small.

In some cases portions of the liver are found extremely soft, and the secreting cells in them completely destroyed. The observation of Dr. Handfield Jones (Case 9) tends to show that this process of disorganization begins in the centres of the lobules. In two or three of the cases related, in which the secreting cells in portions of the liver were completely destroyed, the adjacent tissues were so softened that they were reduced to a soft pulp by the slightest pressure of the finger. In these cases it is probable that the vessels and other tissues were softened by some chemical agency after death; for it is difficult to conceive how the circulation could be carried on in vessels so rotten, and in none of the cases was there any blood effused in the softened portions. The question then arises, was there not some noxious matter retained in the liver in these cases, which excited a solvent action on its tissues after death?

In one of the cases there were numerous purpuric spots on the omentum, and in one or two others, shortly before death, sanguinolent matter was passed from the stomach and bowels, without other hemorrhage. A tendency to hemorrhage is common in jaundice, and is probably owing to the unhealthy state of the blood; but in these cases the occurrence of hemorrhage in the abdominal cavity solely or chiefly seems to show that the hemorrhage was owing, not so much to the state of the blood, as to a special congestion of the alimentary canal, caused by the arrest of secretion in the liver.

In two or three of the cases urine was secreted plentifully up to the time of death, and the kidneys, on superficial examination, presented no marks of disease. In other cases, after a time, the secreting tubules of the kidneys became diseased, evidently in consequence of the elimination of some noxious matter through them. In Case 7 the softness and frangibility of the kidneys after death, and the microscopic appearances, lead to the inference that the change in those organs was of the same kind as that of the liver.

In all the cases in which the kidneys were diseased the morbid change in them seems to have been consecutive to that in the liver.

The question then occurs, did the disease of the kidneys result from the absorption, and the elimination through them, of matter furnished by the disorganized cells of the liver? or did it result from noxious matter, introduced from without, or engendered by faulty digestion or assimilation, which was first detained in the liver; but which, when the liver had become disorganized, and had consequently ceased to detain it, was carried to those great outlets for noxious matters in the blood—the kidneys?

In considering the details of the cases related above, two circumstances arrest attention as having probably had influence in producing the disease.

1. The first is, that, with the exception of Abdul (Case 5), whose case differed in many respects from those of the others, none of the patients had attained middle age. Of the nine remaining cases seven occurred between the ages of 17 and 30, one at the age of 35, and one at the age of 37. It would seem from this that the disease belongs especially to youth and adolescence.

2. The second circumstance worthy of attention is, that most of the patients had been leading irregular lives, and had been subject to depressing influences just before the jaundice came on.

The subjects of these cases were five women and five men. Of the women, one had been recently separated from her husband, and had been in hospital under treatment for syphilitic sores; one had been recently abandoned by a man with whom she cohabited; one was a poor broom girl, wandering in a strange country, ignorant of its language; one weak and cachectic, with long-standing disease of the heart. Of the men, one had been for some time out of work; one was a sailor who had lately led a dissolute life, and had syphilitic sores; two others were sailors, who had been a short time ashore, and had most probably led the irregular and dissipated life that sailors too commonly do on their arrival in port.

These facts favor the inference, that grief, anxiety, dissipation, and other depressing conditions are influential in producing the disease.

Before the occurrence of cerebral disorder there were in most of these cases no constant or peculiar symptoms that could serve to distinguish them from ordinary cases of jaundice occurring in young persons. In six of the cases there was some degree of pain or tenderness in the region of the liver. In the remaining four no pain or tenderness seems to have existed. In most of the cases there was some gastric or intestinal disorder: in eight, there was vomiting, which in some was very distressing; in two, there was protracted hiccough; in several, more or less diarrhœa. The stools were generally clay-colored; but occasionally, in some of the cases, they were more or less tinged with bile. This is explained by the circumstance, that some parts of the liver continued to secrete bile; and that, in consequence of the gall-ducts being pervious, the bile accumulated in the liver at the commencement of the disease could flow freely into the bowel.

In many of the cases the symptoms for several weeks were not of an alarming character. Some of the patients seem to have walked about; one continued to work hard; one was sprightly and cheerful, until the occurrence of delirium.

This terrible kind of jaundice seems, then, to occur especially in youth or adolescence; in persons of both sexes, *especially in those who are depressed from grief, mental anxiety, or dissipation.* It is generally attended with some pain or tenderness in the region of the liver, with some degree of gastric or intestinal disorder, and with signs of exhaustion, but seldom with active inflammatory symptoms. Often the disease presents no alarming characters till the occurrence of delirium, which happens at various times—from a few days to several weeks—after the appearance of the jaundice.

The head symptoms, in such cases, which are different in kind and more constantly and promptly fatal than those which result from exhaustion, have been generally attributed to the retention of the principles of the bile in the blood; but there is abundant evidence to show that the mere retention of bile in its natural state produces no such effects. Cases have been related in a former chapter in which, in consequence of permanent closure of the common gall-duct, the secreting cells of the liver were entirely destroyed; in which it was clear that no bile could have been secreted for some time before death; and yet no appreciable disorder of the intellect existed. The patients were of an olive-green, from the long-continued jaundice, and grew gradually weaker; and at length died, not from disturbance of the functions of the brain, as in the cases just related, but from sheer exhaustion.

If this supposition be dismissed, two others suggest themselves. The first is, that these symptoms are caused by the *direct* action of the poison which caused the jaundice. A great difficulty in the way of this supposition is the *sudden and unexpected* occurrence of the head symptoms, in some of the cases related above, after the jaundice had lasted for some time. It is clear from the symptoms that some deadly agency—sufficient, in one case, to destroy life in fourteen hours—came then *suddenly* to act on the nervous system. If this were the poison that had before arrested the secretion of the liver, and caused the jaundice, the poison must at first have been retained in the liver, like globules of pus or mercury, and from some cause or other have been suddenly liberated to exert its action on the nervous system. It is well known that poisons which kill by stupefying the nervous system take effect rapidly on their passing into the blood; and in some of the preceding cases there was no sign, for several days or even weeks after the occurrence of jaundice, that the brain was under the action of a narcotic poison.

Another supposition that offers a better explanation of the facts than either of the others is, that, *in consequence of decomposition*, some peculiarly noxious agent is evolved in the lobular substance of the liver, which is the real cause of the malignant symptoms.

Circumstances much in favor of this supposition are, that the cerebral disorder occurs rather suddenly, at very variable times after the occurrence of the jaundice; and that, sometimes, jaundice caused *by fright* proves fatal exactly in the same way.

It has been stated that one of the cases (Case 5) differed in many respects from that of the others. The peculiarities of this case are, that the patient was much more advanced in life; that the disease was of shorter duration; that striking morbid changes recently produced, were found in various organs besides the liver; and that several persons living with the patient, and exposed to the same influences, had jaundice about the same time.

These circumstances render it probable that here the jaundice was produced by unwholesome food, or by some noxious effluvia, to which all these persons were exposed.

Many remarkable instances have been recorded of jaundice from suppressed secretion of bile, occurring in several members of a family in succession, and in some of them proving rapidly fatal, with delirium and coma.

The following instance was published by Dr. W. Griffin, of Limerick, in the *Dublin Journal of Medical and Chemical Science*, for 1834, in the first of a series of excellent papers entitled, "Medical Problems." I give it in Dr. Griffin's own words :—

"A poor woman requested me to visit her daughter, Mary Barry, aged 20 years, who, she informed me, had been three days ill, and was now speechless, and she believed dying. On entering the cabin in which she lived, I saw her make a faint expiration, which proved to be her last, as she was quite dead when I reached the bed. Her skin was still warm, and universally tinged with a deep yellow color. The countenance was hydropic, and the pupils were dilated. On inquiring, I found the girl's ailment had set in with languor and heaviness; on the second evening, she was seized with sickness of stomach, vomiting, and appearances of jaundice, and next morning complained much of her head. She then looked so very ill, that her mother began to get alarmed, and insisted on her going to the dispensary for advice; the poor girl shook her head despondingly, and said she was too weak to walk there, but she would go into the room and lie down on the bed. These were the last words she uttered. When the mother went in afterwards, there was an appearance of stupor about her, from which she endeavored to rouse her, but could get no reply. She was in profound coma.

"In about three weeks after, I was called to see Ellen Barry, a sister of the former, and found her laboring under an affection precisely similar. She had been attacked with languor and heaviness, followed by sickness of stomach and vomiting, with universal yellowness of the skin. She was now in perfect coma; conscious when roused, but unable to speak, and very unwilling to be disturbed. From this very dangerous state she was rescued by active and continued purging; the yellow tinge gradually disappeared, and in a few days she regained her usual health.

"Within a very short period afterwards, another member of the same family was attacked—a boy of about 13 years of age. My brother was requested to see him, and found him moaning, and comatose; his belly tender to the touch, his pulse slow, and his skin of a saffron color; his breathing was not stertorous. This case was more sudden than either of the foregoing; the boy was seized with sickness of stomach and vomiting at night, and in the morning was jaundiced and insensible. In this state he lay until nearly the end of the second day, without medical aid, up to which period his bowels had not been moved. An ineffectual effort was then made to purge him, but he was unable to swallow, and died in a few hours.

"The parents were now, it may be supposed, highly apprehensive for their remaining children, and, the event proved, not without just reason. After the lapse of a few months, their next boy, John Barry, aged 11 years, showed symptoms of jaundice. He grew languid and heavy, and in two days the tunica albuginea and skin were of a deep yellow. There was great sluggishness of the bowels, and slight tenderness of the abdomen, but very little pain. He did not complain of his head, but, like the others, was seized with sickness of stomach and vomiting. I had early notice of this attack, and was vigilant in looking for the supervention of coma, although, from existing symptoms, there was no greater reason to apprehend it than in any common case of jaundice, if I except some slight dilatation of the pupils, and sluggishness in their movements. The boy was up and about, and did not, in fact, appear to be very ill; but the fate of his brother and sister left a lesson not to be forgotten, and I accordingly warned the mother to give me instant notice of the occurrence of the slightest stupor; he was in the mean time actively purged. There was little change in him that night or the next, but on the succeeding morning, I had a messenger with me at an early hour, to say that he had fallen into a state of insensibility in the night, and could not now be roused. I found him quite comatose, with slow pulse, dilated pupils, and almost a total loss of sensation and voluntary motion. On pinching his hand severely, however, he evinced signs of consciousness, moaning slightly, and slowly drawing his hand away. Ten ounces of blood were immediately taken from the temporal artery; the head was shaved, and kept wetted with refrigerant washes, and castor oil was administered every fourth hour. As the bowels were slow in acting, injections were given at night, and large blisters applied to the nape of the neck. These had the desired effect. He was copiously purged for several hours, and in the morning evinced signs of returning consciousness; from thenceforward there was, day after day, a steady and progressive improvement, until his recovery became fully established.

"Some time after, the friends were once more alarmed by a recurrence of the vomiting and jaundice; but the progress of coma was arrested, and the complaint readily removed by purging alone.

"These four cases of jaundice, running rapidly into coma, which in two of them terminated in death, when we consider that they occurred in one family, within a few weeks of one another, and without any unusual or remarkable symptoms which could indicate the impending danger, suggest a very important question with regard to the pathology of the disease: 'On what morbid state did the occurrence of coma in these particular instances depend?'"

Another, and almost parallel instance, except that the different members of the family were attacked after long intervals, and that the jaundice was attended by more fever, is related by Dr. Graves, in his work on Clinical Medicine. The account was sent to Dr. Graves by Dr. Hanlon, of Portarlington, his former pupil, of whose assiduity and zeal he speaks in high terms.

The cases appear to me so interesting, when taken in conjunction with those before related, that, notwithstanding its length, I have ventured to transcribe the account entire.

CASE 1.—Saturday, July 25, 1840, I was called to visit Miss Maria B——, aged seventeen years. On the preceding Wednesday she complained of languor, and in a few hours was attacked with bilious vomiting, which had returned three or four times in every twenty-four hours since. When the vomiting commenced she became jaundiced, and the color increased in intensity until it assumed a greenish-yellow tint. The bowels were constipated for two days before the vomiting began, and had remained so, notwithstanding that the apothecary in attendance had given her repeated doses of purgative medicines. Effervescing draughts and other medicines intended to allay the vomiting, had been given without success.

I found the tongue thickly coated with a yellow mucus; tenderness of the epigastrium and hypochondrium; thirst; abdomen not tender on pressure; urine scanty and high-colored; pulse, 80; slight headache; pupils natural; complains of want of sleep; and appears fretful and anxious.

Calomel, combined with compound extract of colocynth, aided by purgative enemata, caused a small, dark, and offensive motion towards evening. Leeches were applied to the epigastrium and region of the liver, followed by stupes, three grains of calomel every four hours, and a purgative draught, consisting of infusion of senna, and tincture of senna, jalap, and cardamoms, after every second dose of calomel.

Sunday.—Vomited twice since yesterday evening: the bilious matter of a darker color; tongue still loaded; thirst diminished; tenderness of epigastrium and right hypochondrium much less; bowels moved twice in the course of the night; motions larger, but still very dark in color; pulse 80; headache relieved; pupils natural; color of skin the same; slept for two or three hours in the night; same treatment continued.

Monday morning, five o'clock.—I was called up in haste to visit her. It appeared that, two hours before my arrival, she complained of violent headache and intolerance of light, and vomited a dark brown matter resembling coffee grounds; soon afterwards became very restless, and gradually fell into a state of stupor. I found her in imperfect coma, the pupils excessively dilated and insensible to light, the eyelids closed. She flung herself every minute or two from one part of the bed to another, and uttered a faint, subdued scream; she was very unwilling to be interfered with; pulse 60, and oppressed; skin of a still deeper tint of greenish-yellow.

The assistance of Dr. Tabuteau and Dr. J. Jacob was procured in consultation. Fourteen leeches were applied to the temples; the head shaved, and cold cloths applied to it; twelve grains of calomel in the first dose, and five grains every second hour afterwards; purgative enemata were employed every second hour. Cold affusion on the head was subsequently used to a great extent, but without producing any change in the state of the pupils or the coma; mercurial inunction in the region of the liver and insides of the arms was commenced, and a large blister applied to the scalp.

At eleven o'clock A. M., she was seized with violent convulsions, which lasted about a minute, and were accompanied by shrill screams; the right extremities appeared more strongly convulsed than the left, the mouth was drawn to the left side. The convulsions returned every thirty or forty minutes with the same violence and screaming, until three o'clock P. M., when they became less violent, but more protracted, and gradually passed into a continued spasm, or jerking, of the extremities. She threw up occasionally a mouthful of dark matter like that which she had previously vomited. The administration of the calomel was relinquished, as every attempt to give it brought on a return of the convulsions. The mercurial inunction was assiduously continued, but no mercurial fetor could be detected in the breath; the coma became more profound; the pulse rose to 108, small, fluttering, and finally intermitting; sordes collected on the teeth; the urine and feces passed involuntarily; the breathing towards the close became stertorous; and she expired at eleven o'clock the following morning. No examination of the body was permitted.

Case 2.—Monday, March 29, 1841, I was requested to visit Miss Charlotte B——, aged eleven years, sister of the former. She had been previously healthy; for the last two days, has had the usual symptoms of a feverish cold, which is attributed to her having wetted her feet. I found the tongue loaded; tenderness of the epigastrium—none in the region of the liver; thirst; bowels confined; urine scanty and high-colored; pulse 120; no headache; pupils natural; no discoloration of the eyes or skin. Six leeches to the epigastrium, to be followed by stuping; purgatives; diaphoretic mixture and diluents prescribed.

Tuesday morning, nine o'clock.—Appears better; slept some hours in the course of the night; tongue cleaner; thirst diminished; tenderness of the epigastrium much less; no tenderness on strong pressure in the right hypochondrium; bowels have been strongly acted on four times; motions dark and offensive; urine more copious and paler; pulse 92; no headache; pupils natural; no discoloration of the conjunctiva or skin. Having been absent from home during the day, I hastened, on my return at eight o'clock in the evening, to visit; and was greatly surprised to find her in the same state as her sister had been. It appeared that about three o'clock she became heavy and languid, and the skin became slightly jaundiced. She complained of headache and intolerance of light; vomited a dark brown matter resembling coffee grounds; tossed about from one part of the bed to another; refused to answers questions, and fell into a state of insensibility; the bowels had been moved twice, the motions dark, but not offensive. I found her in a state of imperfect coma, the eyelids closed, the pupils excessively dilated, and insensible to light; pulse 64, and oppressed; skin jaundiced. In a few minutes after my entering the room, she was seized with violent convulsions, which were accompanied by shrill screams, and lasted about a minute. Pressure on the right hypochondrium appeared to give her pain. Upon my requesting that additional medical aid should be procured, her friends declined having it, on the ground that the case appeared precisely the same as her sister's, and all our efforts on that occasion had been unavailing. Under these circumstances, I had recourse to the same plan of treatment as that adopted in the preceding case; cold affusion on the shaven head; ten leeches to the right hypochondrium; mercurial inunction on the right side and inside of the arms, in the intervals between the convulsions; strong purgative enemata frequently repeated, and a large blister on the scalp. The disease, quite uncontrolled by these means, pursued precisely the same course, in every particular, as the former one. The convulsions continued most violent for two hours, when they began to be less violent, but much more protracted, until they passed into continued twitchings of the muscles of the extremities. The coma became more profound; the breathing stertorous; sordes collected on the teeth, and she expired at seven o'clock the following morning.

Her friends being now alarmed for the safety of her surviving brothers and sisters, became very desirous that the body should be examined. Dr. Tabuteau, who had seen the former case in consultation, assisted me in making the examination. The following are the results: examination made thirty hours after death; surface of the body jaundiced.

Head.—Pacchionian glands preternaturally vascular; venous turgescence generally over the surface of the brain, with increased vascularity of the middle, and especially the left anterior lobes; substance of the brain much more vascular than usual; great vascularity of the choroid plexus; none of the optic thalami, or corpora pyramidalia; the entire surface of the base of the brain highly vascular, particularly at the crura cerebri, pons Varolii, and medulla oblongata; no fluid found in the ventricles.

Abdomen.—Numerous spots of extravasated blood in the omentum; several small patches of inflammation along the small intestines; stomach apparently healthy.

Liver.—Size natural; color, externally of a dull yellow, with several dark spots about the size of a half-crown piece; consistence, less than usual; structure, minutely granular, and of a very peculiar crimson-orange color, somewhat resembling what might be supposed to result from an intimate mixture of arterial blood and bile; gall-bladder distended with bile of the usual appearance. *Thorax* not examined.

I endeavored to preserve portions of the liver in a dilute solution of corrosive sublimate and diluted alcohol, but they gradually lost their characteristic appearance in both fluids.

CASE 3.—Friday, June 18th, 1841, I was called to visit Miss Jane B——, aged eight years, sister of the two former. I was informed that she had been previously healthy. This morning she appeared languid, and was seized with bilious vomiting. No cause can be assigned for her illness. I found the skin jaundiced slightly; the tongue loaded; tenderness of the epigastrium and right hypochondrium; thirst; bowels confined; pulse 108; no headache; no intolerance of light; pupils natural; urine scanty and high colored. Eight ounces of blood were immediately taken from the arm, which afterwards proved to be buffed and cupped; eight leeches applied to the region of the liver, followed by stuping; twenty grains of calomel given at once, and a strong purgative draught every fourth hour until the bowels are fully acted on; three grains of calomel, and one and a half of James's powder every third hour after purgation; cold to the head.

Saturday.—Slept none; skin more deeply jaundiced; tenderness of the epigastrium diminished; heat of the right hypochondrium still remains; tongue yellowish; vomited twice since yesterday evening; urine tinged with bile, and more copious; bowels moved four times; motions dark and offensive; pulse 110; headache and some intolerance of light; considerable restlessness. Six leeches to the right side; four to the temples; cold to the head; a blister to the nape of the neck; mercurial inunction; five grains of calomel and one of James's powder every second hour. I now watched the case with the greatest interest and anxiety.

Sunday Evening.—Slight mercurial fetor of the breath; tongue beginning to clean; tenderness of the right side diminished; bowels moved three times; motions less dark and offensive; pulse 90, and soft; headache and intolerance subsided; restlessness entirely gone; some return of appetite. Calomel and James's powder were continued every fourth hour until a slight salivation was established, and cold carefully applied to the head. No unfavorable symptoms subsequently appeared. The tongue became clean, the pulse fell to the natural standard, the motions became more healthy in appearance, the appetite returned, and under the use of four grains of calomel at night, and a strong dose of black draught the following morning, repeated every third night for three weeks, the jaundice disappeared, and she has remained quite well up to this period.—*Graves's Clinical Medicine*, p. 459.

The cases that have now been related all bear a certain resemblance to each other. In all of them jaundice occurred, not from any impediment to the flow of bile through the ducts, but because the secreting function of the liver was imperfectly performed; no bile, or but a small quantity of bile, was secreted. In all, with one exception, in which death resulted from exhaustion, the jaundice was followed by delirium, or stupor, which in some soon passed into coma, with or without convulsions. In all in which the body was examined, the liver was found altered in structure, and in the same way; it was diminished in size (in all except the Case 5), soft or flabby, and of a light yellow, or brownish yellow, or crimson orange, or some kindred tint. In none of them were any marks of inflammation noticed in the capsule of the liver, or in the gall-ducts. In some of the cases, where the liver was examined by the microscope, the hepatic cells were found to be in some parts completely destroyed.

But although the cases here brought together present so many points of resemblance, it must not be inferred that the disease under which the patients were laboring was essentially the same in all.

Disorganization of the hepatic cells, or suspension of their secreting power, may be the effect of a variety of morbid causes, essentially different from one another in character, and in their other effects on the system.

In the second case related by Dr. Alison, and in the second of those which I have cited from Dr. Bright, jaundice seems to have been consequent on mental distress, and was probably caused by it. We should not be justified in drawing this conclusion from those cases taken by themselves. But so many instances have been recorded, in which jaundice immediately followed a sudden alarm, or shock, or other strong and depressing mental emotion, that no doubt can remain of the influence of such emotions in producing it. Dr. Watson, in his admirable lectures, after relating some striking instances of this sequence of events, observes: "There are scores of instances to the same effect; and *this* is observable of such cases, that they are often fatal, with head symptoms : convulsions, delirium, or coma, supervening upon the jaundice." Morgagni, in his 37th epistle, has related several cases in which jaundice, soon followed by delirium and fatal coma, came on after mental distress, or fright; and in the first of these cases, which he cites from Valsalva, the liver seems to have presented much the same appearances as in the cases related in this chapter. "Ventre aperto, jecur inventum est *flaccidum*, et ad subpallidum vergens; in ejus vesiculâ, bilis subobscura."

In some of the other cases related above, the disease seems to have been the effect of some peculiar poison introduced from without. It is difficult to explain otherwise the occurrence of several cases of jaundice about the same time, among the crew of a vessel; or, at short intervals, in the different children of a family; more especially when the illness attending the jaundice is so peculiar, and so uniform in character, as it was in the instances recorded by Dr. Griffin and Dr. Hanlon. It is worthy of remark, that the symptoms attending the jaundice, though almost exactly alike in the children of the same family, were in many respects different in the different families. In the instance related by Dr. Griffin, no symptoms are noticed but jaundice and vomiting, with languor and oppression, soon passing into coma. In the instance recorded by Dr. Hanlon, the jaundice was attended by other symptoms like those of a severe form of remittent fever. Now and then jaundice occurs in several members of a family in quick succession, without being attended by any alarming symptoms. An instance of this, in the family of a clergyman, in a country parish in Devonshire, fell under the notice of my brother, Dr. Christian Budd, who has sent me the following account of it:—

"On the 2d of July, 1843, I was sent for to see Miss——, aged 6, who had been for a day or two suffering from general disorder; slight shiverings, headache, listlessness, loss of appetite, and restlessness at night. She had complained of no fixed pain, and had not vomited. When I saw her, she was slightly flushed, her skin was hotter than natural, pulse rather frequent, but not very so, tongue furred; she complained of headache, had a dull, heavy look, and rested her head continually on the sofa or a chair. She had no appetite, and not much thirst. I observed nothing peculiar in the color of the skin. I ordered a purgative—mercury and chalk, and senna. The senna she vomited. The next day, her skin was manifestly yellow, urine porter-colored, and motions clay-colored. I gave her gentle purgatives, and she soon got well. Her skin, however, remained yellow for some little time after.

"The last day or two of the same month, her elder sister, aged 10, fell ill in the same way, and on the 3d of August I visited her. Her symptoms were precisely the same as those just detailed, and a yellowness of the skin could already be discerned. The next day she was completely jaundiced. Her convalescence was much slower than that of her sister, and she remained yellow much longer. Before she was quite well, her brother, aged 11, went to London with his father, but the day after his arrival there, complained of being very poorly: was listless, took no notice of the sights around him, sat down whenever and wherever he could, and ate nothing. This state was at first attributed to the fatigue of the journey, but in a short time he also became jaundiced. His convalescence was more rapid than that of his sisters. He took, I believe, some purgatives merely, and soon got well."

Many other instances have come to my knowledge of jaundice occurring in several children of the same family, or in several persons living in the same locality, in quick succession, without being attended by any unusual or alarming symptoms.

In all these instances the disease was limited to a small space, so that it cannot be ascribed to a peculiar state of the general atmosphere. The miasm, or whatever it was that caused it, had a local source.

Another reason for believing that the jaundice in these cases was the effect of some poison is, that jaundice of the same kind, that is, from suppressed secretion, occurs in other diseases, which obviously depend on poisoning of the blood. I have met with two instances of suppurative phlebitis, with scattered abscesses in various parts of the body, in which slight jaundice occurred, without there being abscesses or other marks of inflammation in the liver, and in which the jaundice clearly resulted from suppressed secretion; for there was no obstruction in the ducts, and the gall-bladder contained a pale citron-colored fluid. In one of these cases I remarked that the liver was extremely soft.

Jaundice, with pain at the stomach and vomiting, is one of the effects of the poison of serpents, and is produced, it would seem, not by obstruction to the flow of bile from inflammation and closure of the gall-ducts, but by suspension of the secreting power of the liver.

Jaundice occurs, too, in some malignant forms of fever, obviously produced by the action of a poison. The yellow fever, which owes its name to the concomitant jaundice, has many points of resemblance with some of the cases before related, especially those recorded by Dr. Hanlon. In Dr. Hanlon's cases there was bilious vomiting, with pain at the epigastrium, and fever, and jaundice, followed by the vomiting of altered blood, which is so characteristic of the yellow fever of the West Indies. In these cases, too, as in yellow fever, the *black vomit* proved the harbinger of speedy death. Epidemics of a peculiar form of fever, of which vomiting and jaundice were frequent symptoms, have at times prevailed in certain districts of this country. A fever of this kind was epidemic in Glasgow in the summer of 1843.

In most of the cases of fatal jaundice recorded in the first part of this chapter, which occurred singly, it is much more doubtful how the disease originated. In some of these cases the jaundice was undoubtedly produced by depressing emotions: in some it may have resulted from fatigue or from exposure to cold and wet, which so frequently disturbs the chemical and vital processes that minister to nutrition; and when we consider the relation of the liver to the intestinal canal—when we consider that the stream of blood from the intestinal canal, charged with all the foreign matters which have been there absorbed, has to filter through the liver before it is poured into the general current—it seems probable that in some, where the stomach and the liver seemed to be the organs primarily and for some time exclusively at fault, the disease was the effect of some noxious matter absorbed from the intestinal canal, and either swallowed with the food, or engendered within the body through faulty digestion.

It appears from some of the instances that have been adduced, that this form of jaundice is not necessarily fatal, even after the patient has fallen into a state bordering on coma. The shipmate of Abdul (Case 5), whose disease was undoubtedly of the same nature as his, was brought into the hospital jaundiced, semi-comatose, and passing blood in considerable quantity from the bowels, but yet recovered. Of the four children of the same family whose cases are related by Dr. Griffin, two recovered—one, after being in imperfect coma, conscious when roused, but unable to speak; the other, after being quite comatose, with slow pulse, dilated pupils, and almost total loss of sensation and voluntary motion.

It is impossible to say what amount of damage had occurred in these cases; or whether in them the cells in any part of the liver had been completely destroyed, as in some of the fatal cases. Still less, therefore, can it be determined what are the ulterior effects of the disease, where recovery takes place. It may be, that in favorable cases the cells are not disorganized, and that they resume after a time a healthy action; or, if some of the cells be disorganized, that others are generated, just as fresh blood-cells are generated in persons who recover from losses of blood or from chlorosis; or the disease may end in flattening and atrophy of a lobe, an alteration which is now and then met with, and is generally supposed to be congenital; or the liver may remain long after, perhaps ever after, somewhat altered in appearance and texture, as seems to happen after severe forms of remittent fever.

The cases related above, numerous as they are, do not exhibit all the varieties of this affection.

1st. Instances of jaundice of the kind we are considering now and then occur in which the patient dies exhausted by gastric hemorrhage, before the occurrence of cerebral disorder. In proof of this, I may cite the following case recorded by Abercrombie:—

A lady, aged about fifty, of a full habit and florid complexion, was suddenly seized in the beginning of June, 1821, with very deep jaundice, for which no cause could be traced. There was no pain, no tenderness, and no fulness, in the region of the liver; the pulse was natural, and rather weak; there was little appetite and some nausea, but no other complaint. The bowels were easily moved, and the motions were dark or brownish. After the free use of purgatives, &c., she began to take a little mercury. For a week after this, she seemed to be improving, but she then became more oppressed, with frequent complaints of nausea, and a feeling of languor; the tongue was white, but the pulse was natural. No other symptom was complained of, and nothing could be discovered in the region of the liver.

On the 16th she began to have some vomiting, which occurred occasionally for three days, without any other change in the symptoms, until the 19th, when streaks of a black substance were observed in the matter which was vomited. The vomiting now became more and more urgent, with increase of the quantity of this black matter, and she died, gradually exhausted, on the morning of the 21st.

Inspection.—The liver was reduced to a little more than a third of its natural size; it was of a very dark, almost black color, and internally soft and disorganized, like a mass of coagulated blood. The gall-bladder was empty and collapsed. The stomach and bowels contained a considerable quantity of black matter, similar to that which had been vomited, but were in other respects quite healthy.—*Diseases of the Stomach*, &c., 2d edition, p. 361.

2d. Softening and discoloration of the liver with partial suppression of bile may take place more slowly than in any of the cases related above, and the disease may prove fatal by inducing gradual exhaustion, without either delirium or hemorrhage. A case which appears to have been of this kind has been recorded by Andral (*Clin. Med.*, iv. p. 322).

3d. Fatal disorder of the brain, having the same character as in the preceding cases, and therefore probably produced in the same way, sometimes comes on in the course of jaundice arising from a mechanical impediment to the passage of the bile through the large ducts. An instance of this, recorded by Dr. Graves, has been cited in the preceding chapter; and another instance is exhibited in the following case, which has also been mentioned in the preceding chapter, in reference to a different subject:—

Henry Varley, fifty-three years of age, was admitted into King's College Hospital on the 2d of May, 1855. He had spent his life in London, latterly employed as a foreman of paviors, and acknowledged that for ten years he had drunk freely of spirits, but mostly in a diluted form. Two years before his admission he first had an attack of gout in the left great toe and left ankle, and since that time had had three other attacks, the last of which occurred in the beginning of the January preceding. He was just recovering from this attack, after a confinement of three days, when he felt one afternoon a sense of tightness, not amounting to actual pain, fixing itself in the hepatic and epigastric regions. He had for some time previously suffered a good deal of mental worry. In the course of the evening the sense of constriction increased to such a degree that, to use his own expression, he "could hardly bear himself." He felt, he said, very much as if a cord were drawn very tightly round his waist, below the ribs. The aggravation of pain appears to have been rather, but not very sudden. Concurringly with this he had some slight pain, not unlike that of rheumatism, referred to the right scapula. He had no sickness or nausea at the time, but felt as if his stomach were full of wind. The pain continued very severe for about eight hours, and then gradually subsided, ceasing altogether in about eight hours more. At the end of this time he found that he was jaundiced.

It appears that for some years he had repeatedly suffered slight attacks of the same constricting pain, but none of these former attacks had lasted more than an hour, and none of them were followed by jaundice.

Since the severe attack in January no fresh attack of severe pain had occurred, but the jaundice had continued, the motions were constantly clay-colored, and he had lost flesh considerably. The bowels, which, before the occurrence of jaundice, were very costive, had ever since been rather relaxed.

At the time of his admission to the hospital, when the jaundice had lasted about four months, he was rather thin, his face and body were of a deep dusky lemon color, and his conjunctiva were deeply tinged with bile. He had no pain, vomiting, or nausea, had a clean tongue, and a fair appetite, but did not eat much at a time, as the food, he said, lay heavy on his stomach. The bowels moved on an average twice a day, and the motions were always clay-colored.

The liver was found to be enlarged, reaching half way between the false ribs and the umbilicus, and its edge was felt to be thin. No tumor could be discovered, and there was no rigidity of the recti muscles.

There was no evidence of disease of the lungs, heart, or kidneys.

During the day, there was absence of fever—the pulse being usually under 70—but about 10 P. M. slight fever came on, which lasted great part of the night, and, while it lasted, prevented sleep.

He was ordered a mixture containing bismuth, hydrocyanic acid, and dill-water, to take before meals; and a dose of morphia, to take at night.

The diarrhœa was checked by these remedies, but in other respects the symptoms underwent no material change until the 14th of May, when he complained of pain in a small space in the situation of the gall-bladder, and an ill-defined swelling was remarked there, which suggested the suspicion that the gall-bladder was distended.

A small blister was applied over the painful space, and kept open for a long time. The swelling increased, notwithstanding, and the pain and tenderness became greater. He complained that if it were much handled the pain lasted for several hours.

From this time, the pulse became higher, being usually above 80 in the minute; feverishness, from which he was free in the day-time, constantly came on in the evening, and continued during great part of the night; and he evidently continued to lose flesh.

He complained of nothing except the tenderness and occasional pain in the vicinity of the gall-bladder, and the nightly accessions of fever: and often told us that if it were not for these ailments he should feel quite well.

On the 1st of June, in the evening, he felt a burning sensation in the stomach, and soon after vomited and brought up, as was reported, a great quantity of bile. After this he slept well, and the next morning felt refreshed, and was free from all pain and uneasiness, except a slight feeling of constriction across the stomach.

For a few days after this he had no feverish attacks at night, and slept well.

The fulness about the gall-bladder continued—he began to complain much of weakness, had often some nausea, and the pulse gradually got higher, being often from this time onward between 90 and 100. He complained occasionally of general pain and uneasiness in the back and loins.

On the 25th of June it was remarked that his legs were swelled from œdema.

Nothing else worthy of note happened till the evening of the 3d of July, when he had a severe attack of shivering, which lasted an hour. During the shivering he was slightly delirious, and the next day he lay in a dozing state, and ate nothing; the pulse was 100, and very weak. In the afternoon he vomited a dark-colored matter, consisting of altered blood. Vomiting recurred at intervals, he became unconscious, and, on the morning of the 6th, died in a state of coma.

On examination of the body there was found to be considerable ascites and some œdema of the legs. The fluid in the belly was considerably tinged with bile. The obstruction of the common gall-duct was caused by a tumor, the size of a small bean, which grew from the mucous membrane of the duct, about half an inch from its duodenal end, and completely blocked up the passage. An examination by the microscope led to the conclusion that this tumor was a simple wart-like growth, and not malignant. The liver was of a dark green. The gall-bladder was distended with dark-colored bile, and the hepatic gall-ducts were enlarged to ten times their natural size. As is usual in cases of long-continued obstruction of the common duct, the cells in the lobular substance were, for the most part, broken up; and scattered throughout the liver were small soft spots—from the size of a pin's-head to that of a pea—in which there appeared to be disintegration of the other tissues.

In the duodenum there was a large ragged ulcer, which was most probably the source of the blood vomited shortly before death. There was no ulceration elsewhere in the intestinal canal, and no disease worth noting was detected in other parts of the body.

In this instance, the jaundice resulted from obstruction of the common gall-duct by a wart-like body growing from the mucous membrane of the duct, near its duodenal end; but the disease did not prove fatal by gradual exhaustion—the usual mode of death in cases of permanent jaundice from obstruction of the common duct. About six months from the accession of the jaundice the patient has a severe rigor, and soon after becomes unconscious, vomits blood, and dies in a state of coma. After death there were found scattered throughout the liver small spots in which the hepatic tissue was softened and apparently disorganized. This circumstance and the mode of death, when considered in conjunction with the cases before related, favor the inference that the state of insensibility, ending in fatal coma, was owing to contamination of the blood by some poisonous matter generated by decomposition in the gland-structure of the liver, and that this case, though differing from the cases before related as regards the origin of the jaundice, resembled them in its result. The mental distress caused in susceptible persons by long-continued jaundice may exert the same kind of injurious influence on the liver, when it is already the subject of any disease, as mental anxiety from other causes occasionally does when the liver was previously sound.[1]

The softness and frangibility of the liver, noticed in so many of the preceding cases, does not depend on destruction of the secreting cells, but on the softness and frangibility of the vessels and other tissues of which the liver is made up. The cells, as has been seen in the preceding chapter, may be completely destroyed from permanent closure of the common gall-duct, and the liver may be small and flabby in consequence, but it will not necessarily be readily broken down or torn: and, on the contrary, the liver may be found after death unnaturally soft and frangible when the cells are entire, and when, up to the time of death, bile enough was secreted to prevent the occurrence of jaundice.

In a woman, who died under my care in King's College Hospital, in June, 1844, of tubercular peritonitis, all the upper part of the liver, thirty hours after death, when the body was examined, could be torn by the slightest effort, like a piece of rotten sponge. The portions near the lower edge were very much firmer. The liver was very large, and throughout of a yellowish-green; but there was no jaundice, and the only symptom that the liver was diseased was its large size, which it owed to the presence of a large quantity of oil.

Andral (*Clin. Med.*, iv. p. 320) has given the case of a man who

[1] I have met with several instances of jaundice, which I took to be of this kind coming on in young and sensitive persons affected with syphilis, and resulting, I imagine, from the mental distress which the primary disease occasioned.

died of phthisis, without jaundice or other symptom of disease of the liver, in whom the liver, which was rather large, was softened to an extreme degree—so that in many points it was a mere pulp.

In the kind of jaundice we have been considering, the shrinking of the liver, the small quantity of bile that passes into the intestine, and the small quantity of bile found in the gall-bladder and gall-ducts after death in the fatal cases, show clearly enough, what we have hitherto assumed, that the secretion of bile is greatly diminished, and that in some cases it ceases almost entirely before death occurs; and the question naturally arises—How does the coloring matter of the bile come in such cases to be present in the blood so as to cause jaundice? Two suppositions may be offered in explanation of the fact. One is, that the coloring matters of the bile are not all formed in the liver, as Lehmann and other physiologists have lately inferred, but that they are formed, at least in part, as a result of the processes of nutrition in other parts of the body; and, consequently, that when the liver ceases to eliminate them, they accumulate in the blood. The other supposition is, that the bile-pigment from which the jaundice results is formed in the lobular substance of the liver, but that, from the secretion being faulty and defective, instead of being taken up and carried away, as it should be, by the radicles of the gall-ducts, it is directly absorbed by the bloodvessels and lymphatics in the liver.

I have brought together from different sources the cases related in this chapter for the sake of showing that the secretion of bile may be suppressed, and the secreting substance of the liver be more or less disorganized in various circumstances, and without the occurrence of any process that we are warranted in designating *inflammation*. There is evidence enough to prove that this suspension of the secreting process and disorganization of the liver may result from various perturbing influences—some acting primarily through the nervous system, others through the blood. It may result from powerful and depressing emotions, or from long-continued anxiety or overwork, and probably from other more local causes of disturbance in the nervous system; and it may also result from some poison, introduced from without or engendered in the body by faulty degeneration or assimilation. It appears, too, that various poisons—pus, the poison of serpents, the poison of some forms of fever, and many others—may alike stop the secretion of the liver, and lead to the same kind of disorganization of its structure, while their other effects on the system are very different. These circumstances may serve to explain the different characters of the illness that attended the suppression of bile in the different cases related. They were many of them cases of essentially different diseases, and having merely this one effect, and the consequence of this effect in common.

Almost all the cases related in this chapter proved fatal; but it must not be inferred from this that jaundice resulting from suppressed secretion has necessarily, or indeed generally, a fatal issue. We collect the fatal cases because they are more impressive, and because an examination of the body after death gives us an assurance, which is wanting in other cases, that the jaundice was thus produced. When jaundice does not prove fatal, who can always pronounce positively that it resulted from defective secretion, and not from inflammation of the gall-ducts, or some other of the various conditions from which it may arise? Who, in many of the cases related above, could have said positively, before the fatal head symptoms occurred, that the jaundice resulted from suppressed secretion?

It has been clearly shown above that jaundice thus produced does not necessarily prove fatal, even after alarming cerebral disorder has come on; and that among many cases occurring at the same time and in the same place, and plainly the effect of the same condition, one or two may be rapidly fatal with the most malignant symptoms, while others may be mild.

There can, I think, be little doubt that in a large proportion of cases where jaundice occurs during youth or adolescence—when gall-stones and organic diseases of the liver are rare—the fault is in the secreting cells, and the jaundice results from suppressed or defective secretion.

The question then arises—How can the jaundice thus produced be distinguished from jaundice arising from temporary closure of the gall-ducts? When the jaundice immediately follows a powerful emotion in a person under the age of thirty, and when it comes on as a consequence of some known poisoning, or in conjunction with other symptoms indicative of a poisoned state of the blood, or where, as in the instances related by Dr. Griffin and Dr. Hanlon, it occurs with peculiar characters in several members of a family, or in several persons living together, in succession, it may confidently be assumed that the jaundice results from suppressed secretion.

In other cases, when the circumstances under which the disease occurs are less insignificant, it is often difficult to pronounce a positive judgment. But when jaundice presents the characters it had in many of the cases related above—when it occurs in a young person, who has lately been leading a dissolute life, or been exposed to depressing influences; when the liver, instead of being enlarged, as it is from many conditions that produce jaundice, appears to be *within its natural limits;* when, during the jaundice, the matters brought up by vomiting, or discharged by stool, are occasionally *bilious*, showing that the common bile-duct is not stopped; when the jaundice is attended with depression, and not with inflammatory symptoms—the probability is very great that the jaundice results from suppressed secretion.

When hemorrhage from the stomach or bowels occurs soon after the accession of the jaundice, or when delirium, or coma, or convulsions, supervene, we may be almost sure that the jaundice is thus produced, because these events seldom occur in jaundice that results from mere obstruction of the ducts.

Another circumstance that may help to distinguish the two forms of disease, is itching of the skin, which is generally much complained of in jaundice that results from mechanical closure of the gall-ducts, but not in that which results from suppressed secretion.

The presence or absence of pain does not give us much information, for there is generally some degree of pain or tenderness in jaundice from suppressed secretion, as well as in that which results from closure of the gall-ducts; but in inflammation of the gall-ducts, the tenderness is probably less diffused, and felt more exclusively in the situation of the common duct, which is open to pressure.

One of the surest signs of the existence of this kind of jaundice would be the diminution in the size of the liver, if it could be satisfactorily made out; but it is much more difficult to estimate diminution of the liver than enlargement. When the liver grows large, it extends below the false ribs and across the epigastrium, and can generally be felt through the yielding walls of the belly;

but when the liver shrinks from its natural size, its lower edge rises under the ribs, and changes in the bulk of the organ are difficult to detect. It is probable that the surest means of distinguishing this kind of jaundice will by and by be found in some peculiar condition of the urine. I have long suspected that the presence of oxalate of lime in the urine will turn out to be an important indication of it. In many cases of jaundice which I have supposed to be of this kind, the urine contained oxalate of lime, which disappeared from it as the jaundice went off. In more than one case of the kind, I have found in the urine, with the oxalate of lime, casts of the secreting tubules, or evidence of the rapid shedding of the epithelium of the secreting tubules of the kidney. But none of these cases have proved fatal, so that the real nature of the jaundice is, in some degree, doubtful.

Jaundice from suppressed secretion, even when unattended with fever, or with weakening disorder of the stomach or bowels, *very soon induces a state of great anemia;* and it seems to me to be much more common in summer than in winter, probably from the depressing influence of summer heat, or because noxious effluvia are then most rife.

Until more is known of the causes of this form of disease, and until its different varieties can be distinguished with more certainty, we cannot expect to have very satisfactory proof of the good or ill effects of particular plans of treatment.

A consideration of the foregoing cases leads, however, to the important and gratifying inference that in two or three of them the terrible head symptoms were prevented or removed, and the life of the patient saved, by active purging. If this inference be true, there can be little doubt that purgatives will generally be productive of benefit in milder cases of the same kind.

The medicine which has seemed to be the most generally useful of any that I have tried, in cases of jaundice which I have supposed to result from suppressed secretion, is from ʒss to ʒj of sulphate of magnesia, in conjunction with gr. xv of carbonate of magnesia, and ʒss of aromatic spirits of ammonia, given three times a day, an hour before food—the sulphate of magnesia to keep up free action of the bowels; the carbonate of magnesia to *neutralize any excess of acid in the stomach or bowels;* and the aromatic spirit of ammonia to support the nervous system and to promote the action of the skin. The ammonia may act, not only through the general nervous system, but also as a direct stimulant to the nerves of the liver itself.

In many instances in which there was absence of fever and the urine contained crystals of oxalate of lime, I have given, apparently with much advantage, the nitro-muriatic acid.

The circumstance that jaundice of this kind often results from depressing emotions, and that it is always attended with depression, suggests the propriety of encouraging the patient with the hope of speedy recovery, and thus removing the mental distress which the mere existence of jaundice sometimes occasions.

Where the patient is still able to walk about, he should carefully avoid fatigue, which is very soon induced, and has great influence in checking the secretion of the liver.

When the disorder results from anxiety or mental shock, it is of course very important that the nervous system should be restored by sound sleep, and all expedients that tend to promote this, and that do not act injuriously on the liver or on the system at large, must be beneficial.

I believe that in jaundice from suppressed secretion much harm is often done by the use of mercury, and that the remedies recommended above—aromatic spirits of ammonia, in conjunction with sulphate and carbonate of magnesia, and the invigorating stimulus of hope—will, if had recourse to in time, almost always prevent the occurrence of the fatal head symptoms, except when the suppressed secretion of bile results from the action of some terrible poison.

SECT. II.—*Fatty degeneration of the liver—Partial deposit of fat in the liver—Waxy liver—Appearances caused by deficiency of fat in the liver.*

IT has been before remarked that the size, and color, and firmness of the liver may be much altered without the agency of inflammation, and without destruction of the cells or impaired nutrition of its other tissues, simply from matter being secreted or appropriated by the cells, which, instead of passing off freely in the bile, is retained in the substance of the liver.

The most common disease of this class is what has been called the *fatty liver*, or *fatty degeneration of the liver*.

The outward characters of this disease have been long familiar to pathologists, and have been rightly ascribed to the interstitial deposit of uncombined fatty matter in the substance of the liver; but it was not known precisely in what state, or where, the fat was deposited, till 1841,[1] when Mr. Bowman discovered, in a specimen of very fatty liver which I requested him to examine with this intent, that it existed in the form of oil-globules in the hepatic cells.

In every human liver there is some uncombined oil or fat, which, in healthy grown-up persons, amounts, perhaps, on an average, to three or four per cent. of the whole mass.

In the spring of 1851, Dr. L. S. Beale was kind enough to make at my request an analysis of two livers presumed to be healthy. The first was that of a gentleman, 31 years of age, well formed and muscular, and above the middle stature, who had led a temperate life, and who, while in perfect health, was killed by falling from a second-floor window; the second was that of a schoolmistress, 40 years of age, who had lived well, but very temperately, and had enjoyed good health until an attack of cerebral hemorrhage, of which she died.

[1] See Lancet, January 22, 1842.

The following are the results of the analysis:—

	I.	II.
Water	68.58	72.05
Fatty matter[1]	3.82	4.28
Extractive, soluble in water and in alcohol; Extractive, soluble in water only, and albumen	10.07	10.40
Alkaline and earthy salts	1.50	1.19
Matter insoluble in water, alcohol, and ether	16.03	12.08
	100.00	100.00

Von Bibra, who has made an elaborate examination of the liver fats, has published the analyses of two livers presumed to be healthy: the first taken from a healthy young man, killed suddenly by a blow; the second taken from an itinerant, the nature of whose illness was unknown. The quantity of fatty matter they contained in 100 parts was 2.50 and 3.65 respectively.

The fatty matter of the liver, when separated by alcohol and ether, has always a brown color, and, according to Von Bibra, contains from one and a half to three per cent. of phosphorus. It consists chiefly of olein, which dissolves the more solid fatty principles; so that it has all the form of globules of oil. In consequence of this its presence is most readily detected by the microscope, through which it may be seen in the hepatic cells in the form of very small globules, having a dark outline. These globules are of various sizes, and are placed irregularly in the cells. Their usual appearance in the healthy liver is represented in Fig. 6 (p. 27).

In the fatty liver the quantity of fatty matter is enormously increased. The hepatic cells are gorged with large globules, which greatly distend them (see Fig. 8, p. 30); and usually a great number of oil-globules of various sizes, not contained in cells and probably set free by the rupture of cells, are likewise seen under the microscope.

In many of the cells thus gorged with oil the nuclei have disappeared or are rendered invisible by the oil-globules.

The quantity of oil in a liver in this state may equal in weight, and more than equal in bulk, all the other elements of the liver put together. M. Vauquelin obtained from a portion of fatty liver,

[1] The figures denoting fatty matter in these analyses were obtained by evaporating a portion of the liver over a water bath, then treating the dry powdered residue with successive portions of boiling ether, until nothing further was extracted, and, finally, weighing the matter left on evaporation of the ether.

by boiling, as much as 45 parts of oil in 100 of liver. Nearly half the liver, in weight, consisted of uncombined oil.

A liver still more remarkable for the large amount of fat it contained fell under my observation in King's College Hospital, in the spring of 1850. It was taken from a drunkard, and was in a state of cirrhosis, as well as of fatty degeneration, and in consequence presented a very remarkable "hob-nailed" appearance, from the nodules of cirrhosis being enlarged by the accumulation of oil. A portion of it blazed when thrown into the fire, and a particle from the lobular substance had under the microscope almost the appearance of ordinary fatty tissue, from the number and size of the oil-globules it contained. Dr. L. S. Beale made an analysis of a portion of it for me, and found that 65 parts in 100—about six-sevenths of all the *solid* matter in the liver—consisted of fat.[1]

The following are the particulars of the analysis :—

Water	24.930
Solid matter	75.070
Fatty matter, with a trace of extractive matter and salts	65.190
Fixed salts	.395
Animal matter and extractive	9.485
	100.000

The fatty matter consisted of saponifiable fats, the greater part of which was oily fat. The man had ascites and slight jaundice, but was reported to have died without medical attendance, after two days' illness. A coroner's inquest was in consequence held, and the body was carefully examined by the physician's assistant at the hospital. No tubercles existed in the lungs, and no organ

[1] The result of this analysis is so extraordinary, that I subjoin, in Dr. Beale's words, a statement of the method employed in making it :—

"A portion of the liver was evaporated to dryness, and then treated with a mixture of alcohol and ether. The solution thus obtained was evaporated to dryness, and the dry matter, which consisted of fat, with a little extractive matter and salts, was weighed. The residue, insoluble in alcohol and ether, was dried and weighed. It was attempted to separate the extractive matter and salts from the fat, by treating the mass with water, but, in consequence of the large quantity of fat, this proceeding was found not practicable. After the fats had remained for two or three days on the surface of the water, they separated into two portions : the lighter, yellow, oily, and perfectly fluid at the ordinary temperature ; the heavier, white, granular, opaque, and crystalline—the crystals forming dense, radiating, striated, globular masses."

was found notably diseased except the liver. The kidneys appeared to be healthy.

A liver that has undergone the fatty degeneration is larger, paler, softer, and more greasy than natural. These changes in its sensible qualities depend chiefly, if not solely, on the interstitial deposit of the oil-globules, and their degree may give us some estimate of the quantity of oil the liver contains. When this is very large, the liver is large in proportion, sometimes twice its natural size, and is somewhat altered in shape, being thicker than natural, and having its edges blunter or more rounded. The capsule of the liver is stretched and smooth, and, when divided, its edges recede. The tissue of the liver is pale, and, generally, throughout of a soft buff color, dotted with brown or red. The brown or red dots mark the centres of the lobules, which are unusually large and distinct, and are buff-colored near their margins. The liver is very soft, and greases the hands or the scalpel like common fat.

When the quantity of oil is less, the liver is not so large nor so soft, and is less uniformly pale. The cells near the margins of the lobules contain, as was, I believe, first observed by Mr. Gulliver, a much larger quantity of oil than those near the centres; and, as the blood almost always collects after death in the central parts of the lobules especially, there is a striking contrast between the pale buff-colored margins of the lobules and the red or brownish central portions. Sometimes more of the vessels forming the capillary network of the lobules are filled with blood, so that the red portion, instead of being in isolated spots, forms a continuous band connecting contiguous lobules (see Fig. 10, p. 37), and a section of the liver presents the appearance described as the *nutmeg*-liver. The liver may not feel greasy, but an unusual quantity of fat may be at once detected by placing a thin slice of the liver on a piece of paper and exposing it to the action of heat. Some of the oil or fat exudes, and greases the paper. The best way, however, of ascertaining the quantity of fatty matter is by examining a small particle of the lobular substance of the liver through the microscope. The oil-globules are objects of sight, and from their form and their dark outline are at once distinguished.

When the fatty degeneration occurs in a liver previously healthy, the different parts of the organ are commonly affected in pretty equal degree; but the existence of previous disease of the liver sometimes prevents the even distribution of the fat. When, indeed, an accumulation of fat takes place in what is termed the "scrofulous liver," where the lobules are infiltrated with a soft albuminous substance, the fatty matter is deposited very unevenly. The greatest quantity usually exists in the parts of the liver which are subject to the least pressure—namely, the left lobe, and towards the lower edge of the right; and in those parts the fat is deposited especially in the marginal portion of the superficial lobules, and in the lobules lining the portal canals, sometimes giving a distinct whitish or yellowish rim to the superficial lobules, and forming whitish lines along the portal canals; while in the upper part of the right lobe, which is compressed by the ribs, the liver may contain but little fat, and have the compact texture and the uniformity of aspect that characterize the scrofulous liver.

Few observations have been made on the bile secreted by the human fatty liver. That found in the gall-bladder after death is sometimes unusually pale, and, it is said, less bitter than natural (Andral, *Clin. Med.*, iv. p. 212; and Meckel, *Anatomie*, t. iii. p. 470); but it has generally the greenish or olive color proper to cystic bile. Not unfrequently, indeed, in persons dead of phthisis, with fatty liver (which is very apt to occur in this disease), the bile is unusually dark-colored and thick;[1] but this is doubtless owing to its having remained long in the gall-bladder and become concentrated, in consequence of the repugnance to food, and the empty state of the stomach and intestines, so common in the advanced state of phthisis.

An accumulation of fatty matter in the lobular substance of the liver, notwithstanding it so changes the appearance and other sensible qualities of the liver, causes no obvious derangement of health. There is no jaundice as the result of this condition, and the discharges from the bowels may be properly stained; there is no congestion of the veins that feed the vena portæ—no obstruction, therefore, to the circulation through the liver; no pain, or even tenderness. The absence of jaundice while the discharges from the bowels are properly stained, shows that the coloring matter of the bile is secreted, and passes off, as usual.[2] The absence of other

[1] See Louis, Recherches sur la Phthisie, 2ième édition, p. 122.

[2] In the fatty state of the liver artificially induced in ducks and geese, the proportion of sugar contained in the liver-tissue appears to be not diminished. Bernard

symptoms seems to depend on the softness of the oil-globules, and the readiness with which they change their form and yield to pressure; on their being deposited gradually and evenly, so as not to cause sudden stretching of the capsule of the liver; and on their having no tendency to excite inflammation of the capsule, or of the veins.

This fatty condition of the liver is not always, however, without manifest ill effects. When it exists in high degree, the liver, from its mere bulk, causes distension of the belly, and a sense of weight and fulness on turning in bed from the right side to the left; and sometimes, by compressing the pyloric end of the stomach or the upper part of the duodenum, it prevents the stomach from completely emptying itself, and thus causes vomiting and other gastric disorder, and leads to the enlargement of the stomach, which is so common in phthisis.

The liver becomes fatty in very different states of the body.

1st.—It is often fatty in persons who lead indolent lives, and are at the same time gross feeders—eating largely of fatty substances, and drinking freely of porter and other heavy malt liquors; and in such persons there is generally with the fatty liver an excess of fat under the skin, and in other parts of the body in which fat is usually deposited.

It is sometimes, as in an instance mentioned above, extremely fatty in men who take little exercise, and drink immoderately of ardent spirits.

The fattening effect of food depends much on climate, but in man, still more on individual peculiarities of constitution. Some persons can take no fatty substances without being disordered by them; others take them with apparent impunity, but still remain lean—the fat is not digested, or not assimilated; others, again, take them freely, and grow fat in consequence.[1] In our domestic ani-

found that the fatty liver of a duck contained 1.4 per cent. of sugar, while that of another duck in the ordinary state contained 1.27 per cent.—(*Leçons de Physiologie Expérimentale*, 1855, p. 126.

[1] Prout, Stomach and Urinary Diseases, 3d edition, p. 242. Some important remarks on these points, and valuable hints for future inquirers, will be found, in the chapter here referred to, in Dr. Prout's work; to which we are so deeply indebted for our knowledge of the various effects of faulty digestion and assimilation.

mals the fattening influence of fatty substances taken as food is far more constant. It was well exhibited in some experiments performed by Majendie, for the purpose of ascertaining the nutritive powers of different kinds of food. In one of these experiments, a dog was kept entirely on fresh butter, which it continued to eat, though not regularly, for sixty-eight days. "It then died of inanition, although remarkably fat. All the while the experiment lasted, the animal smelled strongly of butyric acid, its hair was greasy, and its skin covered with a layer of fat. On dissection, all the organs and tissues were found infiltrated with fat. The liver, to use the common phrase, was *fatty;* and, on analysis, it was found to contain a very large quantity of stearine, but little or no oleine. *It had acted as a kind of filter for the butter.*"

Many other experiments of the same kind were made with hog's-lard and other fatty substances, and with a like result. The dogs became loaded with fat, but their muscles wasted; in many the cornea sloughed; and, at length, they died of inanition. In all of them the liver was fatty.

Greasiness of the skin and the smell of butyric acid, which were remarked by Majendie in his dogs, may be likewise noticed in men who, from gross feeding and indolent lives, have their livers and other tissues loaded with fat. It has been rightly remarked by Rokitansky that the fatty condition of the liver in these men is attended with sallowness of the skin and with a greasy sweat of peculiar odor.

The fatty matter passes off by the skin, as well as by the liver, and in precisely the same way—through the agency of the secreting cells. In a state of health, the secreting cells of the sebaceous glands, like those of the lobules of the liver, contain small globules of oil. There can be no doubt that where the body is loaded with fat, the quantity of oil in the former cells, as well as in the latter, is enormously increased. This observation is important, because it gives optical proof that some of the matters eliminated by the liver may also be eliminated through the skin, and because it tends to impress on us the importance of attending to the skin in all cases in which the functions of the liver are deranged.

In the cases under consideration, it is clear that the liver is not primarily in fault, any more than the skin. Both of them are fulfilling their proper office in getting rid of an excess of fatty matter in the blood.

2d.—But the liver is often found fatty in persons dead of *phthisis*, who, instead of being loaded with fat are generally much wasted.

The frequency with which the liver undergoes this change in phthisis was, I believe, first pointed out by M. Louis, in his celebrated work on Phthisis, published in 1825. M. Louis there states that he had detected the fatty degeneration, by the altered look and feel of the liver, in 40 cases of phthisis out of 120—or, in one-third of the subjects he had examined.

It appears from his researches that this change in the liver, in pulmonary consumption, is irrespective of age, and equally frequent whether the consumption is rapid or lingering. The only condition which he ascertained to have a marked relation to its frequency is sex. It was nearly four times as frequent in the women he had examined as in the men. From his subsequent experience he was led to rate still higher the difference between the sexes in this respect. In the second edition of his work, published in 1843, he states that in twenty-four fatal cases of phthisis in men, which had come under his observation at the hospital *La Charité* since the publication of the first edition, the liver was not fatty once, while in thirty fatal cases in women it was fatty thirteen times.

These results have been confirmed by observations made in other countries.

Dr. Home, out of sixty-five persons who died of phthisis in the Edinburgh Infirmary, found the liver fatty in ten, and *waxy* in five others. These fifteen instances, with one exception, occurred in women.[1]

In twenty-three of these sixty-five cases the liver presented different forms of the early stage of cirrhosis. This condition, which is not noticed by Louis in his account of the morbid appearances in phthisis, is, no doubt, more common in Edinburgh than in Paris, in consequence of the habit of whiskey-drinking which prevails among the lower classes in Scotland. But it is probable that in some of the cases Dr. Home mistook the nutmeg appearance of the liver caused by the deposit of fat in moderate quantity for the early stage of cirrhosis. Making a trifling allowance for an error of this kind, it would appear that a fatty condition of the liver is just as frequent in persons dead of phthisis in Edinburgh as in Paris. Its relative frequency in different countries probably de-

[1] Lib. of Med., iv. 163.

pends in some degree on climate, national habits, and race; but no evidence has yet been collected showing the influence of these conditions.

Fatty degeneration of the liver in a high degree is not only frequent in phthisis, but, setting aside the persons in whom the liver is loaded with fat in common with the areolar tissue and other parts of the body in which fat is liable to be deposited, is almost peculiar to this disease. Frequently, indeed, in subjects dead of various diseases, an unusual quantity of fat is found in the liver, which is at once discovered by the microscope, and which may be detected by a practised eye, by merely looking at the liver, but the quantity of fat is seldom so great as to cause a very striking change in the appearance of the organ, except in persons dead of phthisis. M. Louis states that, in the course of three years, he met with forty-nine instances of fatty liver, and in forty-seven of these the patients were phthisical.

In speculating on the cause of this peculiar tendency to accumulation of fat in the liver in phthisis, it is important to remark that it does not depend on tuberculous disease of the liver itself. M. Louis states that there were no tubercles in the liver in any of the cases in which he found it fatty; and that in two cases in which there were tubercles in the liver, the liver was not fatty. He even infers that the one state may preclude the other, and cites in support of this opinion a remark made by M. Reynaud, in his essay on Phthisis in Monkeys—that although in the monkeys he dissected the liver very frequently contained tubercles, it was in no instance fatty. My own observation tends, in some degree, to confirm this remark. The natives of the South Sea Islands, when they come to this country, like the monkeys brought to Paris and London, are extremely liable to phthisis, and to the deposit of tubercles in many organs besides the lungs. I have found the liver and various organs studded with tubercles in several of these men who died in the Seamen's Hospital of phthisis; but in none of these instances did I remark that the liver was fatty.

It has been imagined that fatty matter accumulates in the liver in phthisis, in consequence merely of the office of the lungs being greatly and gradually interfered with—that hydro-carbonaceous matters, passing off in less quantity than natural through the lungs, are, in consequence, eliminated in larger quantity by the liver.

This opinion is rendered very improbable by the circumstance, that in organic diseases of the heart, and in asthma, where the office of the lungs is not unfrequently as much interfered with as in phthisis, the liver does not undergo this change. Still stronger refutation of it is afforded by the fact, noticed by Rokitansky, that fatty degeneration of the liver is found in conjunction with tuberculous disease of other organs—the mesentery, the serous membranes, the bones—when no tubercles exist in the lungs.

These facts show that we must seek the explanation of the fatty degeneration of the liver in phthisis in some other conditions than mere diminished function of the lungs.

It has been already remarked that the fatty condition of the liver, independent of excess of fat in other organs, is seldom met with in such degree as to cause a very striking change in the appearance of the liver, except in persons dead of phthisis. Now and then, however, the liver is just as fatty after other diseases, and we may naturally expect to find the conditions on which the accumulation of fat in the liver really depends in some points of resemblance which these exceptional cases bear to cases of phthisis. These exceptional cases demand, then, great attention in our present inquiry.

The most fatty liver that has fallen under my own observation for several years was that of a man who died in King's College Hospital, in April, 1844, at the age of thirty-six, of extensive cancerous ulceration of the groins.

He was a chimney-sweep, and had good health till about nine years before, when he noticed a pimple on the left side of the scrotum, which gradually grew larger. The pimple was cut out, and the wound healed. He then gave up chimney-sweeping, and became a coal-porter, and from this time enjoyed good health till February, 1843, when another pimple, like that which had been cut out, appeared on the opposite side of the scrotum. He was admitted into St. Bartholomew's Hospital, where this tumor also was removed. The wound healed, as after the former operation. About a month after this the glands in the right groin enlarged and became painful, and shortly afterwards suppurated and burst, leaving a ragged deep ulcer in the course of Poupart's ligament. A glandular swelling soon appeared in the left groin, and burst, leaving a similar ulcer, but less extensive. In this state he was admitted into King's College Hospital, under Mr. Partridge, on the 14th of

September, 1843. He was then much emaciated, and his liver was felt to be enlarged. His complexion was somewhat dusky, but not sallow. He had no cough or difficulty of breathing. His appetite was very good, and he was free from thirst. He was ordered full diet, with a pint of porter; and a watery solution of opium was applied to the ulcers. The ulcers gradually spread till they were of frightful extent; but even then his appetite continued tolerably good. He gradually sank, and died on the 8th of April. Sweating is not mentioned in the notes that were taken of his case.

The liver was very large and very *thick*, and throughout of a pale buff color, from extreme fatty degeneration. It greased the scalpel, and under the microscope the hepatic cells were found gorged with oil-globules. The bile also contained a great number of oil-globules, visible under the microscope, together with distinct particles of greenish coloring matter. The capsule of the liver presented no trace of inflammation. Except this change in the liver, there was no disease but the frightful ulceration of the groins. There were no cancerous tumors in any of the viscera. The lungs were congested, but otherwise perfectly healthy.

A case, in some respects similar, is recorded by Cruveilhier, in which a high degree of fatty degeneration was found in conjunction with disseminated melanotic cancer, and with a large psoas abscess that resulted from caries of the lumbar vertebræ.

CASE.—The patient, a woman thirty years of age, was brought into the Hôtel Dieu, in a state of extreme exhaustion, and died the next day.

Cruveilhier has given a plate representing the front of the body, which was thickly studded with melanotic tubercles in or under the skin. There were also a great number of gray melanotic tumors in the lungs and in the mesentery; many adhering to the kidney, and in the areolar tissue about it; many along the iliac and hypogastric arteries and veins. There was likewise an enormous medullary tumor, growing from the sacrum, which filled the cavity of the true pelvis, but all the organs of the pelvis were sound. In the upper, or expanded portion of the pelvic cavity there was a very large abscess, under the iliac fascia. The matter of this abscess came from the last lumbar vertebræ, which were carious. It extended in the sheath of the psoas muscle as low as the little trochanter. The liver was yellow, and had undergone complete fatty degeneration (*avait passé complètement au gras*), but contained no cancerous tumors. (Liv. xxxii. pl. 3.)

This case presents many striking points of resemblance with the cases of phthisis in which the liver is fatty. The patient was a woman, and much emaciated. From this last circumstance, and from the wide dissemination of cancerous tumors, it may safely be inferred that she was in a state of cancerous cachexy, and probably subject to the profuse sweating common in this state. Lastly, the liver was completely fatty, but, what is very unusual when cancer is so widely disseminated, contained no cancerous tumors.

In the following case, which I have copied from Dr. Bright's Hospital Reports, fatty degeneration of the liver was found in conjunction with chronic dysentery, which had led to the perforation of the lower part of the large intestine, and the consequent formation of a large abscess behind it:—

CASE.—A. B., a young man about twenty-eight years of age, originally stout, vigorous, and active, who had been regular in his diet and very temperate in the use of wine and other fermented drinks, but had frequently been the subject of syphilis. Some years before his death he labored under a dysenteric affection, on the subsidence of which his bowels became habitually constipated. This state appeared to be in part attributable to a stricture of the rectum, which was felt at no great distance from the anus; a bougie was passed, and a considerable dilatation of the stricture was effected. His health continually declined, and symptoms of stricture higher up in the intestine became evident. An abscess was formed just above the crista of the ileum posteriorly, which, on its opening, proved to have communication with the intestine. Pain was felt in the upper part of the left iliac region. Leeches were applied, and their bites produced sinuous ulcers. He had no cough, or obvious chest affection; latterly, he had some diarrhœa, and wasted rapidly.

The head was not opened. There was some old pleuritic adhesion on the left side, but none on the right. The lungs and heart were quite healthy. In the left iliac region the intestines were glued together by peritoneal adhesions, and firmly bound down on the iliacus internus muscle. The cellular membrane below the peritoneum was very firm and much thickened. The mucous membrane of the stomach was free from rugæ, rather firm, and not easily separated from the subjacent coat; towards the cardia it was of a diffused dusky livid color; that of the duodenum was pale, but its mucous glands were enlarged; that of the rest of the small intestines was tolerably healthy. The same was the case with the first part of the large intestines; but in the sigmoid flexure of the colon, and more particularly in the lower part of it, there were numerous traces of old ulcerations; these were of a lightish leaden color, of an uneven surface; and the structure of the intestine at this part was thickened and condensed, and its calibre greatly contracted; there were three or four small perforations through the intestine at this part. Inside, the last part of the colon and the whole of the rectum appeared healthy; but a little above the anus there was a decided thickening with induration. This evidently depended on an old ulcer, which had occupied about half an inch of the intestine. Like those of the colon, it exhibited a leaden hue, an uneven surface, an apparent deficiency of the mucous coat, and thickening of the subjacent structure. The *liver* was remarkably enlarged, and of a yellowish-brown color; it was very exsanguine, and had universally undergone the fatty degeneration. It felt soft and plastic under the fingers, soiled the clean blade of a scalpel which was thrust into it, and yielded an oily fluid on the application of heat. The gall-bladder was small and contained no bile, but a little dirty-colored somewhat puriform mucus. The patient, however, had some bilious vomiting but a few days before his death. The spleen was of moderate size and firm, and the kidneys were healthy. (*Bright's Reports*, vol. i. p. 117.)

In the spring of 1844 Mr. Busk sent me a portion of liver extremely fatty, taken from a lad aged seventeen, who died of chronic dysentery. The lad was much emaciated, but had no disease of the lung, other than recent bronchitis. He died a few days after he was brought to the hospital, and, while under treatment there, had no sweating.

In the autumn of 1843 I found a very fatty liver in a woman who died in King's College Hospital of gray hepatization of the left lung. Her illness lasted a month, and towards the end she had much hectic and sweating. There were no tubercles.

It is stated by MM. Biett and Rayer, that a fatty condition of the liver is very common in persons with chronic pemphigus—persons almost invariably very low in condition.

It would seem from these instances that the fatty condition of the liver so common in phthisis does not result from the office of the lung being interfered with, or from the presence of tuberculous matter in any particular organ, but rather that it is connected in some way with the general constitutional disturbance—the abundant suppuration, the wasting, the hectic—so common in advanced stages of phthisis.

The opinion was many years ago advanced by the late Baron Larrey, that the fatty condition of the liver in these cases results from solution of the fat previously laid up in the body. He considered this opinion strongly supported by the method then employed in France to make the livers of geese fatty, and of which he gives the following account: "To procure the large livers of geese for the making of patties, fatted birds are confined in close cages, and then exposed to a graduated heat, being kept at the same time entirely without food, even without water. They become feverish, the fat undergoes a kind of fusion, and the liver grows enormously large. The liver is considered to be in the desired state when the animal is *extremely wasted*, and the fever increases."[1]

It is quite clear that if the liver be rendered fatty in this way, the fat which accumulates in it is derived from that previously laid up in the body. It is extremely probable that the same thing happens in phthisis, and in the other wasting diseases in which fatty degeneration of the liver occurs in man: that, in the process of wasting, the fat stored up in the body is largely taken up by the veins, so that it comes to be in excess in the blood, and is then laid hold of by the hepatic cells, which have a natural affinity for it.

If this opinion be correct, it follows that in this class of cases, as in those before spoken of, the liver is not primarily in fault, any more than the kidneys are in fault in saccharine diabetes. In certain states of the system the liver eliminates an unusual quantity of fat, just as in certain other states the kidneys eliminate sugar. But the fat in the liver, being in the form of large oil-globules, which are perhaps only slowly dissolved in the bile, is long pent up in the close meshes of the capillary network of the liver, and of course adds to the size of the liver, and alters its texture—while sugar, from its solubility and from the large quantity of water secreted with it, is at once carried out of the system, and may leave the kidneys unaltered.

When oil has accumulated in the liver beyond a certain amount, it probably impedes the proper action of the liver and lessens the secretion of bile; but in cases of phthisis, when the liver is fatty—if we may judge from the usual clearness of complexion, and from the appearance of the intestinal discharges, and from the fact that the bile found in the gall-bladder after death is often dark green or olive-colored—bile continues to be secreted in considerable quantity, and the oil in the liver offers no impediment to its escape

[1] Baron Larrey was a native of the South of France, and the account cited above was probably derived from personal observation: but at present, as far as I can learn, there is in the fattening of ducks and geese in France only one method employed—which consists in keeping the birds in a dark place, with little space to move in, and in cramming them with a paste of maize or some other farinaceous food, allowing them water to drink at will. Under this treatment there is at first a general increase of fat in the body: but when the fat stored up throughout the body has reached a certain amount, the further increment of fat appears to be deposited chiefly in the liver, which soon passes into the fatty state that is so much prized. The color of the fat in any particular bird varies with the color of the maize on which it was fattened.

through the ducts. The liver seems, at least at first, not to be in fault, but to be merely performing its allotted task in withdrawing an excess of fatty matter from the blood. The question then comes to be, Why is the fat taken up by the blood in such quantity in phthisis as to be present in great excess in that fluid? If it be to serve as fuel for respiration, why is not the liver fatty in all chronic diseases which prove fatal by slow emaciation? Why does the liver become fatty so much more frequently in women affected with phthisis than in men? As yet no satisfactory answers have been given to these questions.[1]

But although in the class of cases already considered the liver may not be primarily in fault, it is probable that fat may also accumulate in the liver, as in other organs, from local causes—causes affecting directly the nutrition of the part.

It now and then happens that a very small portion of the liver—the size, it may be, of a walnut—is completely fatty, while the rest of the organ is quite sound. In the year 1843, when my attention was directed to this subject, I met with three instances of this. One was in a portion of liver sent me by Mr. Busk, taken from a man who died in the Seamen's Hospital with enormous cavities in the lungs, which were probably tuberculous. The only morbid appearance on the surface of the portion of liver sent me was a pale drab-colored spot, the size of a shilling. When this was sliced across, a portion of the liver immediately beneath, as large as a walnut, with an irregular outline, was found to be of the same pale color, contrasting strongly with the color of the rest of the liver, and completely fatty. The appearance of this portion was precisely like that of extreme fatty liver in phthisis; and under the microscope the hepatic cells were seen to be filled to bursting with oil, while the cells in the rest of the liver had scarcely more oil than natural. There was another spot in the same state and about the same size in a different part of the liver.

The second instance was in the liver of a woman who died in King's College Hospital of diseased heart. She was reported to have drunk freely of spirits. At the surface of the left lobe, near the suspensory ligament, was an irregular portion, the size of a

[1] The greater frequency of fatty liver in women may be partly accounted for by the circumstance that women are, in general, fatter than men.

small walnut, soft, and of a pale yellow color, in strong contrast with the color of the other portions. The cells in this pale portion were gorged with oil-globules; in the rest of the liver they were healthy. In another portion of the left lobe there was some atrophy, and the surface was slightly puckered, from obliterated branches of the portal vein.

The third instance was in a girl, aged 20, who died also in King's College Hospital, of chorea. The capsule of the liver was united to the diaphragm and the abdominal parietes by threads of old false membrane. On the surface of the liver were two or three pale spots, like those before described, of about the same size, and having the same irregular outline. Under the microscope, the hepatic tissue forming these spots exhibited a few cells gorged with oil-globules, and an immense number of free oil-globules. Throughout, the liver contained more oil than natural. In these two last cases, there was no tuberculous disease of the lung. From the fat being deposited so partially, and from the presence of marks of former inflammation of the liver, we are perhaps justified in inferring that the complete fatty degeneration resulted here, not so much from general or constitutional causes as from some local cause affecting the nutrition of the parts in which it occurred.

In other parts of the body, in persons even much emaciated, accumulations of fat are often found in wasted parts, especially where a certain form must be preserved for the due exercise of their functions. This is especially the case with the heart.[1] Fat is almost always found about the heart in persons above the age of infancy, gradually increasing in quantity as the two sides of the heart become more unequal in bulk. This fat, as Mr. Paget has shown, serves a mechanical purpose, and allows the different cavities to assume readily the changes of volume and position, which the entrance of the blood and its forcible expulsion require. In phthisis, where the muscles of the heart, like other muscles, waste, and where the fat of most parts of the body disappears, an unusual quantity of fat is sometimes deposited about the heart;[2] in obedience, it would seem, to the law which determines the deposit of fat about

[1] For an account of the manner in which fat is deposited about the heart, see an elaborate paper by M. Bizot, in the first volume of Mémoires de la Société Médicale d'Observation.

[2] For an account of the fatty state of the heart in phthisis, See Louis *sur la Phthisie*, second edition, pp. 61 and 63.

the heart in health, as, by the progress of age, the inequality of the two sides of the heart increases.

Accumulation of fat about the heart, in phthisis, is associated with accumulation of it in the liver. Like the latter, it is almost exclusively met with in women, and is seldom found in persons who die of other wasting diseases. In phthisis, as in the process before described, that was formerly employed to make the livers of geese fatty, the fat previously laid up in the body seems to be absorbed by the vessels in greater quantity than is requisite to combine with the oxygen inhaled. The excess of fatty matter thus present in the blood is, in part, eliminated by the glands destined to excrete fat; in part, deposited about the heart, where, from the wasting of other tissues, an additional quantity of it seems to be required to serve an important mechanical purpose, and where forces have been placed which strongly favor its accumulation to the extent requisite for that purpose. The difficulty that before presented itself meets us again here. Why does the fat laid up in the body become absorbed, so as to be in excess in the blood, in phthisis, and not also in other chronic diseases equally wasting?

The bones of persons very advanced in life always contain a large quantity of oil, which accumulates in them (as the vascular part of their structure shrinks), it would seem, for no other end than to occupy space.

Another situation in which fat accumulates, and apparently for the same end—to occupy space—is under the integument of the belly in women who have had many children. In a woman who died in King's College Hospital, in the autumn of 1842, of stricture of the pylorus, although the body generally was *extremely emaciated*, there was a layer of fat, an inch thick, on the abdominal muscles. Andral, from the observation of similar facts, was led to imagine that the fatty state of the liver in phthisis might result from atrophy of its proper tissues. (*Clin. Med.*, iv. p. 174.) There is, at present, no evidence to support this opinion.[1] The liver becomes fatty without any previous diminution of size; and the accumulation of fat, so far from being intended merely to fill up a void, may go on till the natural volume of the liver is doubled.

[1] This opinion is likewise advanced by Dr. Thompson, in an excellent article on Diseases of the Liver, published in the Library of Medicine. (*Lib. of Med.*, vol. iv. p. 190.)

It is probable, however, that in some of the cases in which fat is found in less quantity, or in parts only of the liver, the fat may merely take the place of other tissues.

But occasionally fat is deposited in great quantity in particular parts from causes that affect their nutrition without previous wasting of their proper structure, and where no beneficial mechanical purpose seems to be answered by it. This frequently happens in the neighborhood of cancer. Cancerous tumors of the breast, and cancerous glands in the axilla, are often surrounded by a large quantity of fat. The frequent accumulation of fat about cancer has been particularly noticed by Cruveilhier, who has given a striking instance of it in a case of colloid cancer of the stomach with cancerous tubercles in the mesentery. (Liv. 27, Pl. 3, p. 1.)

In examining the bodies of sailors who have died much reduced by chronic dysentery, I have been often much struck with the large quantity of fat in the *appendices epiploicæ*, and elsewhere in the neighborhood of the diseased intestine. In the dissections of persons dead of chronic dysentery, related by Annesley, in his work on the diseases of India, a fatty condition of the omentum is also frequently noticed.

An unusual quantity of fat is sometimes found about a diseased joint; but this perhaps results, in part, from wasting of the adjacent muscles.

Fat is sometimes deposited in the liver, in the same partial manner, about other disease, especially cancer. The hepatic tissue just round a cancerous tumor has often a nutmeg appearance from containing an unusual quantity of fat, and not unfrequently is for a short distance, completely fatty, when, in other parts of the liver, fat does not exist in sufficient quantity to produce any striking changes.

In all the cases in which I have yet ascribed fatty degeneration of the liver to local causes affecting the nutrition of the part, the accumulation of fat has been partial. It may be, however, that the entire organ may be damaged by some acute disease, or in other ways, and may become fatty in consequence. I strongly suspect that this happens in yellow fever and in the severe bilious remittents of tropical climates. These fevers greatly disturb the secreting function of the liver, and without leaving any permanent marks of inflammation, and apparently without exciting inflammation at all, may permanently alter its condition. It often happens that the office of the liver is not adequately performed for the future, and that years after, when the person dies, perhaps from some disease quite independent of this, the liver is found unusually pale. The pale color of the liver depends, I imagine, on fat, which is not present, however, in such quantity as to increase the size of the liver and to cause the striking appearance of the extreme fatty liver in phthisis. It is not unlikely that long courses of mercury, and other medicines that directly affect the nutrition of the liver, may, now and then, have a similar result.

Hitherto we have considered merely the ordinary form of fatty liver, in which the fatty matter consists chiefly of olein. Various forms of fatty matter—olein, margarin, cholesterine—have been found in human bile; and it might have been expected, therefore, that the deposit in the liver would occasionally consist mainly of the more solid forms of fat. It has been proved that in some animals kept exclusively on fatty substances, the fatter matter may be deposited in the form of stearin. In the dog that Majendie kept exclusively on fresh butter for sixty-eight days, the liver was found, on analysis, to contain a large quantity of stearin, but little or no olein. But no analogous observations have been made on man. The relative proportions of the different kinds of fat in the liver are difficult to ascertain by chemical analysis, and cannot be discovered, even approximately, by the microscope, because the solid fats, though microscopic objects, and readily distinguishable when separate, are soluble in olein, so that all the fat in the liver appears as globules of oil. In examining fatty livers under the microscope, I have, however, occasionally seen within some of the oil-globules a crystallized mass, like a small star, which probably consisted of margarin;[1] but have never observed a scale of cholesterine, and am not aware that an interstitial deposit of cholesterine has ever been seen in the substance of the liver. This is the more remarkable, as cholesterine, which seems to be a normal constituent of bile, forms a very definite microscopic object, and is often found in large quantity in the gall-bladder in the form of gall-stones, or in glistening scales floating in the cystic bile.

[1] In most animal fats, stearin and margarin exist together; but human fat contains no stearin.

In the fatty degeneration of the *gall-bladder*, considered in a former chapter, cholesterine is generally secreted in very large quantity by the diseased coats of the bladder.

Now and then a liver is enormously enlarged and thickened, and its lower edge is rounded, as in the common fatty liver, evidently from the interstitial deposit of some foreign matter; but its substance is more compact than that of the common fatty liver, and does not feel greasy, and the cut surface is somewhat glistening, and occasionally has a rich yellow color from the retention of bile. These characters are well expressed by the epithet "waxy," which has been applied by many pathologists to livers in this state. This condition of the liver, like the common fatty degeneration, comes on gradually, often without pain or other striking symptom of hepatic disease, and the liver presents no marks of inflammation on its capsule. All these points of resemblance between the "waxy" liver and the "fatty" liver have led Laennec,[1] and many pathologists since his time, to consider the former to be a mere variety of fatty liver, caused by the deposit of the more solid forms of fat. Such may, in some instances, be the case; but in the most striking examples of "waxy" liver which I have met with, the foreign matter in the liver was *albuminous*, and not fatty. They were examples, not of fatty degeneration, but of what may be termed, from the most common cause of the condition, the *scrofulous* enlargement—a condition which forms the subject of the next chapter.

Our knowledge of the frequency of fatty degeneration of the liver in phthisis enables us often to discover it during the life of the patient. In a woman laboring under phthisis, considerable enlargement of the liver, without jaundice or ascites, or much pain or tenderness, is evidence enough, especially when she has been of temperate habits, that the liver is fatty. But as this condition of the liver usually causes but little inconvenience in itself, and as the disease with which it is associated is generally fatal, it is not an object of treatment.

When the liver becomes fatty from gross feeding and indolent habits, the excess of fat will, doubtless, disappear from it, as from other parts, on the person adopting an opposite mode of life. If he will rise early, take active exercise, live chiefly on lean meat,

[1] See Traité de l'Auscultation, tom. ii. p. 36.

with plenty of salt, and drink water, and will abstain from butter, bacon, oil, beer and other fermented drinks, and not eat too largely of sugar and starch,[1] he will not only get rid of much of his fat, but generally his muscles will be better nourished, and his strength be increased.

There are some states of the system in which the quantity of fat in the liver, instead of rising above the standard of health, falls much below it. One of these states is diabetes. In advanced stages of diabetes, scarcely a particle of true fat can be found in the limbs, in the cavity of the belly, or even about the heart.[2] The brain, too, is generally somewhat shrunk, probably from deficient supply of fatty matter to repair its waste; and the oil-globules in the liver are few and small. As excess of fatty matter renders the liver large, and pale, and soft, and the individual lobules large and distinct, a deficiency of it must tend to produce contrary effects. Where the cells contain but little oil, and are small, or fewer in number than they should be, the lobules of the liver, unless they are distended by some other foreign matter, are usually small and indistinct, and a cut surface of the liver is smooth and uniformly red. The whole liver is, of course, small in proportion to the small size of the individual lobules, and its lower edge is thin and sharp. In the scrofulous disease of the liver, to be noticed in the next chapter, the liver likewise contains an unusually small quantity of fat; but in this disease, as has been before observed, the liver attains a very large size, and its lower edge is rounded, as in the common fatty liver, from the interstitial deposit of foreign matter of a different kind.

[1] Starch and its chemical equivalents contribute directly to the formation of fat, and furnish besides a material for respiration soluble in the blood, and more readily acted on by oxygen than the insoluble fat, which is thus protected, and laid up in the system. Alcohol has a still stronger protecting power, for similar reasons.

[2] See Observations by Dr. Percy, in the Medical Gazette, April 7, 1843.

SECT. III.—*Scrofulous enlargement of the liver, and other kindred states.*

A CONDITION, resembling the fatty liver in many respects, but differing from it in the character of the matter deposited in the liver, is sometimes met with in persons who have long suffered from scrofulous disease, *especially of the bones*, and may be described as the *scrofulous enlargement* of the liver.

In the spring of 1844, I had an opportunity of examining a very striking specimen of this disease obtained from a boy who was a patient of my brother, Dr. William Budd, of Bristol, from whom I procured the following brief notes of the boy's illness:—

CASE 1.—The boy had suffered many years from scrofulous disease of the hip, and pieces of bone had come away through permanent fistulous openings. About six months before his death he became dropsical. There was general anasarca, but dropsy of the belly predominated, and, on account of this, he was tapped three times. After tapping, the ascites returned very rapidly to the same degree as before. There never was any jaundice. There was great emaciation at last, but it came on very slowly. Throughout the illness very little fever had existed; and the appetite continued good up to a late period. The urine was of low sp. gr., and much loaded with albumen. The boy had been always sickly, and in consequence much indulged by his parents; having been allowed, among other things, to drink, for a child, large quantities of beer.

The liver was immensely enlarged, its edges were rounded, and its peritoneal coat was remarkably smooth and tense, from stretching. When the liver was sliced, the cut surface was smooth, presenting no appearance of lobules. It was of a very pale red, mottled by white lines and spots. The pale red portions were of close uniform texture, and semi-transparent, having much the look of bacon-rind; the white lines and spots were opaque. The opaque white matter consisted almost entirely of fat. Under the microscope, it exhibited a mass of large oil-globules—some free, others in hepatic cells. In the interior of the liver the fatty matter was deposited chiefly along the small twigs of the portal and the hepatic veins, forming very distinct white lines. Near the surface it was in greater quantity; and in this portion of the liver some lobules were completely fatty, and large and very distinct to the eye, as in ordinary fatty degeneration. In the pale semi-transparent portions the hepatic cells were distinct, and contained no oil-globules at all. No other objects were visible. The fat was not in sufficient quantity to cause the great increase in the size of the liver, and the liver contained hardly any blood.

It was clear that the increased size of the liver and the semi-transparency resulted from some peculiar matter deposited in the lobules—in the cells or between them. After the fat was dissolved out with ether, the tissue of the liver had still a very peculiar appearance—in many parts the compact, uniform aspect of bacon.

On the surface of the peritoneum covering the intestines there was a deposit of granular lymph, having much the appearance of the semi-transparent granulation of tubercle, the result probably of inflammation of the peritoneum set up by the "tappings."

Several of the bronchial glands were tuberculous, and there was one encysted tubercle in the left pleura; but there were no tubercles in the substance of the lungs.

The kidneys were in a state of granular degeneration.

Here the liver was immensely enlarged, and its capsule stretched, from an accumulation, not of oil, but of some other matter, which rendered the organ pale, almost effaced the appearance of lobules, and gave to great part of its substance the close uniform texture and the semi-transparency of bacon-rind. Notwithstanding these remarkable changes, there was very little fever, the appetite continued good, and there was no jaundice.

The scrofulous disease of the hip had existed many years, but there is no evidence to show when the disease of the liver came on. The circumstance that there was very little fever and no jaundice, and the immense size of the liver, tend, however, to show that the enlargement was very gradual; and the predominance of ascites over other dropsy, six months before death, would alone render it probable that disease of the liver then existed. Other cases of the same kind, to be presently related, leave little doubt that it existed long before that time.

It will be remarked that the kidneys were diseased as well as the liver; and, from the occurrence of general dropsy, there can be little doubt that they were diseased at least six months before death. All that was noted respecting them is, that they were in a state of granular degeneration; but a more minute examination of the kidneys made in one or two of the subsequent cases renders it probable that the foreign matter choking the gland was like that in the liver, and somewhat peculiar in kind.

In November, 1844, I had an opportunity of examining a more remarkable specimen of the disease, taken from a woman who died in St. Peter's Hospital, Bristol, under the care of my brother, Dr. Wm. Budd. The following are notes of the case:—

CASE 2.—The patient was a single woman, rather above thirty, who at the time of her death had been about twelve months in St. Peter's Hospital for scrofulous *caries* of the metatarsal bones of both feet, and of one ankle-joint. She had several scrofulous sores besides, but there was no enlargement of the glands of the neck or groin. At the time of her admission to the hospital, it was discovered that her liver nearly filled the belly. All that was recorded of her former history is, that she had been living for several years in London—it was believed on the town, though she would not confess as much; that she had been intemperate there; and that it was there her health broke down.

Throughout her illness there was no ascites or other dropsy; and she appeared to die, at length, from the mechanical effects of the enormous enlargement of the liver. For the last fortnight of her life she could retain nothing on her stomach.

The *liver*, which was nine pounds in weight, occupied the whole belly, and a great part of the chest, especially on the right side, where it rose to the third rib.

In consequence of this, the right lung, which was universally adherent, was compressed into a space not much bigger than one's hand; the heart was displaced, and lying quite across the chest; and the greater part of the stomach was in the pelvis.

On the right lobe there was a large space which had been formerly the seat of peritonitis; and the gall-bladder was distended with rather thick, dark olive-colored bile.

The substance of the liver did not burn or grease paper, and was compact and tough, having much the appearance of yellow wax.

On microscopic examination, the cells were found to be for the most part imperfect, their outline being more or less irregular, and to contain oil-globules and a much more coarsely granular matter than is contained in normal cells. Beside the cells was seen a granular matter (the granules being of very irregular form and size), and a quantity of oil.

From the "waxy" appearance of the liver, I thought that it probably contained some solid form of fatty matter, and requested Professor Miller to analyze a portion of it for me. He found that a small proportion of yellow oily fat could be extracted by digesting thin slices of the liver in ether; but that the foreign matter to which the liver owed its large size was not fatty, but *albuminous*. The albumen was not in a soluble form, as cold water merely took up a portion of albumen, such as might have been expected from the serum contained in the gland.

The *spleen* was of an enormous size, and there were extensive adhesions between it and the diaphragm.

The *kidneys* were in an early stage of granular degeneration.

The greater part of the stomach, as has been already observed, was in the pelvis. Its cardiac end was singularly drawn out into a tube, nearly as narrow as the œsophagus. The intestine, and especially the colon, was very much contracted.

In the summit of each lung there was a tuberculous deposit, about the size of a walnut, not yet broken down, and having no active disease about it.

The heart was somewhat enlarged, but had no valvular disease. There were no tubercles in the mesentery or intestines.

In this case, as in the last, the patient had long suffered from scrofulous *caries;* and the liver was enormously enlarged by the accumulation of an albuminous matter in its substance.

The history of the case, incomplete as it is, and the enormous size of the liver, make it certain that the enlargement had been coming on for a long time.

It is remarkable that, notwithstanding the liver was so changed, in size and texture, no pain in the side was noted, there was no ascites, and bile was secreted to the last. After death, indeed, the gall-bladder was found *distended* by thick olive-colored bile.

Great enlargement of the liver was known to have existed for at least twelve months, but it was only when the body was examined that it was discovered that the kidneys were likewise diseased.

The appearance of the kidneys, which was taken for the early stage of granular degeneration, and the absence of dropsy, render it probable that the kidneys became diseased only a short time before death.

In November, 1848, I witnessed a striking instance of the same disease in a young man who died in King's College Hospital, under the care of Mr. Partridge, with scrofulous disease of the bones, and tubercles in the left lung. The following particulars of the case were recorded:—

CASE 3.—John Shaw was admitted into King's College Hospital, under Mr. Partridge, in 1846, with numerous small abscesses in the left arm—the result, he imagined, of a fall he had not long before. He was a native of London, had never had very good health, and was then nineteen years of age.

Portions of the *radius* were removed by Mr. Partridge, and Shaw left the hospital. The discharge from fistulous openings in the arm continued, and two years afterwards, on the 28th of June, 1848, he again came into the hospital under Mr. Partridge.

At that time, in addition to the disease of the arm, there was a small circular wound in the left side of the chest, and an abscess on the side of the great toe of the left foot.

After staying in the hospital a few days, he was sent to the Margate Infirmary.

On the 19th of November, not having received any benefit from his visit to Margate, he was taken again into the hospital; and it was then observed that he had marked symptoms of phthisis, and that his liver filled the whole abdomen.

On the 25th of November he died. There had been no jaundice. At the time of death the left leg was puffy, but there was no ascites or dropsy of other parts of the body.

The *liver* was enormously enlarged, extending down to the crest of the ilium, over all the viscera of the abdomen, and was much thickened. There was no contraction of the surface, and no mark of inflammation on the capsule. The substance was paler than usual, and contained very little blood. It was not *indurated*, as in cirrhosis, and a considerable quantity of serous fluid could be squeezed out of it, which coagulated on the application of heat and nitric acid.

The cut surface presented only faint traces of lobules, and had a uniform "waxy" appearance. On microscopic examination, it appeared that the liver owed its large size and its "waxy" appearance to the deposit of a whitish matter throughout its substance. This matter, which seemed to have taken the place of the secreting cells, and to have no organization, had, under the microscope, a peculiar white glistening appearance, very like semi-fluid size. In parts of the liver where the deposit was less abundant, the secreting cells were visible, and contained about the usual amount of oil.

Mr. L. S. Beale was kind enough to make for me an analysis of the liver, and found that in 100 parts it contained—

Water	80.600
Solid matter	19.400
Animal extractive, soluble in water only	1.391
Animal extractive, soluble in water and alcohol	.885
Albumen (soluble)	1.933
Alkaline salts	.850
Earthy salts	.120
Fatty matter	1.119
Animal matter	13.100

A small piece of the liver, when boiled in water or submitted to the action of dilute nitric acid, became quite white, almost like white of egg.

The *kidneys* were of the natural size, but presented in some parts an irregular, puckered appearance, as if from the contraction of a white deposit like that found in the liver.

On microscopic examination, in making which I had the valuable assistance of my friend and colleague, Dr. George Johnson, it was found that the greater number of the tubes in each kidney, with their epithelial lining, were quite healthy, but that some of them were filled with a material having the same appearance as that in the liver. The tubes thus filled *contained no epithelial cells.* It seemed as if the unorganized product had exuded from the basement membrane, and had taken the place of the normal secreting cells.

The *radius* of the left arm was found to be extensively carious for about three-fourths of its extent, and two pieces of dead bone, each about an inch in length, lay loose in its substance. The *ulna* was quite sound. The *joints* of the arm were unaffected, except that the bone was a little softened.

The phalanges of the great toe, and half of the metatarsal bone of the left foot, were also carious, and the metatarso-phalangeal joint was extremely diseased. The seventh rib on the left side was carious for about two inches over the pericardium.

On opening the chest, a great quantity of yellowish serum was found in the sac of the pericardium, and a large quantity of lymph was spread on the heart. The inflammation of the pericardium, of which these were traces, most probably resulted from the disease of the rib immediately above.

The upper part of the left lung was filled with tubercles. The lower and posterior part was carnified, apparently from the pressure of the fluid in the pericardium.

The right lung and pleura were quite healthy.

The state of other organs was not noted.

The main facts of this case are very like those of the case immediately preceding. Extensive scrofulous *caries* had existed for a long time; a deposit of tuberculous matter, not very extensive, had taken place in the lung; and the liver was enormously enlarged, and much thickened, not by an accumulation of oil, as so often happens in cases of simple tuberculous disease of the lung, but by the presence of a large quantity of foreign albuminous matter, diffused pretty evenly throughout its substance. The presence of all this foreign matter in the liver did not very much impede the passage of blood through it, for there was no ascites; and it probably did not prevent the secretion and escape of bile, for the discharges from the bowels were not remarked to be white, and there was no jaundice.

Here, as in the former cases, the kidneys were diseased; and a microscopic examination showed that some of their secreting tubes were filled by a foreign matter, which had much the same appearance as that in the liver.

The disease of the kidneys was, however, in this case only partial, and, to judge from the puckering at certain parts of the gland, must have occurred some time before death.

In 1850, another very remarkable instance of the same kind fell more immediately under my own observation, and for some time before death the progress of the disease was carefully watched. The following were the main facts recorded :—

CASE 4.—Frederick Woodman, a fair-haired lad, fifteen years of age, small in stature and crippled by scrofulous disease of the right hip, but very intelligent, applied to me as an out-patient of King's College Hospital, in June, 1850.

He was an orphan, and had spent all his life in London.

Four years before this time he came under the care of Mr. Fergusson, on account of disease of the right hip-joint, with abscesses in the upper part of the thigh. The abscesses broke or were opened, leaving fistulous openings, which continued to discharge matter up to the time of his death.

Some time in the course of the first year after he became afflicted with disease of the hip, his belly began to grow large. He noticed nothing further respecting it till about two years before I saw him, when he observed a definite swelling, the result of a large liver, in the epigastric and right hypochondriac regions.

When he first applied to me, his belly was greatly distended, obviously in consequence of enormous enlargement of the liver and spleen, the lower edges of which could very readily be traced. In the upper part of the right thigh there were two fistulous openings, which discharged freely. He was pale, but not at all jaundiced, and not much wasted in flesh.

There seemed to me little doubt that the large size of the liver was owing to that peculiar change in its texture which existed in the foregoing cases, and I prescribed, in succession, the oil of almonds, as a substitute for cod-liver oil, nitro-muriatic acid, and muriate of ammonia.

These medicines gave him no marked relief, and on the 30th of October he came into the hospital.

At that time he was very pallid, but not particularly thin.

The belly was enormously distended, and large veins were seen on its surface, passing up from the flanks. There was evidently a small quantity of liquid in the peritoneal sac; but the large size of the belly was owing to the liver and the spleen, the lower edges of which could still be very readily traced.

His appetite was tolerably good, and his tongue clean, and he slept pretty well; but his skin was dry, his pulse was above 100, and he complained constantly of thirst. For a few days he had been troubled with diarrhœa, which, he said, had made him feel weak. There had never been any jaundice, but there was now a faint sallow tinge in the conjunctiva.

The urine was acid, and contained a large quantity of albumen, being rendered almost solid by nitric acid. When it was examined under the microscope, a few transparent and slightly granular casts of the tubules of the kidney, without any oil-globules, were seen.

It was now plain that the kidneys were likewise diseased, and there could be little doubt that they had undergone much the same change as the liver.

For more than a month after he entered the hospital no striking change in his condition occurred. He had occasionally a feeling of nausea, and frequently complained of thirst; but his appetite remained tolerably good, and his tongue clean, and he generally slept well. The pulse was always rapid; never under 100, and sometimes as high as 120. The diarrhœa he had on his admission to the hospital soon ceased, but more than once afterwards it recurred and lasted a few days.

He now and then complained of slight pain at particular parts of the liver, which were then also slightly tender on pressure.

The urine was throughout in good quantity, of sp. gr. about 1008, and contained a considerable quantity of albumen. At times it contained, also, a large quantity of lithic acid.

About the middle of December the urine began to diminish greatly in quantity. The following are the quantities noted as passed on the successive days, reckoning from 7 P. M. of one day to 7 P. M. of the next:—

	Ounces.		Ounces.
Dec. 6	54	Dec. 10	48
" 7	42	" 11	47
" 8	45	" 12	44
" 9	54	" 13	44

During this time, then, the quantity did not vary much. The real variation was doubtless less than it appears to be from this table; for, whenever the quantity of urine is thus measured on successive days, it almost necessarily happens that what belongs to one day gets now and then placed to the account of the next, and there is an apparent variation, even though none may really exist.

After the 13th of December, the following quantities were noted:—

	Ounces.		Ounces.
Dec. 14	54	Dec. 19	30
" 15	42	" 20	22
" 16	36	" 21	17
" 17	36	" 22	12
" 18	40		

During these nine days, therefore, there was a rapid and progressive diminution in the quantity of urine, which at length became reduced to one-fourth of its former amount. The kidneys seemed to be rapidly blocking up. As the quantity of urine diminished from fifty-four ounces to twelve, its specific gravity rose from 1010 to 1015.

During the latter part of this time Woodman's appetite failed, and he was much purged, and frequently vomited. He complained also, at times, of headache.

He gradually sank, and died, apparently from exhaustion, on the 29th of December.

The *liver* was enormously enlarged, weighing eight pounds and a half avoirdupois, and reaching in the body as low as the pubis. It had no unnatural adhesions, and there were no false membranes upon it; but its convex surface presented a few short linear fissures, which resulted, I believe, from the obliteration of small twigs of the portal vein, near the surface of the liver, and the consequent atrophy of the portions of the liver which those twigs supplied.

The gall-bladder was filled with bile, which was viscid and of an olive color, as bile usually is which has become concentrated in the gall-bladder. It was not analyzed, but there was nothing unusual in its appearance. The large gall-ducts were apparently healthy, as were the large branches of the portal and hepatic veins.

The morbid changes were confined to the substance of the liver, which was of a pale yellowish color, and pitted when pressed by the finger.

In all its upper broad and thick portion, the liver presented no appearance of lobules, and seemed composed of a uniform, grayish, compact, and in some degree transparent substance; its cut surface looking not unlike that of firm bacon.

In some parts, however, near the edges of the liver, the lobules were very conspicuous. They were enlarged, as in the fatty liver, and had yellow opaque margins, contrasting strongly with the central portions, which were grayish and compact, and somewhat transparent, as the entire substance of the liver was in its upper portion.

On examination under the microscope, the gray compact substance exhibited a few gland-cells, which contained a good deal of granular matter, and were in consequence somewhat opaque, but were not enlarged.

The opaque yellow matter composing the margin of the lobules was more readily torn up for microscopic examination than the gray substance, and exhibited under the microscope a greater number of detached cells, and more oil-globules, both in the cells and out of them.

A portion of the liver was analyzed for me by Mr. Beale, as in the case of Shaw, before related, and the following is the result:—

In 100 parts there were—

Water	80.150
Animal matter, with much albumen	16.098
Extractive matter, soluble in water	1.986
Fatty matter	.575
Alkaline salts	.784
Earthy salts	.407
	100.000

So that there was little more than half a grain of fatty matter in 100 grains of the liver.

The *kidneys* were slightly nodulated on the surface, and their texture was changed, like that of the liver.

They were of a yellowish white color, and the capsular surface presented very little appearance of vascularity, or of lobular structure. They were not, however, much increased in size; the two, together, weighing ten ounces.

In making a microscopic examination of them, I had the assistance of Dr. Johnson.

Some of the tubes were filled with a material like that in the liver; and this, in some places, being squeezed out, formed large casts, which, like those observed in the urine during life, had somewhat the appearance of "wax."

The tubes which contained this waxy-looking material had no epithelial lining.

In some of the other tubes, not thus blocked up, the epithelium was opaque and granular, having undergone a change like that of the liver cells. Microscopic examination confirmed, then, the opinion which the first sight of the two organs suggested—that the liver and the kidneys had undergone the same kind of change.

In some of the medullary cones of the kidneys, near their apices, were opaque white lines, plainly seen by the naked eye. Under the microscope, this opaque white matter was found to consist of crystals of a square prismatic form. I could not tell by their shape what they were composed of, and sought the aid of Mr. Beale, to make out this point by chemical analysis. The result of this analysis is, that the matter was—

Insoluble in boiling acetic acid, and in alcohol, and in potash.

Insoluble in cold water, but soluble to a great extent in boiling water.

Soluble in strong nitric acid, with effervescence. When this solution was evaporated to dryness, the dry residue, treated with ammonia, gave the purple color of murexide.

After incineration, it left no appreciable residue.

The inference from all this is, that the salt was some "lithate." It will be recollected that during life the urine often contained abundance of lithic acid.

The *spleen* was very large and very firm, and weighed one pound and a half. It had no unnatual adhesions.

As had been inferred during life, there was a small quantity of serous fluid in the peritoneal sac.

The head of the right thigh-bone was completely destroyed by caries. All that remained of it were two fragments that were lying loose in the socket of the acetabulum.

There was not much else found amiss in the body.

The right lung was everywhere united to the pleura costalis by adhesions, which were readily broken through. The left lung was free from adhesions.

The lungs themselves, and the heart, were sound.

The stomach and intestines were small and contracted, but presented no marks of disease; and the mesenteric glands were little, if at all, enlarged.

In this case, the patient died after scrofulous disease of the hip had lasted four years, and the following striking changes were found:—

1st. The liver was enormously enlarged, as in the preceding cases, by the interstitial deposit of a whitish and glistening matter.

2d. The kidneys, though not much enlarged, had undergone an analogous change. Their secreting substance presented the same general appearance as that of the liver, and many of the secreting tubes were blocked up by a foreign matter, looking like that in the liver.

3d. The spleen was greatly enlarged and very firm.

The disease of the liver seems to have come on in the course of the first year after the occurrence of the disease of the hip; for it was then remarked that the belly was growing large.

There are no means of fixing the date of the disease of the kidney. It certainly existed on the 30th of October, two months before death, for the urine then contained a large quantity of albumen. It is probable, however, that it had not then long existed, *in any great degree*, for there had been no dropsy, and the daily examination of the urine which was made subsequently, showed that the kidneys were rapidly blocking up in the last fortnight of life. The enlargement of the spleen was detected six months before death. There is no evidence to show how long it had existed.

It will be seen that in all the four cases related, this peculiar change in the liver was found in conjunction with protracted *caries*, and that in all of them, at the time of death, the kidneys were diseased as well as the liver.

In the last two cases, simple inspection of the kidneys, as well as the more minute examination by the microscope, showed that the disease of the kidneys was analogous to that of the liver—that the secreting part of the gland was blocked up by a foreign matter having the same general appearances as the matter in the liver. There can be little doubt that the disease of the kidneys was of the same kind in the former cases in which they were not so carefully examined.

In every instance, the disease of the kidney appeared to be much more recent than that of the liver. It seems probable, therefore, that in such cases the liver becomes generally blocked up first, and then the kidneys.

The disease of the kidney is, however, much more fatal than that of the liver, so that it is possible that it may sometimes come on first, and may destroy life before the liver is so much enlarged and changed in texture as to excite attention. The patient may die of what may be termed granular disease of the kidney, and the condition of the liver be unnoticed.

In this scrofulous disease, the liver increases in size in much greater degree than the kidney. In the case of Woodman, last related, where, by the progress of the disease, the kidneys had almost ceased to perform their office, the liver reached to the pubis, and almost filled the belly, while the kidneys were not very much larger than they should be. The same thing happens in the "fatty degeneration" of these organs: the liver enlarges in much greater degree than the kidneys, and contains a very much larger proportion of fatty matter.

But although the foreign matter is relatively in much smaller amount in the kidney, it does, apparently, much more mischief.

To take merely the case of Woodman. Notwithstanding the large size of the liver in him, there was no decided jaundice; and after death, the gall-bladder was found filled with dark-colored, viscid bile, as it usually is in persons who have taken no food for some time before death. Bile, then, of the usual appearance, continued to be secreted to the last, and its passage through the ducts was not sufficiently impeded to cause serious disorder of health. There was, indeed, some obstruction to the passage of the blood through the liver; but it was not sufficient to cause much ascites.

The disease of the liver most probaby induced an impoverished state of the blood, but there is reason to believe that if it had existed alone, Woodman might have continued to live for a long time. It was the disease of the kidneys that brought his life to a close.

This disease of the kidneys caused a constant drain of albumen, and thus gradually exhausted the strength; and, in the end, destroyed life quickly, by preventing the proper excretion of urine.

A similar difference is observed in the effects of the fatty degeneration of these two organs.

The liver, from fatty degeneration, may be doubled in weight, and more than doubled in bulk, but may still perform its office tolerably well; the blood, at least, may pass freely through it; there may be no jaundice; and, after death, the bile found in the gall-bladder may present no unusual appearances.

Fatty degeneration of the kidney, however, although the organ is increased in bulk in much less degree, and the fatty matter forms a much smaller proportion of the entire weight, leads to albuminous urine and dropsy, and destroys life.

It will be seen that in two of the four cases, *without any history of ague*, the spleen was very large and very firm. No minute examination of it was made; but it is probable that it had undergone a change analogous to that of the liver and the kidney, and that its increase of size was due to the interstitial deposit of a foreign albuminous matter.

The details of the preceding cases show the changes which the liver undergoes in this disease.

1st. It becomes enormously enlarged, and, as happens in the fatty degeneration, in which the foreign matter is likewise retained in the lobules, it becomes at the same time much thickened, and its lower edge much rounded.

2d. Like a liver that is much enlarged by fatty degeneration, and probably from the same mechanical condition, it contains after death but a small quantity of blood, and is consequently pale.

3d. When the disease is far advanced, the lobules can scarcely be distinguished, especially in the centre and in the upper broad part of the liver, where they are most compressed; and the hepatic substance is uniform and compact, and at the same time somewhat glistening or semi-transparent, so that the cut surface looks very much like that of compact bacon. It is very tough, so as not to be readily broken down, and is generally whitish; but, now and then (as in Case 4), from the retention of bile, has a yellowish cast.

Livers in this state have been often described as "waxy" livers, and their peculiar appearances have been wrongly attributed to the interstitial deposit of one of the solid forms of fat.

4th. The foreign matter, to which the liver owes its large size, is *albuminous*, and, when not stained by bile, is whitish and somewhat glistening. It does not become hard, and, unlike the lymph that is poured out in ordinary inflammation, it seems to have no tendency to contract; so that after the disease has lasted for years, the liver pits on pressure, and its surface is smooth. These circumstances explain the fact, that the foreign matter, though large in amount, does not much impede either the passage of the blood through the liver or the escape of the bile through the ducts.

5th. The foreign matter is situated within the lobules, and from one of the cases (Case 4), it would seem that it is deposited first in the central portions of the lobules.

In the parts of the liver which are most diseased, the secreting cells are few in number, and they are not enlarged. The foreign matter is not within the cells, but between them, and, in advanced stages of the disease, seems, in some parts of the liver, completely to take their place, filling up the interstices of the capillary vessels that form the lobular network.

In some of the cases the cells were observed to contain much granular matter, and to be in consequence more opaque than natural; but it must be remembered that this was after the occurrence of disease of the kidney, which might in some degree have changed the secreted product of the liver-cells.

The absence of decided jaundice, the natural appearance of the bile found in the gall-bladder in two of the cases, notwithstanding the disease of the liver had lasted so long, and the fact that the cells contained nearly their natural quantity of oil, tend to show that the cells performed their office tolerably well.

6th. Chemical analysis showed that in two of the cases the liver contained a small proportional quantity of fat. In one of them (Case 3), it contained rather more than a grain of fatty matter, and, in the other (Case 4), little more than half a grain in 100 grains of liver: whereas, it would appear, from cases related in the preceding chapter, that the normal quantity of oil in the liver is three or four parts in 100.

It must be borne in mind, however, that the liver was doubled in weight by the interstitial deposit of a foreign albuminous matter; so that the total quantity of oil in the liver was only half as much below the natural standard as the figures above would at first seem to denote. It is probable, also, that by the long presence of the foreign matter the cells had become much less numerous than in a healthy liver; and we have thus an explanation of the fact, that while the liver contained a very small relative amount of oil, the quantity of oil seen by the microscope in the cells did not seem to be much smaller than natural.

7th. All the cases related above were striking examples of the disease. The same changes, in less degree, not unfrequently occur among such of the poor in our large cities as are scrofulous or cachectic, and, at the same time, intemperate—causing more or less enlargement of the liver, and giving it a somewhat "waxy" appearance, but without otherwise attracting particular notice.

8th. This peculiar condition of the liver, in its highest degree, is most frequently found in young persons who have long suffered from scrofulous caries. There is some circumstance connected with caries—most probably the protracted suppuration resulting from it, or the continual loss of earthy matter—that disposes to this peculiar form of disease.

In the following case it occurred in a man of middle age, who exhibited no marks of the scrofulous habit, and was not afflicted with caries, but who had long suffered from disease of the left kidney, attended with constant suppuration.

Case 5.—Henry Warner, a printer, aged thirty-seven, who had always lived in London, was admitted into King's College Hospital on the 26th of August, 1849, suffering severe pain in the left loin, passing pus with his urine, and having other symptoms indicating the existence of suppuration in the left kidney. He was rather short in stature, but well-formed and muscular, and presented no marks of the scrofulous habit. He confessed that of late years he had drunk gin rather freely; but stated that his health had been good until the accession of the illness he then had, of which he gave the following account:—

About four years before he was taken with severe pain in the left loin, extending to the pubis and scrotum; attended with difficulty in passing his water, which was red and turbid. The pain subsided after a time, but the water continued to be more or less turbid.

Between two and three years after this illness, in the summer of 1848, he received a severe blow in the back by a trap-door falling on him while he was in the act of stooping. On account of this accident he was taken to St. Bartholomew's Hospital, where he remained a fortnight. About a month after this he had severe pain in the left loin, with rigors and vomiting, and applied as an out-patient at King's College Hospital. He was there under treatment, as an out-patient, for four months, during which time there was constantly pus in his urine

In August, 1849, soon after he was admitted into King's College Hospital, it was discovered that there was an abscess in the left loin, making its way to the surface. The abscess was opened, and a great quantity of pus escaped.

From that time, with the exception of a few weeks during which the opening in the back was closed, there was constantly a discharge of pus through a fistulous opening in the loin. He was a patient at the hospital, off and on, for several months, constantly suffering pain in the loin, and having a constant discharge of pus in the urine, and also through the fistulous opening in the loin.

In this state he at length resumed his work, and I lost sight of him. No enlargement of the liver had been then noticed.

On the 15th of October, 1851, he was again brought into the hospital, considerably reduced in flesh, and suffering much in the same way as before, with pus still escaping with his urine, and through the loin. The liver was now found to be enormously enlarged, reaching below the umbilicus and into the right iliac region, and greatly distending the belly. The superficial veins of the belly were enlarged, and there seemed to be a small quantity of fluid in the peritoneal sac. The liver was slightly tender, and he occasionally felt pain in it when lying on the right side. Its lower edge was felt to be rounded.

He stated that the belly had been growing gradually larger for twelve months.

He remained in the hospital till the 28th of November, when he left at his own request. During the last fortnight of his stay there the urine, which was constantly acid, ranged in quantity from two to three pints a day, and in sp. gr. from 1017 to 1010. It always contained a small quantity of pus.

On the 19th of January, 1852, he came into the hospital again—more emaciated than before. His complexion was now slightly sallow; there was distinct ascites; and the legs and scrotum were slightly œdematous. Pus still escaped in the urine, and through the loin. The pulse was frequent; the tongue brown; and he had frequent vomiting. The urine now averaged little more than a pint daily, and its sp. gr. was about 1016.

He died in the hospital on the 29th of January.

The body was examined thirty-two hours after death.

It was much emaciated, and the skin had a faint yellow tinge.

The peritoneum contained a large quantity of straw-colored fluid of sp. gr. 1017; and the legs and scrotum were slightly dropsical.

The liver, which had no unnatural adhesions, was enormously enlarged, and weighed eight pounds and three-quarters.

Its surface was smooth, except near the lower edge, where it was slightly nodulous, as in cirrhosis. It was tough, and pitted on pressure, and when cut into presented the compactness and the same uniform glistening appearance as in the preceding cases. In its upper part there seemed to be but little fat, and the lobules could nowhere be distinguished.

Towards the lower edge fat was deposited in greater quantity, and formed a distinct yellowish rim round many of the lobules.

A portion of the liver from the upper part, and a portion from near the lower edge, were analyzed for me by Mr. Beale, and were found to contain in 100 parts 2.1 parts and 4.7 parts of fatty matter respectively.

The gall-bladder contained a pale orange-colored bile, which reddened litmus paper.

The left kidney, which was imbedded in a dense mass of fat and adventitious tissue, was distended into pouches filled up by irregular calculi of phosphate of lime. Its interior communicated with the fistulous opening in the back.

The right kidney was enlarged, and presented changes of structure like those noticed in some of the preceding cases. All the secreting tubules were more or less diseased; in some the epithelium was only slightly granular; in others it was entirely disintegrated; in others, again, it was replaced by cells in size and appearance like pus-globules. In a few tubules the epithelium contained pretty numerous but minute oil-globules.

There was no disease worthy of note in other parts of the body.

In this case, the change in the liver was of precisely the same kind as in the preceding cases, but the circumstances under which it occurred were different. The patient, instead of being young and affected with scrofulous caries, was of middle age, and his primary disease was abscess of the left kidney, which seems to have nothing in common with scrofulous caries, excepting *protracted suppuration.*

By the nature of the matter choking the liver, the disease we are considering is closely allied to cirrhosis, and in the instance just related the patient was known to have drunk spirits to excess. It seems probable, therefore, that in this instance spirit-drinking contributed to produce the disease; and it is not unlikely, although no evidence is adduced to this effect, that in some of the former cases ardent spirits were taken, according to the custom which prevails among the poor in this city, with the view of supporting the strength under the protracted suppuration, and that in them, too, it may have contributed to induce the disease.

It will be seen that in the case just related, as in many of the preceding cases, there was disease of the secreting tubules of the kidney. The disease of the liver, indeed, in such cases, almost necessarily leads, in the end, to disease of the kidney. In consequence of the primary chronic disease, and the unhealthy constitution, and, it may be, the faulty habits of life, the blood becomes charged with impurities, which, as they can no longer be retained in the liver, or cast off through it, are thrown upon the kidneys. An attempt is made by the kidneys to eliminate them, in addition to the ordinary principles of the urine, and the result is disease of the secreting tubules.

In most of the preceding cases it was noted that the patient, even when not much wasted in flesh, was in a state of anemia. The state of anemia in these cases may have resulted, in part, from the loss of albumen, in consequence of the disease of the kidney; but this disease of the liver itself, as does every disease of the liver that causes much atrophy of its secreting element, induces after a time a state of anemia, most probably by lessening the amount of those changes which the blood naturally undergoes in its passage through the liver, and which, doubtless, contribute in some way or other to the reproduction of its colored corpuscles.

It seems strange that, notwithstanding the striking change in the size and texture of the liver, which must often be attended with great diminution in the number of its secreting cells, there should be no jaundice in this disease, and after death, often no tinge of bile in the liver itself. The circumstance may, like the state of anemia, be owing in some measure to diminution in the amount of those changes which the blood naturally undergoes in its passage through the liver, which diminution probably lessens the quantity of biliary coloring matter that has to be cast off. The absence of jaundice affords, therefore, a strong argument in favor of the opinion that much of the coloring matter of the bile is formed in the liver itself, as a result of the changes which there take place in the blood.

The bile found in the gall-bladder after death presents, as in cirrhosis, different appearances in different cases. In some cases (as in Case 4) it is viscid and of a dark olive color, like healthy bile that has been concentrated; in others, on the contrary (as in Case 5), it is thin and unusually pale. It might be expected that it would occasionally contain albumen; but no observations, that I am aware of, have been made showing that it has any peculiar or constant characters.

The scrofulous enlargement of the liver may sometimes be distinguished when the patient is living. It occurs in its highest degree in scrofulous persons suffering from caries, and, like the enlargement from accumulation of fat, it comes on insidiously, without much pain or even much tenderness—a circumstance accounted for by the gradual and even manner in which the foreign matter accumulates, and by its having no tendency to cause inflammation of the capsule of the liver. As happens with the fatty degeneration, the first evidence that the liver is diseased is generally furnished by its large size. The belly is observed to be large, and, on examination, the liver is found to extend much below its natural limits. The intestines are seldom much distended with gas, and, if the walls of the belly be thin, the surface of the liver may be felt to be smooth, and its lower edge to be rounded. The effects are, so far, like those of the fatty degeneration; but in the scrofulous enlargement, the passage of the blood through the liver is more impeded than in the fatty degeneration—probably from the foreign matter being firmer and less yielding than oil-globules—and the escape of bile from the liver is also somewhat more impeded, so that, after a time (as happened in Case 4), the superficial veins of the belly sometimes grow large, a small quantity of fluid collects in the peritoneal sac, and there is a slight tinge of yellow in the conjunctiva and the skin. The effects of this disease at this stage are intermediate between the effects of the fatty liver and those of cirrhosis.

If, in a young person, who has long suffered from scrofulous disease of the bones, there is great enlargement of the liver, with a *small* quantity of liquid in the peritoneal sac, and *very slight* sallowness of the conjunctiva, and if the surface of the liver be smooth, and its lower edge rounded, and it be occasionally slightly tender at certain spots—there can be little doubt that the liver does not owe its large size to an accumulation of fatty matter, but to the peculiar disease we are considering.

If, after a time, the urine becomes albuminous, and if, when the urine is examined under the microscope, waxy-looking casts of the secreting tubules are seen, there can be no doubt of the existence of this peculiar change in the liver, and of corresponding disease in the kidney.

The cases related above furnish no satisfactory evidence on the subject of treatment. In the last but one of the series (Case 4), the patient was under treatment for many months after the nature of the disease of the liver was known; and almond oil, nitro-muriatic acid, and the muriate of ammonia, were given for some time in succession, without lessening the size of the liver, or doing any essential good. From the failure of these medicines, in this instance, we should not, however, be warranted in inferring their complete inefficacy to remedy or prevent this disease in all other cases. It must be borne in mind that the scrofulous disease of the hip, which was, seemingly, the primary cause of the changes in the liver and the kidney, was not remedied; and it can hardly be expected that any such changes will be arrested while their cause continues in active operation.

If the diseased limb could have been removed, or the caries of the bone stopped, before the kidneys became seriously damaged, it is not impossible that the effect of some of those medicines might have been more satisfactory. I have more than once known a large liver, which I supposed to have undergone the change we have been considering, diminish very much in size under the prolonged use of *muriate of ammonia.*

Enlargement of the liver, which seems to be identical with the scrofulous enlargement, sometimes occurs in persons whose health is broken from the combined effects of mercury and syphilis. The fact that *enlargement* of the liver is apt to occur in such persons, was, I believe, first distinctly noticed by Dr. Graves, who gives the following account of a case of it: "About two years since, I was consulted by an English gentleman, who had been ill for a considerable time. The history of his case from the commencement was this: Three years previously, he had venereal—used and abused mercury—was exposed to cold, and got periostitis. He now got into a bad state of health, used mercury a second time; obtained some relief, and then relapsed again; finally, after having used mercury three or four times, he was attacked with mercurial cachexy, became weak and emaciated; the periostitis degenerated into ostitis, producing superficial caries and nodes of a bad character; he had exfoliation of the bones of the cranium, and rupia, and was reduced to a most miserable state. Under our care, the symptoms gradually disappeared; he recovered to all appearances, and even got fat. He then caught cold, and relapsed again. At last, his liver became engaged; he was attacked with hypertrophy of the liver, ascites, and jaundice, and died soon afterwards." "While this gentleman's liver was enlarging, there was no tenderness of the right hypochondrium on pressure." "What is equally remarkable, he had no fever, and the tongue was perfectly clean and moist during the whole course of the hepatic affection."

Dr. Graves says that he has since witnessed a similar train of phenomena—syphilis, abuse of mercury, periostitis, enlargement of the liver—twice in private practice, and once in hospital practice. In not one of these cases was the liver tender on pressure.

This account alone would render it extremely probable that the change which the liver undergoes in such cases is very like that which occurs in scrofula. Mere fatty degeneration of the liver does not cause ascites, which occurred in the case of which Dr. Graves has given the details.

My own experience furnishes more positive evidence on this point. Some time ago I had an opportunity of minutely examining a liver, which had all the characters of the scrofulous enlargement in a striking degree, and which was taken from a man of middle age, who had long had syphilitic caries of the bones of the skull. Severe and protracted syphilitic disease of the bones, like scrofulous disease, often leads after a time to fatal disease of the kidney, which, like the enlargement of the liver, comes on gradually without pain or any active inflammatory symptoms. Suspicion is excited by the gradually increasing paleness, and an examination of the urine leads to the discovery that it is highly charged with albumen. I could cite from my own experience many examples of this sequence of events.

It has been truly remarked by Dr. Graves, that the mercurial and syphilitic cachexy very closely resembles scrofulous cachexy. There is the same impaired nutrition, irritability and feverishness; and the skin, the glands, and the bones, which principally suffer in the one, suffer also, and in much the same way, in the other. I believe, however, that when arising from syphilis, as when arising from scrofula, the highest degree of this peculiar change in the liver will be generally found associated with *caries, or with some other disease of the bones.*

It is stated by Rokitansky, that enlargement of the liver, with the same anatomical characters, is sometimes produced by prolonged attacks of ague. I have met with one instance in which severe and long-continued ague in a boy was followed by scrofulous disease of the glands of the neck and of the bones, and subsequently, by great enlargement of the liver, and ascites. But here, the enlargement of the liver was attributable to the scrofula, and could not be considered the immediate effect of the ague. The liver very seldom gets much enlarged from ague. I have examined, in the Seamen's Hospital, a great number of bodies in which the spleen was enormously enlarged from ague, caught in China, in the West Indies, or on the west coast of Africa; but in none of those cases did I remark the liver to be much enlarged. After remittent or yellow fever, the liver remains for a long time of a pale slate color, but it is not generally enlarged.

Enlargement of the liver presenting the characters of the scrofulous enlargement now and then occurs, without our being able to trace it to any of the circumstances specified.

The diseases we have been considering were at one time regarded as *simple hypertrophy* of the liver; the term *hypertrophy* meaning, as when applied to muscles, mere increase of bulk, without change of structure. But, as we have seen, this is an erroneous view. The increased size of the liver, in the fatty liver, in the scrofulous liver, and in other kindred states, depends on the presence of some peculiar matter which, instead of passing off in the bile, is retained in the substance of the organ. The pathologists, who looked upon the enlargement of the liver in these cases as due to simple hypertrophy, were at times much perplexed to account for the symptoms attending it. Andral, in his remarks on a case of great enlargement of the liver, consequent on syphilis and the use of mercury, which he has given as an instance of simple hypertrophy of this organ, expresses much surprise that there was not a corresponding increase in the quantity of bile secreted. He says: "One would have thought, *à priori*, that when the nutrition of the liver was increased in so extraordinary a degree, the secretion of bile would have been more abundant in proportion. Such, however was not the case. During life but little bile was discharged, and after death the gall-bladder held only a small quantity, and this containing, seemingly, more water and albumen than usual, as if, while the nutrition of the liver became more active, its force of secretion diminished. The case to be next related will serve, perhaps, to confirm this conjecture. It furnishes, in fact, an instance of jaundice, without other change in the liver than simple hypertrophy." (*Clin. Med.*, iv. 305.)

The thin and pale bile in one of the cases related by Andral, and the complete suspension of secretion, as evinced by the complete jaundice in the other, lead to the conclusion, that the malady was not simple hypertrophy, in the sense usually given to that term.

The liver, if it be called on to do for a long time somewhat more than its ordinary work, may perhaps become somewhat enlarged from simple hypertrophy—that is, from increase in the number of the secreting cells, and a corresponding increased development of the other tissues of which the liver is made up; parts of the liver may doubtless undergo this kind of hypertrophy when other parts are wasted; but in such cases the functional power of the organ will be increased in proportion to its increased bulk, and the hypertrophy will not be disease.

The *treatment* in the class of cases considered in this chapter should in some degree be directed by reference to the primary disease, or the peculiar *cachexy*, on which the enlargement of the liver depends.

When the enlargement of the liver is consequent on scrofula, our chief reliance must be on warm clothing; sea air and sea-bathing; a light nourishing diet, comprising a liberal allowance of animal food; cod-liver oil; the muriate of ammonia; the preparations of iodine and iron, separate or combined; and if the enlargement of the liver should be associated with caries, *those surgical or other means which tend to arrest the disease of the bone.*

When the health has been broken by the combined effects of syphilis and mercury, warm clothing, a tonic regimen, *iodide of potassium*, iron, nitric acid, hot sulphur baths, sarsaparilla, and guaiacum, are the appropriate remedies.

In either case, when the liver is thus oppressed, the patient should entirely abstain from *ardent spirits*, and be very sparing in the use of the less injurious fermented drinks. Reasons have, indeed been already given for thinking that spirit-drinking is often, if not generally, instrumental in producing the disease.

However the disease may originate, it must be important, with the view of relieving the oppressed liver and of preventing the similar, but more serious disease of the kidney, that the bowels should be rightly regulated; that the action of the skin should be kept up; and that the patient should breathe the fresh air.

There is great reason to hope, that, if we can cure the original malady before the enlargement of the liver has attained a very great degree and before the kidneys have become likewise diseased, we shall be able, in many cases, if not in all, to remedy, in great measure, the unnatural condition of the liver and other secondary ailments. The matter deposited in the liver does not become organized, like the lymph poured out in common inflammation; and if the general health should mend, it may, in time, all pass off with the bile, or be removed by absorption.

I have met with more than one instance of considerable chronic enlargement of the liver, with impairment of health, in which, after a time, the liver returned to its natural size, and the health was restored.

In July, 1846, I was consulted by a lady, forty-four years of age, on account of considerable enlargement of the liver, which had been detected by her former medical attendant in the March preceding. She had been much out of health more than six months, and had lost flesh, and had a craving appetite, and a constant sense of weight and fulness in the right side; but there was no jaundice. She remained under my care for three months, at the end of which time, contrary to my anticipation, her health was re-established, and the liver had returned nearly, if not quite, to its natural size.

The amendment seemed to result from properly regulated diet, and the prolonged use of the *sesquicarbonate of ammonia*, in doses of five grains twice a day. This was ordered, at first, without direct reference to the liver, and persevered in, from the fact that her health continued to improve under its use.

In December, 1847, a young lady, twenty-six years of age, was placed under my care, with great enlargement both of the liver and the spleen. The enlargement of the liver had been detected nine months before. She had lost flesh much, and was pallid and slightly sallow, and had a good deal of irritative fever. Mercury to salivation, iodine, taraxacum, and nitro-muriatic acid, had been tried in turn, without success. Her health greatly improved under strict diet, with abstinence from all stimulants, and the *muriate of ammonia*, in doses from five to ten grains, three times a day. In

1850, the spleen was still large, but the liver had returned to its normal size; and, though still looking very delicate, she considered herself well.

The salts of ammonia probably relieve the liver, and do good in such cases by promoting the action of the *skin* and the kidneys.

Dr. Graves has given very strong testimony to the fact that considerable enlargement of the liver, having the characters of the fatty or the scrofulous enlargement, may after a time disappear. He says:—

"In persons below thirty, the liver may become enlarged to a very considerable extent, and yet return again to its natural size under proper treatment. I could point out several persons, in Dublin, in whom the liver had been so much enlarged that I thought their cases hopeless, and yet they have recovered, and are at present in the enjoyment of good health. The process by which the organ returns to its natural state and dimensions is generally slow; in two or three cases it occupied a space of time varying from one to two years. I attended a gentleman some time ago, with Mr. Carmichael, and, from the history of the case, as well as from the symptoms present, we were induced to look upon it as incurable, and yet the patient has completely recovered. The late Mr. Macnamara and I attended a lady who had a very remarkable enlargement of the liver, but, in the course of a year, the viscus diminished so much in size as to be very little above the normal dimensions. Within the last year (1842), Dr. Stokes and I have treated successfully an old gentleman, between seventy and eighty years of age, who had an enormously enlarged liver and ascites. We agreed to try a combination of blue pill and hydriodate of potash. This he took for nearly six months, and its use was attended by visible, almost daily, decrease in the size of the liver, and his general health gradually improved. He took the pills for a couple of months before his mouth got a little sore; but full salivation was not produced. He called on us, a few weeks ago, to thank us for our successful treatment, and took no small pleasure in directing attention to his altered appearance and renovated health. This is a matter of no common interest, for cases of this description have been generally looked upon as beyond the reach of medical aid. You should, therefore, be very careful in your prognosis of such cases, and not give them up at once as incurable." (*Clinical Medicine*, p. 568.)

A paper has recently been published by Virchow (*Archiv. f. Pa-*

tholog. Anatomie und Physiologie, Bd. viii. p. 364), and transferred to the pages of the *Microscopical Journal* (*Quarterly Journal of Microscopical Science*, No. 14, for January, 1856), in which he announces that the matter infiltrating the liver, in what I have called "the scrofulous enlargement," gives, with a solution of iodine, the chemical reaction of starch, like the so-called *amyloid* bodies, occasionally found in the brain; that, when treated with a solution of iodine, it acquires, like starch, an intense reddish-yellow color, turning, on the addition of sulphuric acid, to a beautiful violet and blue, and he, therefore, proposes to call this condition of the liver the *amyloid degeneration*. Virchow observes that, as I have before stated, the peculiar matter in the liver is deposited first in the centres of the lobules, and that the liver, spleen, and kidney, undergo, in succession, the same change. He likewise confirms the remark that this peculiar change is in some way or other connected with disease of the bones, especially with caries. If the announcement —that the matter which infiltrates the liver is starch—should turn out to be true, this disease of the liver may be cited to show how unexpected are the changes and relations sometimes disclosed, as medicine advances, and how imperfect and transitional our knowledge of most subjects of pathology still is.

SECT. IV.—*Excessive and defective secretion of bile—Unhealthy states of the bile.*

FROM the diseases just considered, we pass, naturally, to a very important class of disorders—namely, those functional disorders in which too much, or too little, bile is secreted, or the bile secreted is not healthy.

It has been shown by Bernard (see p. 56) that two distinct processes of the nature of secretions go on in the liver—the secretion of bile, and the formation of sugar. The bile flows through the gall-ducts into the bowel; the sugar is absorbed by the veins and lymphatics in the liver, and thus passes directly into the blood which is about to traverse the lung.

Both these secretions are no doubt connected with the reparative and other changes which the blood undergoes in its passage through the liver.

The manner in which the functions of the liver are performed may, therefore, be investigated with reference to three points—

1st. To the changes effected in the blood.

2d. To the formation of sugar.

3d. To the secretion of bile.

In living human beings we have no means of ascertaining the degree in which the regeneration of the blood in the liver is affected by various morbid conditions; but the facts related in the preceding pages show clearly enough that any great destruction of the lobular substance of the liver, or any condition that arrests the secretion of bile, causes a state of *anemia*—that is, lessens the proportion of the red corpuscles in the blood.

Our knowledge of the formation of sugar in the liver, and of the various conditions that lessen or increase it, is entirely due to the researches of Bernard. The sugar formed in the liver, except it be in excessive amount so as to cause the diabetic state, is all transformed in the blood, and does not appear in any secretion open to our inspection, so that its relative amount at different times in ordinary cases cannot be determined, even approximately, by mere clinical observation.

It has been ascertained by Bernard that, in the animals that were the subjects of his experiments, the production of sugar is lessened by subjecting them to extreme heat or extreme cold; that it is lessened by prolonged fasting, by severe pain, and, generally, by acute diseases attended with fever; so that, in persons who die of disease, the liver after death seldom contains sugar; and that it is completely arrested by division of the pneumogastric nerves in the neck, and by cutting across the spinal marrow just below the brachial enlargement.

The secretion may be increased, so as to cause for a time the diabetic state, by lacerating the floor of the fourth ventricle, between the origins of the pneumogastric and the auditory nerves; and it is somewhat increased by the apoplectic state, whether this result from disease or physical injury of the brain, or from the action of some narcotic poison upon it.

The increased formation of sugar in the apoplectic state is, according to Bernard, but a particular exemplification of the general law, that, "when the voluntary movements and sensation are extinguished, all internal organs—the liver, intestines, glands—all the viscera, in short, which are not subjected to the influence of the will, present a greater activity than in the normal state. The vital energy, which has ceased for all the actions of *animal* life, seems to concentrate itself upon the acts that are purely organic."

The most striking and suggestive circumstance disclosed in these remarkable researches, is the controlling and governing power over the secretion of sugar which the nervous system exerts.

It appears, from Bernard's experiments, that although these two secretions—the secretion of sugar and the secretion of bile—go on together in the liver, the variations in the one do not correspond in time or degree with the variations in the other.

The secretion of bile may be disordered from organic disease of the liver, which renders it incapable of adequately performing its functions; or, without this, when the portal blood, from which the materials of the bile are drawn, is rendered unhealthy by medicines, by unwholesome food, by faulty digestion or assimilation, or by defective action of some other excreting organ. It may be disordered, too, by the direct influence of anxiety or strong mental emotion. In any case, the disordered secretion of bile is the effect of some other disease, or of some condition that deranges other organs as well as the liver.

But the bile has a long course before it passes out of the body, and serves an important office in the intestinal canal; and on these accounts, if it be in undue quantity, or unhealthy, however the change in its quantity or quality may have been brought about, it may cause various secondary disorders. In the first place, it may inflame or irritate the gall-ducts, or the parts of the intestine with which it is brought into contact. There is reason to believe that most of the diseases of the gall-bladder and gall-ducts are produced by irritating bile; and there can be no doubt that disorders of the bowels sometimes arise from the bile being in improper quantity or unhealthy. But besides these mere local effects, a faulty state of the bile may render digestion imperfect, and in this way may impair nutrition; and the noxious products of imperfect digestion may be absorbed into the blood, and from this, again, many secondary evils may spring.

Unhealthy states of the bile are analogous to unhealthy states of the urine, and may result in the same way, either from fault of the secreting organ, or from an unhealthy state of the blood. Unhealthy states of the urine have excited more interest, because, from our being able to collect and analyze the urine, we can distinguish them, and trace them to the disease of the kidney, or to the faulty digestion and assimilation, on which they depend. They are some of them, as albuminous urine and saccharine urine, almost pathognomonic of certain fatal diseases which we might not otherwise detect. Unhealthy states of the bile have less importance in this sense, because we cannot distinguish them, and thus trace them to their source; but in another sense they are more important, from the bile serving an important office, and not being merely excrementitious, like the urine.

From our not being able to collect the bile during the life of the patient, and from the difficulty of analyzing what may be found in the gall-bladder after death, we have little knowledge of unhealthy states of this fluid. It is often easy to say, from the symptoms, that too much bile, or too little bile, is secreted, and something is known of the effects of this redundant or deficient secretion; but we have little knowledge of changes in the composition of bile, except what is derived from mere inspection.

We may therefore first consider excessive secretion of bile, and deficient secretion of bile.

Excessive secretion of bile.—The quantity of bile secreted, like the quantity of urine, no doubt varies very much, without disorder of health, according to climate, season, and habits of life. In certain circumstances, pointed out in a former part of this work, an unusually large secretion of bile is necessary for the maintenance of health. It can only be considered morbid, when, from the abundance of the bile, and perhaps from its being at the same time altered in quality, secondary disorders arise. This frequently happens to persons on their first going to a hot climate. It is of very common occurrence among Europeans in India, and has been well described by Annesley, under the head, *Excessive Secretion of Bile.*

In the slighter degrees of this bilious disorder the patient has purging of bilious matter, which soon produces scalding of the rectum, with slight sickness, a bitter taste in the mouth, and a foul tongue, but without much fever, or the pulse being much quickened. These symptoms rapidly subside, when the redundant bile has been got rid of by an emetic and by purgatives.

In a more severe form of the disease, together with purging of bilious matter, and vomiting, and foul tongue, there is a good deal of fever, with pain and tenderness in the region of the liver; and the complexion is bilious, or dusky. The illness resembles a slight form of bilious fever, and is attended with much congestion of the liver, and, it would seem, with inflammation of the gall-ducts, caused by the bile, which, while it is increased in quantity, is doubtless also altered in quality, and irritating to the lining membrane of the ducts as well as to that of the bowel.

In such cases, Annesley recommends bleeding from the arm, or cupping over the liver, calomel and saline purgatives, and copious draughts of hot water to dilute the irritating bile. Under this treatment, the patient in most cases soon regains his former health.[1]

[1] Diluents must have a most beneficial action in such cases, because water is readily excreted by the liver, and thus tends to dilute the bile at its source. It has been shown by Lehmann that the blood of the portal vein contains much more water than the blood of the hepatic vein, especially after drinking. (Lehmann's *Physiological Chemistry*, vol. ii. p. 99.)

In this country a similar form of illness is often seen, especially among men of middle age who have long been in the habit of living freely. Such persons go on for some time without apparent indigestion or other inconvenience, but, at length, get what is called a *bilious* attack. This is marked by sickness and bilious diarrhœa, a certain degree of fever, with a feeling of general disorder, often with headache, and by a foul tongue and turbid urine. In some instances there is likewise a sense of fulness, or uneasiness, in the region of the liver, and the complexion is bilious. These complaints are, in most cases, readily removed by brisk purging with calomel and salts, and the patient enjoys again, for some time, his former health. If he returns to his former habits, he, by-and-by, gets a similar attack, which perhaps is removed as before. In this way, he may go on for years, his general good health being only interrupted by an occasional bilious attack of this kind, which, like a fit of gout, seems to clear the system for a time. As was remarked by Dr. Prout, the acid and unassimilated matters seem to accumulate in the system, and to be thrown off periodically.

The readiness with which these attacks are removed, often makes people regard them lightly; but they are not unimportant, as evidence of disorders, which, aggravated by time and by continuance in the habits under which they have arisen, may end in some organic disease, or in the total failure of those assimilating processes on which nutrition depends. During the attacks, signal relief is produced by a dose of calomel, or blue pill, followed by saline purgatives. If there should be pain or tenderness in the region of the liver, and the patient can well bear it, blood may be taken by leeches, or by cupping. These measures are generally sufficient for the time, but they do not strike at the root of the evil. Exemption from future attacks, and from the manifold and greater evils to which these disorders may lead as age advances, can only be procured by a change of habits. One of our objects in directing this should be to increase the amount of oxygen inspired, and thus to consume in respiration, or burn off, materials that would otherwise be left for the liver to excrete. The means most efficacious for this purpose are sea-voyages, riding, or other exercise in the open air, well-ventilated rooms, early rising, the cold or shower bath, &c. Too much indulgence in sleep, which so much reduces the activity of both respiration and circulation, must be especially injurious, more particularly in rooms that are ill ventilated, as most bedrooms are.

Another object, of equal or still greater importance, should be to limit in the food the supply of those materials—such as spirituous liquors, butter, cream, fat—which, in persons in the condition we are considering, embarrass the secreting function of the liver, and, at the same time, if they do not contribute directly to form bile, tend, by serving as fuel for respiration, to increase the quantity of matter which the liver is called on to excrete.

Plainly enough, it must be especially injurious for persons who suffer from this class of disorders, to indulge in sleep immediately after a full meal. To lessen by sleep the activity of respiration at the very time when the materials consumed in this process are being poured in large quantity into the blood, must lead, in a twofold way, to an accumulation of excrementitious matters in the system, and favor the occurrence of a bilious attack. In this way may be explained the ill effects of suppers in disorders of this class, and the well known fact that a single indulgence of this kind may bring on a bilious attack in a person predisposed to it.

The medicines that are most efficacious are such as tend to promote digestion, and to keep up a regular action of the bowels. A few grains of rhubarb, alone, or in conjunction with a grain of ipecacuanha, taken habitually at dinner, or, if the patient be plethoric, occasional small doses of saline purgatives, taken in the morning, are often of service.

Fluids taken in large quantity, in the form of mineral waters, or pure water, have also often much efficacy in these disorders.

But our most effective resources are those hygienic regulations, before pointed out, which have relation to the great conditions of air, exercise, and temperature, on the one hand, and to the quantity and quality of the food, on the other. In the degree of confidence he places in these resources, and in the preponderance he gives them over mere drugging in the treatment of disorders of this class, the practitioner will give the best evidence of his real insight into their nature, and of practical skill founded upon it. It adds not a little to the value and importance of these means that they are so free from hazard, and that they act in a way in which no others can act, and therefore have no perfect substitute in any direct medication. By appropriate purgatives, we may temporarily drain the liver and intestines of redundant bile; but by the means here pointed out, we attack the evil at its source, and prevent the occurrence of the bilious state.

Deficient secretion of bile.—But disorder may likewise result from the bile being secreted in too small quantity.

In secreting bile the liver serves two purposes—it purifies the blood by freeing it from the excrementitious principles of the bile and from other excrementitious substances that are eliminated with it; and, by means of the bile, it aids the work of intestinal digestion. The secretion of bile may therefore be deficient in two respects. Too little bile may be secreted to purify the blood, or without this, too little may be secreted to perform the necessary part in digestion.

The simplest form of disorder arising from deficient secretion of bile is where, while the blood is not tinged with the biliary pigment, and the complexion remains clear, too little bile is secreted for the purposes of digestion. In such cases, digestion is usually slow and imperfect; the bowels are irregular, and generally confined; the contents of the large intestine often become too acid, or otherwise irritating, and produce headache, or depression of spirits, or occasional diarrhœa.

Disorder of this kind is sometimes the effect of the spare diet to which weakly and nervous persons are often condemned by painful digestion or uneasiness in the stomach after meals. Many of the evils of this state may be lessened by supplying the place of the bile, as a purgative, by aloes or colocynth; but the disorder will not be removed until the patient is enabled to live more freely.

Another form of disorder, attended with a very scanty flow of bile into the intestine, if not with diminished secretion of bile, and of which I have met with several well-marked examples, is this: a young person, delicate, and easily upset by any imprudence in diet, has three or four times a year an attack of diarrhœa, which lasts three or four days, or, it may be, a week, and which, during that time, no sedatives or vegetable astringents will stop. The diarrhœa is attended by smarting at the anus, and by great languor and debility, but not by sickness; and while it lasts the intestinal discharges are not at all colored by bile. As soon as the bile flows the diarrhœa immediately stops of itself. In these cases, the diarrhœa and the general disorder cannot be ascribed merely to defective secretion of bile, or to the bile's not flowing into the intestine. It is probable that the illness begins in disordered digestion, and that acid and irritating matters produced by this check the secretion of bile, or stop the flow of bile into the intestine by causing spasm or inflammation of the mouth of the common gall-duct, at the same time that they cause diarrhœa. While the disorder lasts, the contents of the bowels seem to be unnaturally acid, and the most effectual remedies are, magnesia, bismuth, and chalk.

Dr. Prout has ascribed a variety of similar disorders to excess of acid in some part of the intestinal canal, especially the cæcum.

He says: "Excessive acidity of the cæcum is generally accompanied by a deficient secretion of bile; and sometimes by a complete temporary suppression of the bilious discharge, apparently from spasmodic constriction of the common gall-duct; or, it may be, of the biliary ducts themselves. In this state of things all individuals feel more or less of uneasiness; but the point we wish to mention is, that certain individuals under these circumstances experience what is called nervous headache. This species of headache is frequently accompanied by nausea; is confined to the forehead; and, when severe, produces complete intolerance of light and sounds, and a state of mind bordering on delirium. After a greater or less period the pain ceases, sometimes quite suddenly; and the remarkable circumstances to be mentioned here are, that this sudden termination is preceded by a peculiar sensation (sometimes accompanied by an audible clicking noise) in the region of the gall-ducts; that immediately afterwards a gurgling sensation is felt in the upper bowels, as if a fluid was passing through them; and that in a few seconds, when this fluid, which we suppose to be bile, has reached the cæcum, the headache at once vanishes like a dream. One of the greatest martyrs to this species of headache I have ever seen, invariably experiences the train of symptoms above described; and I have witnessed it in a greater or less degree in many instances; indeed, I have experienced it in my own person." (*Stomach and Urinary Disorders*, 3d ed. p. 75.)

During attacks of this kind, our object should be to neutralize the excess of acid, and to carry off this and other offending matters by a mild but effectual purgative. Dr. Prout recommends the compound decoction of aloes, with magnesia, as well adapted to fulfil these objects. He says: "Drastic purgatives, in general, should be avoided; for, though they sometimes give immediate relief, they usually leave the patient more inveterately disposed to the disease."—(*Id.*,

p. 88.) I have lately had striking proof of the truth of this remark. A healthy-looking man, near fifty, who has habitually difficult digestion, and costive bowels, with occasional heartburn, has had for a great number of years frequent attacks of headache, like those described in the passage just cited from Dr. Prout. The headache generally comes on at night, and is confined to the forehead. It is extremely severe, and while it lasts the brow feels hot, the eyes water, and the urine is turbid. If let alone, its always lasts two or three days; but for many years he was in the habit of getting rid of it by Morrison's Pills. In the evening, as soon as the headache came on, he took sixteen of Morrison's Pills. In the course of three hours these purged him violently, and the headache was relieved at once. He continued to treat himself in this way for several years, but gave the plan up at last, from the headaches becoming more severe and more frequent. Under a restricted diet, and by taking daily at dinner a few grains of rhubarb, with a grain of ipecacuanha, and, now and then, a little magnesia or potash, to correct acidity, the headaches have become again much less frequent. In all diseases of this class, resulting from faulty digestion or assimilation—which manifest themselves now and then in a bilious attack, or a severe headache, or a fit of gout—our object must be, not merely to remedy the present disorder, but to change those habits of life by which recurrence of the disorder is favored.

Another class of disorders is where the secretion of bile is deficient, not with reference to digestion merely, but as regards the blood—where the blood is not sufficiently freed from the excrementitious principles which it is the business of the liver to excrete.

This may even happen where a large quantity of bile is secreted. The bile may be in excess as regards the intestines, and cause the bilious diarrhœa before described, and yet may be eliminated in too small quantity to purify the blood, and the complexion be bilious or sallow. Disorder of this kind is, in general, of short duration. A dose of calomel and a few brisk purgatives carry off the redundant bile; and if no mischief have been done to the gall-ducts, all is soon well. The malady depends, not on defective power in the liver, but on heat of climate, or too rich living, or indolent habits, which render necessary a more than commonly abundant secretion of bile.

But it often happens that, in consequence of some structural change in the liver, too little bile is habitually secreted both to purify the blood and to forward digestion, even when the habits of life, and other circumstances, are most favorable to health. Where there has been adhesive inflammation of branches of the portal vein, or where adhesive inflammation in the areolar tissue about the vein has obliterated many of its small twigs, and the parts of the liver which those branches or those twigs supplied are atrophied; or where, from the more interstitial deposit of lymph, in cirrhosis, the original substance of the liver is divided into small masses of lobules, which, by the subsequent contraction of the effused lymph, get more or less atrophied; or where by a different agency, and, it may be, without inflammation at all, the number and power of the secreting cells have been permanently lessened—the liver may be inadequate duly to perform its office, and the health be permanently impaired in consequence.

The various forms of adhesive inflammation which lead to induration and atrophy of parts of the liver are brought on, in almost all cases, by spirit-drinking. The more direct injury to the secreting element of the liver is more commonly the effect of mental anxiety, of some form of protracted indigestion, or of long residence in a hot climate and of the various bilious disorders incident to it. Habitual defective secretion of bile is therefore met with most commonly in persons who have been hard drinkers, and in persons who have been subject to the other influences injurious to the liver that have been just named. The condition of the liver in these two classes of persons differs in this, that in the former class there is an impediment to the passage of blood through the liver, in consequence of a deposit of lymph about the vessels, and its subsequent contraction; while in the latter class no such impediment exists. But the condition of the liver is so far alike in the two classes, that the secreting element has been damaged in both, and what is left of it does not suffice for the purposes of health.

In effect of the injury done to the secreting element of the liver, and the consequent inadequate secretion of bile, digestion is slow, and imperfectly performed; the bowels are habitually costive; the blood contains less than its natural proportion of globules; there is a falling-off in flesh and strength; and usually the skin is more or less sallow and dry. In this state a person may go on for years, with very little effective liver left. When a state of great anemia is induced, comparatively little liver, as well as comparatively little lung, is required to maintain the blood at the diminished standard. In the advanced stage of consumption, the blood is sometimes perfectly arterialized, and, while the patient is at rest, there is no distress of breathing, when not more than one-third or one-fourth of the lungs is left in an effective state. The reason of this is, that the muscular tissue and the quantity of blood in the body are almost as much diminished as the respiratory power. So it is with the liver. Many of the persons who return from India with dry wrinkled skins and greenish complexions, who, if we consider the liver merely as a secreting organ, have truly, to use the common phrase, very little liver left, may yet, with proper care, enjoy moderate comfort for years. In the advanced stages of cirrhosis, too, a person may still live on, when but a comparatively small portion of the original secreting structure of the liver remains; and here there is an additional cause of wasting, in the impediment to the passage of the portal blood. But, in all such cases, where, from some damage done to its secreting element, the liver is permanently very inadequate to its office, though life may continue, digestion and nutrition are imperfect, *a state of anemia exists*, the person grows gradually thinner, and at length dies, much wasted.

In disorders of this class, which result from organic disease, the health cannot be perfectly re-established; but it may be very much mended, and life may be much prolonged. Nothing contributes to this so much as strict attention to diet. A sufficiency of light nourishing food should, of course, be taken; but all rich dishes should be avoided, and, as much as possible, fermented drinks, as they tend to induce a bilious state of the system, and thus to render the liver still more inadequate to its office. The bowels should be regulated by some mild, but effectual, purgative. A pill of aloes, or of aloes and rhubarb, taken habitually at dinner, answers the purpose well. The patient should have the advantage, when possible, of a pure, moderate cool air, which has great efficacy in bilious states of the system. When the weather permits, airing in an open carriage, or, if it can be borne, riding on horseback, short of fatigue, will be productive of good. These simple hygienic measures—regulation of diet, and provision for free respiration—are the more important, because, as has been before remarked, there is no substitute for them.

A medicine that is often of much efficacy in cases in which there is deficient secretion of bile from injury to the secreting structure of the liver, is the so-called nitro-muriatic acid, which has long been extensively used in India in the treatment of chronic hepatic derangements. When it acts favorably, it increases the secretion of bile, and at the same time strengthens digestion, promotes the action of the bowels, and has a tonic influence on the system at large. From eight to fifteen minims of each of the dilute acids in a wineglass of water may be given twice a day, half an hour or three-quarters of an hour before the principal meals; or, as is a common practice in India, the nitro-muriatic acid may be applied *externally* in the various forms of bath and lotion. The most convenient forms for general use are foot-baths, and fomentations or lotions to the side.[1]

Of medicines that have a special action on the liver to increase the flow of bile, or, as they have been termed, *cholagogues*, the most energetic is mercury. In the occasional bilious disorders of persons who have no organic disease of the liver, a dose of calomel or blue pills, followed by a brisk saline purgative, produces more speedy relief than anything else, and is more likely, therefore, to prevent inflammation or ulceration of the gall-ducts, which seem generally to result from the irritation of unhealthy bile. Occasionally, and under these circumstances, and especially in persons of full habit, mercury may be given with great advantage. But its frequent use, in any case, may lead to much mischief. When the liver has been accustomed to the stimulus of mercury, no other medicine will sufficiently excite its action. The person is thus led to the habitual use of this medicine, and, after a time, the constitution is seriously injured by it. In the class of cases we have just been considering, where, from organic disease, the liver is inadequate to its office, and nutrition has suffered much in consequence, mercury, although even here it may relieve for the moment, almost invariably does harm. It increases the activity of the liver at first, but seems

[1] Annesley directs f℥iv of nitric acid, and f℥iv of muriatic acid, of the strength of the London Pharmacopœia, to be added to f℥viij of pure water, and the mixture to be labelled, "*the nitro-muriatic solution.*" From fʒj to fʒij of this solution to a pint of water is the strength used for lotions and foot-baths. For a foot-bath, the water should be nearly the temperature of the blood, and the feet should be kept immersed in it for twenty minutes or half an hour, every night, at bedtime. When used as a wash, it should be of an agreeable temperature, and should be applied assiduously to the trunk and insides of the thighs for a quarter of an hour daily.

to leave it weaker than before; and if frequently resorted to, the nutrition of the patient, impaired by the original disease, is still further impaired by the drug. In all such cases we should be content with milder medicines, which promote the secretion of bile without having any permanent deleterious effect on the system. One of the best medicines of this class is taraxacum, which may be given alone, or in conjunction with the nitro-muriatic acid. Cholagogue medicines, especially mercury and soda, are, like diuretics, uncertain in their action; and if given in too large doses when the secreting organ has been damaged, or when any extraneous condition exists interfering with its action, they sometimes lessen or even altogether arrest secretion instead of increasing it.

In all organic diseases of the liver, where the secretion of bile is habitually deficient, and nutrition is impaired in consequence, the person should be warmly clad, and should avoid all avoidable causes of exhaustion. Fatigue, and lowering remedies, exhaust the strength, and draw, as it were, upon the *capital* of the patient, when this is very difficult to recruit. The disease destroys its victim, not by sudden illness, but by gradually wasting the strength. The more, therefore, this is economized, the longer will life be preserved.

The bile altered in quality.—The bile found in the gall-bladder after death varies much in color and consistence in different cases. In some it is of a light yellow, and thin, or watery; in others, it has a reddish cast; in others, again, it is of a dark olive, and thick, and viscid—but little is known of the changes in its chemical composition that correspond to these changes in its outward characters. Few analyses have been made even of healthy human bile. The attempts of chemists to ascertain the composition of bile have most of them been made on ox-bile, which can be more readily obtained fresh, and can be obtained in larger quantity than human bile. It cannot, therefore, excite surprise that little is yet known by chemical analysis of the changes produced by disease in human bile. The chief morbid states of bile ascertained in this way consist in the presence of a free acid, in the presence of urea, in the presence of some medicines that pass off in the bile, and in an excess or a deficiency of the water, biliary matter, or mucus of the bile.

The presence of a free acid in bile found in the human gall-bladder after death is not a very uncommon occurrence. Instances have been related above in which it occurred:—

1st. In a woman who died, in the month of July, of jaundice from suppressed secretion, with symptoms of cerebral poisoning. (See page 273.) Rapid decomposition of the body took place, and when it was examined thirty-six hours after death, the gall-bladder contained about a drachm of chocolate-colored bile, which, to judge by the reaction of blue litmus-paper, was intensely acid. Litmus-paper placed in contact with the liver itself was immediately changed to a bright red.

2d. In a man (p. 245) who died in January, 1852, in a state of great exhaustion, from scrofulous enlargement of the liver and chronic abscess of the left kidney. The bile in the gall-bladder was of a pale orange color, and had a distinct acid reaction. The body, which was examined thirty-two hours after death, presented no striking marks of decomposition.

In the first edition of this work, reference was made to the case of a woman who died in the autumn of 1843, in King's College Hospital, of cancerous ulceration of the rectum and granular kidney, in which this condition was observed. The bile reddened litmus-paper distinctly, and from its being of a pale amber color, no doubt could exist that the change of color in the paper was owing to the action of an acid.

In the autumn of 1849 I met with very pale-colored bile, distinctly acid, together with three gall-stones, in the gall-bladder of a man who died in King's College Hospital of chronic granular disease of the kidney, with recent inflammation of the pericardium and pleura. The bile in this instance presented other unnatural appearances, containing numerous flaky masses which were found to consist of epithelium, and many amorphous masses which seemed to consist chiefly of biliary coloring matter.

I have met with several other instances in which the bile, and the liver itself, had a very distinct acid reaction; and in most of them the bile, as in the instances noticed above, was unnaturally pale. Deficiency of the proper biliary coloring matter seems to promote the occurrence of an acid condition in the bile.

The immediate cause of this acid condition of the bile is most probably decomposition of the bile, or of the mucus it contains.[1]

[1] Since the preceding observations were published in the second edition of this work, the third volume of Lehmann's elaborate work on *Physiological Chemistry*

When ox-bile is allowed to decompose exposed to the air, it becomes after some days distinctly acid; and if it be then neutralized, it becomes, on further standing, acid again. It is a curious circumstance, tending to show the complementary relation that exists between the bile and the urine, that decomposition, which renders the urine alkaline, renders the bile acid. The decomposition of the bile takes place, of course, more rapidly in hot weather, and is much promoted by the mucus it contains, which acts as a ferment. There can be little doubt that in the bodies of persons who die of disease, a process of decomposition goes on constantly in the liver after death, although for some time it may produce no striking change. In animals that were killed, M. Bernard constantly found sugar in the liver, when the liver was analyzed immediately after death; but if some hours only were allowed to elapse before the analysis was made, no sugar was found. In this short time the sugar had been changed into some other substance.

We may expect then most frequently to find the bile acid when it is unnaturally pale, or contains a large proportion of unhealthy mucus, and is thus unnaturally prone to decomposition; when death occurs from exhaustion, and rapid decomposition of the body ensues; and when the body is examined a considerable time after death, in hot weather.

We may expect, also, sometimes to find it acid in those cases of jaundice from suppressed secretion, in which the unexpected occurrence of fatal head symptoms, the softened state of the liver after death, and the early putrefaction of the body,* evince the existence of some noxious agent which seems (see page 273) to be developed in the system by decomposition of the broken-up hepatic cells, or of the retained elements of the bile.

In some instances the bile may be rendered acid, as Gorup-Besanez has suggested, by the presence of pus, generating lactic acid.

It is possible, however, that under certain circumstances, bile may be acid when first secreted.

Dr. Prout seems to have imagined that in consequence of great development of *lactic* acid, either in the stomach from imperfect

has appeared, in which it is stated that the juices of the liver, spleen, thymus, supra-renal capsules, and the smooth muscles, all contain free acid.—(Lehmann's *Physiological Chemistry*, translation of the Sydenham Society, vol. iii. p. 223.)

digestion, or in the blood from constitutional diseases, especially those produced by malaria—the portal blood might become black and *acid;* and that this unnatural blood passing through the liver might disorder its secretion, and the bile might thus be deprived of its neutralizing properties, "if not actually rendered acid."[1] I am not aware that any attempts have been made, by chemical analysis, to settle this important point.

Urea has been found in the bile, only, I believe, in persons dead of cholera. It was first detected by Dr. O'Shaughnessey, in bile which he analyzed at the request of Dr. Roupell, and which was taken from a person who died of cholera, after having made very little urine for eight days. The bile did not differ in appearance from ordinary bile, but contained in one thousand parts, six of salts, and *three of urea.* (*Roupell on Cholera*, p. 84.)

Various medicines have been found in the bile, but our list of those which pass off in this way is, doubtless, very imperfect. It is probable that most of the medicines which increase the secretion of bile pass off, in part, either bodily or more or less changed, through this channel.

The observations made by chemical analysis on the altered qualities of the natural constituents of bile are very few and of little value. They are sufficient to show that some of the natural constituents of bile become changed in disease—which might have been anticipated from the readiness with which the principles of bile enter into new combinations—but they do not tell us in what these changes consist.

The difficulty of analyzing bile, and the circumstance that human bile can only be obtained in small quantity and many hours after death, when the bile in the gall-bladder is probably already changed by decomposition, sufficiently account for the observations of this kind yet made being so few and so little to be relied on.

The most valuable observations that have been made on altered qualities of the bile—and these are few and imperfect—relate to changes that can be at once recognized by the senses.

In some cases, the coloring matter is deficient, the bile, found even in the gall-bladder, is pale and thin, and has not its usual bitterness, and the lining membrane of the gall-bladder and gall-

[1] See Prout on Stomach and Urinary Diseases. 3d edition. Introduction, p. 45.

ducts is hardly stained by it. This condition of the bile is frequently found in those diseases which change the structure of the whole liver. It is not uncommon in cirrhosis, and is now and then remarked where the liver is much enlarged from the interstitial deposit of fat, or other morbid products.

But occasionally the bile has these characters when there is no apparent disease of the liver itself, and when the unnatural quality of the bile results from an unhealthy state of the blood. I have found bile of this kind several times in persons dead of granular kidney, and twice in cases of suppurative phlebitis, with scattered abscesses in the lungs and other parts of the body, without there being any abscess or other marks of inflammation in the liver.

The elaborate researches of M. Louis have shown that in persons dead of typhoid fever, the bile in the gall-bladder is often (in more than one-half the cases) more thin and watery than healthy bile, and often has a reddish or *rust* color, instead of the yellow or greenish tints proper to bile. It has been remarked in a former chapter that, in typhoid fever, suppurative inflammation of the gall-bladder sometimes comes on, doubtless in consequence of the retention, and it may be the decomposition, of unhealthy and irritating bile.

The observations of M. Louis, on the condition of the cystic bile in persons dead of typhoid fever, have been confirmed by the late researches of Gorup-Besanez, who states that he analyzed many specimens of bile taken from the gall-bladders of persons who died of this disease, and found that not one of them contained more than half the usual quantity of solid matter.

In persons dead of inflammation of the lungs, according to Gorup-Besanez, the bile in the gall-bladder has often the outward characters so common in typhoid fever, and contains an unnaturally small proportion of solid matter.

The same thing happens not unfrequently in dysentery.[1] But in none of these cases do the color and consistence, and the relative proportion of the solid constituents, of the bile in the gall-bladder afford very trustworthy evidence respecting the characters of the bile when first secreted, because the bile undergoes concentration in the gall-bladder, and consequently its color and consistence depend very much on the time it had been in the bladder when death occurred.

[1] See Parkes on Dysentery, &c., p. 46.

In other cases, and sometimes even in the diseases referred to above, the bile, instead of being pale and thin, is unusually dark-colored and thick. This may be from mere long retention in the gall-bladder. If the bile remain long in the bladder, much of its water is absorbed, and it becomes very dark-colored and viscid. This is usually found to be the case in healthy persons who die from some accident after long fasting. In persons who die during the cold stage of malignant cholera, where the whole body is drained of its water, the bile in the gall-bladder is always of a dark olive and viscid. In persons who die of phthisis, the bile in the gall-bladder, even when the liver is fatty, is often very dark-colored and viscid, most probably from remaining there long, and becoming concentrated, by reason of the repugnance to food, and the consequent emptiness of the stomach and intestines, that is common in the advanced stages of phthisis.

But the bile may be *secreted* unusually viscid, and unusually dark-colored, and may present these characters in the hepatic ducts when the passage of the ducts is free. This is, perhaps, most common in hot climates, where the essential principles of the bile are formed in large quantity in the system. Annesley states that very commonly in India, in persons who die of diseases of the liver, or of other organs, the gall-bladder is found distended with thick, acrid bile, and the hepatic ducts are completely gorged with bile of this character, without any apparent organic change sufficient to account for the circumstance, and without other impediment to the escape of the bile than that which arises from its own viscidity. Where the secretion of bile is very abundant, a partial obstruction of short continuance may cause great accumulation of it in the gall-bladder and in the liver itself. Annesley believes that in India this accumulation of bile occurs, not only in the course of other disorders, but as an ailment of itself, the disturbance in the system resulting solely from the retention of bile in the liver, and the subsequent irruption of the long retained bile into the intestinal canal. He says: "The earliest symptoms of which the patient generally complains, when he attends to his sensations and state of health, are, clamminess and foulness of the mouth, fauces, and tongue, with a bitter taste, particularly in the morning; a sense of distension and weight at the epigastric region, and at the precordia, frequently with a sense of coldness and sinking in the same situations; slight anxiety; acid and acrid eructations about three or four hours after a full meal, with painful fulness at the epigastrium, and difficult digestion. The patient often complains of headache, pain in the back or loins, uneasiness under the shoulder-blades, fulness and pain in the region of the liver, particularly when pressure is made at the time of his taking a full inspiration, and of aching in his knees, shoulders, and limbs, his countenance being pale, sallow, or muddy, and the conjunctivæ more or less tinged of a yellowish hue. The state of the pulse is different in different cases. It is often slow and full, and sometimes it is irregular in frequency and strength; occasionally it intermits, and not unfrequently becomes quick, but oppressed upon the least motion or exertion. The urine is generally high-colored, and deposits a brownish sediment. The stools are often costive, sometimes light or clay-colored, and frequently tenacious. When the accumulated bile is discharged into the alimentary canal, much constitutional disturbance generally arises, according to the qualities which this fluid may have acquired from its retention. The pulse now becomes quick, and often irregular; vomiting and purging, with griping pain and anxiety, often supervene, sometimes with spasms. Thirst becomes urgent, and the tongue, which was before foul, is now excited, often dry, and its papillæ large, distinct, and erect." (Vol. i. p. 329.)

"It sometimes occurs that the inordinate flow of morbid bile into the duodenum, particularly when it has been long retained, and during close, warm, and moist states of the air, occasions faintness, the most alarming state of sinking, and prostration of the vital energies." (Id. p. 331.)

In this country, a bilious disorder attended with symptoms very like those described by Annesley, is now and then met with, and is probably occasioned, as Annesley, supposes, by temporary retention of viscid or unhealthy bile.

But the retention of thick and unhealthy bile may lead to other mischief. When healthy bile even is much concentrated, it throws down irregular, solid, green or yellow particles—consisting of biliary pigment in combination with bases—which may be distinctly seen under the microscope, and which, if the concentration be carried far enough, render the bile gritty, or even form a complete *magma*. If the bile be unusually dark-colored and thick, and otherwise unhealthy, when first secreted, and especially if it remain long in the gall-bladder, such a precipitate may take place *in the bladder*, and lead to the formation of gall-stones.

In man, gall-stones have almost always a dark nucleus of concrete biliary matter, which is surrounded by cholesterine, mixed with variable proportions of the coloring matter of bile; and they are almost always found in the gall-bladder or in the cystic or common ducts, obviously because the bile, during its stay in the gall-bladder, becomes concentrated, and perhaps decomposed, and is, in consequence, more apt to be precipitated in solid form there than in the hepatic ducts.[1]

Another morbid state of bile, of great importance from its contributing largely to the formation of gall-stones, is where the bile contains sparkling scales of cholesterine. I have never found this in the hepatic ducts. Cholesterine seems in most cases to be formed in the gall-bladder, or at least to be there deposited in crystals, and its presence in visible scales in the bile is generally associated with disease of the gall-bladder. When the coats of the gall-bladder have undergone the fatty degeneration before spoken of, the cystic bile always abounds in crystals of this substance. But crystals of cholesterine are now and then formed when the coats of the gall-bladder seem healthy.[2]

These considerations lead us to gall-stones, which, from their palpable form, their frequency, and the distressing symptoms they often occasion, have excited more attention than any other result of unhealthy bile.

[1] In stall-fed oxen, whose bile, from the nature of their food, is perhaps richer in coloring matter, gall-stones, composed entirely of the coloring matters and the resinous principles of bile, are frequently found in the hepatic ducts.

[2] Cholesterine may doubtless be secreted by any part of the mucous lining of the biliary passages. The "knotty tumors" described in the next chapter prove an abundant secretion of it from the hepatic ducts under certain circumstances.

SECT. V.—*Gall-stones.*

GALL-STONES, as already remarked, are usually formed in the gall-bladder, where the bile becomes concentrated from absorption of part of its water, and often otherwise altered by unhealthy secretions from the coats of the bladder, and where it is longer stagnant than in the ducts. But it now and then happens that gall-stones form in the substance of the liver, in branches of the hepatic duct. These *hepatic* gall-stones are always very small, of irregular, tuberculated form, and of a dark olive color, approaching to black. They probably originate, in most cases, in inflammation of the hepatic ducts. In consequence of this, a duct becomes closed at some point. The bile then accumulates in the portion beyond, and after being some time stagnant, is inspissated by the absorption of part of its water, and some of its constituents are precipitated, forming solid dark-coloured granules. These granules and the inspissated bile that remains are cemented by mucus secreted by the coats of the duct, so as to form a small calculus.

The way in which gall-stones in the substance of the liver are formed explains the circumstance, remarked by Cruveilhier and others, that they are often *encysted.* The cyst, like some other varieties of cyst occasionally found in the liver, is formed of the coats of the gall-duct. The duct is distended into a pouch by the foreign matter, and, being closed on each side of this by inflammation, forms, if the foreign body be not absorbed, a permanent cyst.

Gall-stones of the same kind are now and then found in the gall-bladder. They are usually small, and are at once distinguished from ordinary gall-stones by their irregular, tuberculated form, and their almost black color—circumstances which have led to their being compared, and not unaptly, to black pepper. They are heavier than ordinary gall-stones, and do not burn so readily, and, when burnt, sometimes leave a considerable quantity of carbonate and phosphate of lime.[1] They are composed chiefly of biliary coloring matter, some salts of lime, and mucus. The bile-pigment forms insoluble compounds with the alkaline earths, and the pigment and lime are consequently precipitated together, forming minute dark-colored nodules, which become cemented by mucus.

Little is known of the circumstances which lead to the formation of this kind of gall-stone. Dr. Prout has hinted that they are associated with a tendency to the formation of oxalic acid, and to that of malignant disease, more especially of the liver.

I have met with gall-stones of this kind in two cases, of which I have kept notes. The first was that of a sailor, fifty-four years of age, who died of fever, in the Seamen's Hospital, in July, 1827, and who for seven months previously had been employed on the Thames. The liver appeared healthy, and no marks of disease were noticed in the gall-bladder. There were some small serous cysts in the cortical substance of each kidney; and at the back part of the upper lobe of the left lung, the surface, for the breadth of a half crown, was puckered, and the pulmonary tissue beneath indurated, the consequence of a cavity which had formed there at some former period, and which was not quite closed. There were no tubercles, or other marks of former disease, and the only recent changes of structure were ulcers in the lower part of the ileum, the result of the fever. The gall-bladder contained a great number of very dark mulberry-looking calculi, all of them about the size of small peas. When dried, they were very friable, and were found to be composed of solid black grains, cemented by a greenish matter, which consisted of mucus and inspissated bile.

The second case was that of a man, aged sixty-two, who died in the summer of 1838, also of fever. The gall-bladder contained three irregular black calculi, apparently composed of biliary matter and mucus, the smallest of the size of a cherry-stone. There was a calculus of the same kind in one of the hepatic ducts. The mucous membrane of the gall-bladder was somewhat thickened, but was not ulcerated. Besides the calculi, there was in the bladder a small quantity of yellow gritty bile.

In the Museum of King's College is a dry preparation, left to the College by the late Dr. Hooper, showing a great number of

[1] Prout on Stomach and Urinary Diseases. Third edition. Introduction, p. 65; and Lehmann's Physiological Chemistry.

gall-stones of this kind in the bladder in which they were found. (See Plate I., Fig. 1, in which some of these gall-stones are represented.) The coats of the bladder seem to have been healthy.

A healthy state of the gall-bladder seems to be requisite in order that stones of this kind may continue to exist for any considerable time in it. When its coats are much diseased, cholesterine is usually formed, or at least takes the solid form, in large quantity in the gall-bladder, and if there be a small mass of inspissated bile, to serve as a nucleus, cholesterine collects around it, and produces the more common kind of gall-stone.

Gall-stones composed for the most part of precipitated biliary pigment are seldom found in the human gall-bladder, and when found there, are usually very small, on account of the great tendency to the formation of cholesterine; but in the gall-bladder of the ox, cholesterine seems less apt to be formed, and gall-stones, composed almost entirely of the coloring matters of bile, are not unfrequently met with. The gall-stones found in the bladder of the ox have been long esteemed as a pigment. (Prout.)

Gall-stones from the human gall-bladder are almost always composed in great part of cholesterine, mixed with a certain quantity of the coloring matters of bile. They have all a nucleus, which is generally of a dark olive or black, and which, like the small, irregular, dark-colored gall-stones, described above, is in most cases composed chiefly of biliary coloring matter and lime, cemented by mucus. Late researches have shown that dark-colored gall-stones often contain also an appreciable quantity of copper.

The shape, and size, and appearance of gall-stones vary very much, according to the circumstances under which they are formed.

When there is only one gall-stone in the bladder, it may grow to the size of a hen's egg, but is seldom found so large. While it remains small, and can move freely in the bladder, it is generally spherical; but when it becomes so large that it is girthed by the bladder, or can no longer roll freely in it, it grows most at the ends which are not subject to pressure, and so becomes somewhat egg-shaped.

Large solitary gall-stones, with the exception of their nuclei, are composed almost entirely of cholesterine, and are, consequently, whitish and crystalline. They have a soapy feel, and when placed in the flame of a candle, readily melt, and burn with a bright flame.

Sometimes the cholesterine is deposited after closure of the cystic duct, and when all the bile previously in the gall-bladder has been absorbed, and the stone is then quite white, like a ball of camphor, or of white marble. The surface is generally a little rough and dull, but it readily takes a fine polish. When these round or oval stones are sawn through the centre, they are seen to be crystallized in rays, which converge towards the nucleus. (See Plate I., Fig. 2, which represents the section of a gall-stone of this kind.)

It sometimes happens that two round or oval gall-stones are found in the bladder, when, by some constriction at its middle, the bladder is divided into two distinct pouches.

When the cystic duct has been closed, and the coats of the gall-bladder are healthy, the stone is sometimes closely embraced by the bladder and marked by its rugæ, so that it has its surface tubercular, like the mulberry.

But it is much more common to find many gall-stones in the bladder than a single one; and occasionally they are found in almost incredible numbers. As many as three thousand have been counted in a single bladder.

When there are many gall-stones in the bladder, they differ in form and appearance from solitary gall-stones. Instead of being round or oval, they have, usually, plane, polished faces—the effect of the mutual attrition of the stones, which polish each other the more from the presence of the minute crystals of cholesterine contained in the bile.

When the stones are few in number, and can shift their relative positions in the bladder, they may attain a considerable size, and sometimes become very irregular in form, often, as remarked by Haller, very much resembling the bones of the wrist.

In other instances, their forms are strikingly regular. In the spring of 1837 I found in the gall-bladder of a man, who died of scurvy, at the age of sixty, eight gall-stones, little larger than peas, all of them very regular tetrahedrons. It is difficult to imagine how forms so regular are produced.

Gall-stones which have smooth, flat faces, generally contain more of the coloring matters of bile than large solitary gall-stones, and are usually of a variegated greenish and brownish color. When sawn through the centre, they are found to be laminated, and to have a nucleus, which generally contains traces of mucus and earthy phosphates, but consists principally of a combination of the bile-pigment with lime.[1] The successive laminæ are sometimes very fine; but, even then, when the face is polished, they are generally distinctly visible from being of different shades of brown and green. When a section is made through the centre, and its surface polished, together with the concentric laminæ, rays may still be seen converging towards the centre, as in the white oval calculi of cholesterine. (See Plate I., Fig. 3.) In both varieties of calculi the cholesterine is deposited in the same way, but in the pure cholesterine calculi the appearance of concentric laminæ is not produced, because the successive layers are not tinged of different colors by the bile.

Gall-stones, which appear distinctly laminated, have sometimes a crust of pure cholesterine, which was formed after the entrance of bile into the bladder had been prevented by one of them becoming impacted in the cystic duct. (See Plate II., Fig. 2.)

Now and then, but rarely, for obvious reasons, this order is reversed. A gall-stone almost of pure cholesterine, and therefore uniformly white, has a crust, of which the successive layers are differently colored by bile, and which therefore appears laminated.

The different gall-stones found in the same bladder have almost always the same characters. They are laminated alike; their nuclei have the same appearance; and if one of them have a crust of pure cholesterine, they all have it. From this it is probable that they are generally formed at the same time, and not in succession.

A circumstance that seems almost necessary to the formation of gall-stones, is the presence of a small mass of biliary gravel, or inspissated bile cemented by mucus, or some other substance about which the cholesterine may collect. An excess of cholesterine is not, of itself, sufficient for the formation of gall-stones. In a case related in a former part of this work, the mouth of the cystic duct seemed to have been long blocked up by a gall-stone, and the gall-bladder, whose coats had undergone the fatty degeneration, was filled with viscid mucus sparkling with scales of cholesterine, yet no other gall-stones had formed in the bladder. Another specimen, precisely of the same kind, was sent to King's College Museum, in

[1] The nucleus sometimes contains copper, and probably other metals, which, in the state of oxide, combine, like the alkaline and earthy bases, with the coloring matter of bile. Occasionally uric acid has been found in gall-stones. (See Lehmann's *Physiological Chemistry*. Translation by Dr. Day, vol. ii. pp. 74–5.)

the summer of 1843, by Mr. Lingen, of Hereford. (King's College Museum, Prep. 268.) Gall-stones are formed in numbers in the gall-bladder, only when the bile can flow into it through the cystic duct. But the presence of bile, even of dark-colored bile, and a plentiful formation of cholesterine, are not alone sufficient. On more than one occasion I have found in the gall-bladder very dark-colored viscid bile, sparkling with scales of cholesterine, when there were no gall-stones. It seems necessary for the formation of a gall-stone, that there should be a nucleus of some other substance, about which the cholesterine may crystallize. It would appear, from some of the published descriptions of gall-stones, that a particle of cholesterine may of itself serve as a nucleus of a solitary gall-stone, but this happens very seldom. In almost all cases the nucleus is of a dark color, and consists chiefly of biliary coloring matter, lime, and mucus. The nucleus presents different appearances in different gall-stones. In some it is round and compact, even when the gall-stone has been long kept, and is perfectly dry; in others, in which it is composed in great part of *mucus*, it is of irregular outline, and, in drying, contracts, so as to leave a hollow in the centre of the stone. (Plate I., Fig. 4.) In some, the nucleus is a mere point; in others, of the size of a small pea. But, as before remarked, when there are many gall-stones in the same bladder, their nuclei have, usually, all the same characters. If one nucleus is small, all are small; if one is compact, all are compact; if one stone have a hollow in the centre, all have it.

A few instances have been recorded in which some other substance than those mentioned above formed the nucleus of a gall-stone.

Bouisson states that he has a small solitary gall-stone, whose nucleus seemed to be formed of blood (Bouisson, p. 243); and one the size of an almond, which he found in the hepatic duct of an ox, in which the nucleus is a fragment of a fluke. He cites an instance, represented by Lobstein in his plates of morbid anatomy, where a large gall-stone had formed about a dried lumbric worm. The gall-stone was found in the common duct of a woman, sixty-eight years of age, who died of colliquative diarrhœa, in a hospital at Strasburg. There were one hundred and eighty-five worms of this kind in the stomach, and thirty in the branches of the gall-ducts, which were very much dilated. He cites another instance where a gall-stone had formed about a pin in the gall-bladder; and another, where the nucleus of a gall-stone is said to have contained globules of mercury. This last gall-stone, which was of the size of a prune, and composed chiefly of cholesterine, was taken from a person to whom mercury had been given for syphilis. The nucleus of the stone, when melted by heat, *is said* to have presented many globules of mercury.

Gall-stones are very light considering their size. When fresh from the gall-bladder, they usually sink if placed in water; but when they have been kept long, and are quite dry, most of them float, until they have imbibed a certain quantity of the water, when they sink slowly. Their specific gravity depends chiefly on the relative proportion of cholesterine and coloring matter. Cholesterine is lighter than water; the bile-pigment and its compound with lime are heavier. The lightest gall-stones are therefore usually those which contain the largest proportion of cholesterine. The weight of gall-stones, especially when dry, will, of course, vary also with the character of their nuclei.

Mr. Taylor has lately described a calculus, which he found among the calculi in the Museum of the College of Surgeons, and which he supposes to be biliary, composed chiefly of *stearate of lime.* It was oval, slightly flattened, an inch and a half in length, rather more than an inch in thickness, and about an inch and a quarter in breadth. Its surface was of a dirty white, and it had the greasy feel of cholesterine calculi. It floated in water, and when applied to the tongue left an impression of bitterness. It yielded readily to the knife, and the cut surface had a polished appearance. It was composed of white and reddish yellow concentric layers, alternating with each other, and easily separable. At its centre there was a small hollow. When heated before the blowpipe it readily fused, and then caught fire, burning with a clear flame, and giving out the smell of animal matter, but nothing of a urinous character. "From cholesterine calculi it is readily distinguished by the absence of any crystalline structure when broken, which, unless the quantity of coloring matter be very large, is always more or less apparent in that variety; also by its insolubility in alcohol and ether, and by readily dissolving in these menstrua, and in a cold solution of caustic potass, after it has been acted upon by an acid. (*London and Edinburgh Phil. Magazine*, 1840.)

There is no account of the source from which this calculus was derived; and it is doubtful, therefore, whether it was taken from man or from one of the lower animals.

Now and then, *chalky concretions*, composed chiefly of phosphate of lime, or of carbonate of lime, are found in the gall-bladder or in the ducts, or, apparently isolated from the ducts, in the substance of the liver. Andral relates the case of a man who died at the age of fifty, in whose gall-bladder were three small calculi of phosphate of lime. The cystic duct was obliterated, and, with the exception of these calculi, the gall-bladder contained nothing but a little ropy mucus. The liver was united to all the adjacent parts by old false membranes, and its substance was remarkably tough and granular. The disease seems to have commenced ten years before death, when the patient had jaundice, which was soon followed by ascites. (*Clin. Med.*, iv. p. 511.)

M. Bouisson states that he once found a calculus, of the size of a pea, composed of carbonate of lime, projecting from the surface of the liver. (*Bouisson*, p. 197.)

I have more than once found a small gall-stone of biliary matter surrounded by a layer of phosphate and carbonate of lime, in a pouch formed by partial dilatation of the cystic duct.

These chalky concretions are not formed from the bile, but originate in disease of the mucous membrane of the gall-bladder or gall-ducts. In sheep that have been infested with flukes, some of the gall-ducts not unfrequently become almost converted in this way into bony cylinders; and, now and then, in the liver of one of these animals a small chalky concretion may be found, apparently isolated from the ducts. These chalky bodies are surrounded by a cyst, which is formed, like so many other varieties of hepatic cyst, from a small portion of a gall-duct, which becomes dilated by the foreign matter, and isolated, by inflammation, from the rest of the duct.

Ordinary gall-stones are composed, as we have seen, of cholesterine, which, with variable proportions of coloring matter, is deposited about a nucleus, which generally consists of biliary coloring matter, some salts of lime, and mucus. The cholesterine crystallizes so as to form rays converging from all points of the circumference of the stone to its centre; but when it is mixed with, or stained by, the coloring matters of bile, which, as is usual, are in different proportions in layers successively deposited, the stone, while it still exhibits the converging rays, appears made up of distinct concentric laminæ.

Two circumstances seem, then, generally to concur in the formation of these cholesterine calculi: the presence of a small mass of concrete biliary matter, lime, or mucus, to serve as a nucleus, and the presence of cholesterine in crystals, to make up the body of the stone. The first step is the formation of the nucleus, which probably results in most cases, especially when many gall-stones are formed together, from an unhealthy state of the bile, or from its decomposition, or undue concentration in the gall-bladder, leading to precipitation of some of the essential principles of the bile, or of some salt of lime, in solid form.[1] The second step is the formation of crystals of cholesterine. This may likewise result from an unnatural state of the bile, especially from a relative deficiency of tauro-cholic acid, or tauro-cholate of soda, which seems to be the chief solvent of the cholesterine in the bile; but it is frequently associated with, and apparently dependent upon, fatty degeneration of the coats of the gall-bladder.

In every case the presence of gall-stones is evidence of an unnatural state of the bile at the time of their formation.

The question then arises—What conditions of life, or what other influences, tend to bring about those unnatural states of the bile on which the formation of gall-stones depends?

The first circumstance to be noticed is, that gall-stones can seldom be traced to structural disease in the substance of the liver itself. Some diseases of the liver seem, indeed, to be almost incompatible with gall-stones. Dr. Prout has made a remark, which

[1] The formation of gall-stones is illustrated by the fact noticed by Dr. Beale, that when ox-bile undergoes spontaneous decomposition exposed to the air, it has usually, at the end of three or four days, a tolerably abundant sediment, consisting of white nodular granules, which seem to be composed of lime in conjunction with a biliary or fatty acid. At a further stage of decomposition, it contains numerous crystals of oxalate of lime. The nuclei of gall-stones taken from the gall-bladder usually contain lime, and occasionally, according to Lehmann, a minute quantity of oxalate of lime: a substance which, from want of oxidizing influences, is much less likely to form when bile undergoes decomposition in the gall-bladder than when it does so exposed to the air. The absence of the peculiar biliary acids in the nuclei of gall-stones may be partly attributable to the readiness with which these substances undergo decomposition, when in contact with organic matter.

my own experience tends to confirm, that gall-stones of cholesterine are seldom found in conjunction with the granular disease of the liver produced by spirit-drinking. They are also, I believe, very seldom met with in the diseases of the liver that occur in hot climates. Among the numbers of bodies that I examined in the Seamen's Hospital, of men who returned from India with abscess or other disease of the liver, very few, indeed hardly any, had gall-stones; but these men, it must be remembered, were sailors, and had probably great immunity from gall-stones on account of their seafaring life.

There is, however, one disease of the liver in which gall-stones are of very frequent occurrence—namely, cancer: but gall-stones are also frequently found in conjunction with cancer of other parts, and seem connected with the cancerous diathesis rather than with cancer of the liver itself, which probably gives no additional tendency to them, except when it involves the gall-bladder, or causes the bile to stagnate in it by narrowing the cystic or the common duct.

The tendency to the formation of gall-stones is much influenced by age. Gall-stones of cholesterine, like the fatty degeneration of the coats of the gall-bladder with which they are frequently associated, are seldom found in persons under the age of 30. Bouisson, calculating from the numerous observations collected by Walter (*Museum Anatomicum*, tom. iii., in 4to., Berolini, 1805), found that among 91 persons who had gall-stones, 1 was 20 years of age, 27 were between 30 and 40, 14 between 40 and 50, 19 between 50 and 60, 8 between 60 and 70, 13 between 70 and 80; while one was 80, and another 90. The ages of the remaining 7 are not mentioned.

The youngest persons in whom I have found a gall-stone composed chiefly of cholesterine were of the ages of 24 and 18. The first was a woman, aged twenty-four, who died in King's College Hospital, in the summer of 1844, of phthisis, with extremely fatty liver, whose gall-bladder contained a single round calculus, of the size of a small marble, composed almost entirely of cholesterine; the second, a girl, aged eighteen, whose case has been related above (p. 206), who died of fever, and in whose gall-bladder six small angular gall-stones, composed chiefly of cholesterine, were found.

Gall-stones are, in this country, much more frequent in women than in men; but in what exact proportion in the different classes of society we have as yet no statistics to determine. Hoffman, Haller, and Sœmmering, found gall-stones more common in women than in men; but the rule does not seem to be universal. Bouisson states that, of the 91 instances of gall-stones collected by Walter, before referred to, 44 occurred in women, 47 in men. Morgagni states that, among the numerous cases of gall-stones he had observed himself, or had collected from others, the number of men was nearly equal to that of women.

The greater liability of women to gall-stones depends, probably, not so much on the peculiar constitution of the sex as on their habits of life, which are different in the different classes of society and in different countries.

Among the conditions of life that dispose to gall-stones, sedentary occupations and confinement seem to have the greatest influence. Gall-stones have been observed to be especially frequent among literary men, and prisoners, and people long bed-ridden; while, on the contrary, they are, like urinary calculi, very rare among sailors, who lead an active and roaming life, and are constantly exposed to a current of fresh air. The sedentary habits of women in this country perhaps sufficiently account for their being so much more liable to gall-stones than men.

The influence of confinement in bringing on gall-stones might almost have been inferred from the circumstance that cholesterine, which is their chief constituent, is a fatty substance, into the composition of which oxygen enters but in very small proportion.

Another condition that seems to me to have great influence in the production of gall-stones, or at least of biliary gravel, is mental anxiety or trouble.

Particular modes of living, which directly alter the qualities of the bile, have, without doubt, great influence in producing gall-stones; but our knowledge on this point is very vague. Gall-stones are most frequent in fat persons, and in those who live richly and lead indolent lives; but they are not unfrequently found in persons advanced in life, especially women, who are lean and have always been extremely temperate. It has been stated that they are especially frequent in districts where the water drunk is rich in lime.

There can be no doubt, also, that a liability to gall-stones often depends on peculiarity of constitution, which, like the tendency to gout or urinary gravel, may be inherited as well as acquired. Instances are not unfrequently met with of several members of a family becoming affected with gall-stones, without any marked peculiarity in their habits of life. At present little is known of the characters, or of the other effects, of this *diathesis.* It probably conduces to fatty degeneration of the coats of the gall-bladder, which is so frequently associated with gall-stones, and to the fatty degeneration of the arteries, so common in advanced life. Dr. Prout has remarked that a tendency to the formation of gall-stones of cholesterine is frequently associated with a tendency to lithic-acid deposits in the urine. It is probable that in London the habit of drinking porter, which frequently leads to lithic-acid deposits and to the most inveterate forms of gout in persons who inherit no disposition to them, may also frequently lead to the formation of gall-stones.

When, from any cause, the bile is prone to form deposits, various circumstances that favor its stagnation in the gall-bladder—such as the habit of sleeping long, long fasting, some obstruction in the cystic or the common duct—that otherwise would be without effect, may lead to the formation of gall-stones. Inflammation or ulceration, of the gall-bladder, by altering the quality of the mucus, or by leading to the effusion of a small clot of blood or a flake of lymph, may also cause their formation.

When gall-stones have formed in the gall-bladder, they may produce various effects upon the bladder and ducts. One of the most common of these is closure of the cystic duct. A gall-stone too large to pass through the duct floats with the current of bile to its mouth, and becomes firmly lodged there. This prevents the flow of bile into the gall-bladder, and not unfrequently, by exciting inflammation, leads to permanent closure of the duct beyond the stone. We have already considered the effect which this closure of the cystic duct has on the gall-bladder. The bile in the gall-bladder gets absorbed, and its place occupied by the secretions of the bladder itself, which consist of a mucous, glairy fluid, in which are suspended glistening scales of cholesterine. Perhaps the closure of the duct may lead to the formation of another gall-stone around an unusually large scale of cholesterine, or a flake of lymph that may be retained in the bladder, or some concrete biliary matter that may be left when the more watery parts of the bile are absorbed. But it never happens that many gall-stones are formed in the bladder after the cystic duct is closed. That many gall-stones may be formed, it is requisite that the bile should flow into the bladder, and that some of its constituents should be deposited in solid masses, to serve as nuclei about which the cholesterine may collect.

Closure of the cystic duct of course destroys the office of the gall-bladder, and by so doing more or less deranges digestion; but when gall-stones have formed, the evils resulting from this are perhaps more than compensated by its preventing for the future the passage of the stones along the ducts, which is the cause of most of the suffering and of many of the other evils which gall-stones occasion.

If a gall-stone pass through the cystic duct, it generally passes also through the common duct, which is larger and straighter than the cystic duct. If it pass slowly, and be large enough completely to block up the duct and prevent the flow of bile into the intestine, it soon causes jaundice and dilatation of the gall-ducts behind and of the gall-bladder. The distension of the gall-bladder may be so rapid and so great, that, on some trifling effort, as that of coughing or vomiting, it may burst, especially if its coats were previously diseased, and its contents be poured into the cavity of the peritoneum. Several instances of this kind have been recorded. The gall-stone may also become *fastened* in the common duct, and may lead to permanent closure of the duct below it, by adhesion, and, consequently, to permanent jaundice and all the other evils which obliteration of the common duct occasions. Sometimes a large gall-stone gets permanently lodged in the lower end of the common duct, without completely closing it. That part of the duct which embraces the stone participates in the dilatation of the ducts behind, and bile still passes round the stone into the intestine. This, however, can scarcely happen without much impeding the flow of this fluid, and leading to occasional jaundice, and, in the end, to great dilatation of the hepatic gall-ducts and more or less destruction of the secreting element of the liver. But, as before remarked, a gall-stone does not often rest long in the common duct. After a time, which seldom extends beyond a few days, it passes into the intestine. One is occasionally surprised, considering the natural size of the common duct, at the large size of a gall-stone which has passed through the ducts, without ulceration, into the intestine. A stone, as large as an almond, or larger, may escape in this way.

The circumstance shows to what an extent the ducts may be dilated by a constant, and gradually increasing, fluid pressure. When the ducts have been much dilated, they return to their natural size very slowly. The common duct has been found as large as the finger, or even larger, a considerable time after the passage of the stone by which its dilatation was caused.

But gall-stones, while lodged in the gall-bladder, may, by mechanical irritation, excite inflammation of its coats, and perhaps hasten the progress of fatty degeneration and ossification of them. The frequent association of gall-stones with fatty degeneration of the coats of the gall-bladder has been already noticed. It is probable that this change in the gall-bladder is generally the effect of that derangement of the animal chemistry which leads to the formation of gall-stones, and that it is often one of the immediate causes of the gall-stones, by rendering the secretions of the gall-bladder unhealthy and causing them to be loaded with scales of cholesterine; but it is probable also that gall-stones, once formed, may, by mechanical irritation, bring about degeneration of the coats of the gall-bladder, or may, in their turn, hasten that degeneration of the gall-bladder to which in part they owe their origin. I have more than once found fatty degeneration and ossification of the gall-bladder which contained gall-stones far more advanced than elsewhere at its under and free surface, near the broad end, where gall-stones must be most apt to rest.

Another occasional and very serious effect of gall-stones is ulceration of the gall-bladder, or of the cystic or common duct. The relation of gall-stones to ulceration of the bladder and ducts has already been considered. Gall-stones are frequently associated with ulceration of the bladder; but it must not be inferred in all such cases, that the ulcers were caused by the stones. Ulcers of the gall-bladder and gall-ducts may be produced by unhealthy bile, and are sometimes found where there are no gall-stones. It is fair, therefore, to infer, that in some cases where gall-stones and ulcers are found together, and where from the very existence of the gall-stones, we know that the bile has been unhealthy, the ulcers, like the gall-stones, are the immediate effect of unhealthy bile. Small, scattered, round ulcers, found in connection with a few small gall-stones, which do not rest on the ulcers and can readily change their place, are probably always produced in this way. But there can be no doubt that a large gall-stone, lodged in the bladder, or in some part of the cystic or common duct, may cause ulceration and sloughing, or may fret a small ulcer produced by unhealthy bile into a large and deep one. The effects of this vary, according to the situation of the ulcer and other circumstances. An ulcer in the gall-bladder or in the cystic or the common duct may eat through the different coats, till the peritoneal coat is laid bare. The contact of the bile then causes this to slough, and the contents of the bladder or ducts escape at once into the cavity of the peritoneum, causing inflammation of the whole surface of that membrane, rapid collapse, and death. If, however, the cystic duct has been previously closed, and the bile that was in the bladder absorbed, the contents of the bladder may escape into the peritoneum by *oozing*, and suppurative inflammation may set up, which is limited to the neighborhood of the gall-bladder by adhesions, thus forming a circumscribed abscess in the cavity of the peritoneum. But either of these events is very rare. In the great majority of cases in which an ulcer in the gall-bladder or ducts is formed, or fretted, by a gall-stone, adhesive inflammation of the peritoneum covering the ulcer is set up before all the coats are eaten through, and lymph is poured out, which glues that part of the gall-bladder or duct in which the ulcer is situated to the part with which it happens to be in contact. When the ulcer is in the common duct, this is generally the duodenum; when in the gall-bladder, the duodenum or the colon. After these adhesions have formed, the process of ulceration may still go on till the coats of the bowel are eaten through as well, and the gall-stone escapes into the intestinal canal. It has been already remarked that, in such cases, the process of ulceration is slow, and that the adhesive inflammation of the peritoneum which it sets up is of small extent, so that there are seldom severe or alarming symptoms, and, now and then, the first clear intimation that anything serious has been going on, is the discharge of a large gall-stone from the bowel. A large gall-stone escaping into the bowel in this way, may cause much less suffering than by passing along the ducts. When an unnatural communication is thus made between the gall-bladder, or duct, and the intestine, the continued passage of the bile may prevent it from being closed, and a permanent biliary fistula be formed. Now and then, the gall-stone passes by ulceration from the gall-bladder into the stomach; or the gall-bladder becomes adherent to the abdominal parietes, and the stone escapes, by ulceration, through them.[1] In either case, unless the cystic duct be closed so as to prevent the bile from flowing into the bladder, a permanent fistula will be formed.

It would also seem, from cases before referred to, that gall-stones, by causing, or by keeping up, ulceration of the gall-bladder or ducts, may lead to abscesses in the substance of the liver: either by setting up suppurative inflammation of a small vein in the neighborhood of the ulcer, or through absorption of ichorous matter from it. Such a result is, however, very rare.

In these several ways, and by their passage through the ducts, gall-stones are, in this country, the cause of a large proportion of the severe and recurring ailments attributable to the liver in persons, more especially in women of the middle and upper classes, who have led sedentary lives and have reached the middle period of life.

Gall-stones may exist in the gall-bladder a long time without giving rise to any symptoms that are noticed. They are not unfrequently found, and sometimes in great numbers, in persons who during life had no ailments referable to the liver that could lead to the suspicion even of their presence. While stationary in the bladder they seldom give rise to striking symptoms, unless they are so large or so numerous as to distend it, or unless there be at the same time ulceration or inflammation of its coats. In such cases they cause a sense of weight or uneasiness often felt in the region of the gall-bladder, or pain, with more or less tenderness, in that part. Not unfrequently they cause also pain in the back, about the angle of the right scapula, which is very significant of irritation of the gall-bladder or gall-ducts, and which sometimes extends even to the right arm. The pain or uneasiness in the site of the gall-bladder is increased by distension of the stomach, by a deep breath, or by certain movements of the body.[2]

The fact that gall-stones often exist without causing much pain, is explained by the circumstance, that the gall-bladder does not contract on the stones, and is perhaps seldom completely emptied,

[1] Andral, Précis d'Anat. Path., i. pp. 187 and 241. Since the first edition of this book was published, three instances have been brought under my own notice, in which a gall-stone had thus worked its way through the walls of the belly.

[2] In describing the symptoms produced by gall-stones, I have freely availed myself of the admirable account that has been given of them by Dr. Prout, in the third edition of his work on Stomach and Urinary Diseases.

and that gall-stones are so light that they are suspended in bile, and in consequence exert no pressure on the coats of the bladder by reason of their *weight*. It may also be owing in part to the little sensibility to pain which the gall-bladder has when not inflamed.

A gall-stone may also remain long impacted in the *cystic* duct, without causing pain or having other ill effect than those obscure disorders of disgestion which result from loss of the natural reservoir of the bile. Some instances of this kind have been related in a former chapter.

A gall-stone fastened in the *common* duct must cause jaundice by impeding the flow of bile, but unless it occasion sloughing or ulceration of the duct, it may cause no other pain than that which results from the mere stoppage of the bile.

The *passage* of gall-stones through the ducts is generally productive of great pain, but, unless there be ulceration or inflammation, it is seldom that much pain results from their mere presence, either in the bladder or in the ducts.

The symptoms of the passing of gall-stones generally come on suddenly and unexpectedly, two or three hours after eating, with severe pain, and what is described, and no doubt rightly described, as *spasm* in the region of the gall-bladder. The pain is not equable, but subsides and again recurs in paroxysms, which are often so excruciating that the patient bends himself double or rolls about the floor, at the same time pressing his hands against the pit of the stomach, which sometimes eases the pain. The severe paroxysms produce great exhaustion; the pulse becomes slow or weak, the face pallid, and the whole body covered with a cold sweat. The pain in the region of the gall-bladder is often attended with pain referred to the angle of the right scapula, and with a sense of *constriction* round the lower part of the chest, as if a cord were tied tightly round it—a sensation not peculiar to gall-stones, but very distinctive of sudden stoppage of the common gall-duct. Together with these symptoms there is sympathetic disorder of the stomach, which varies in degree, according to the intensity of the original irritation and the nervous susceptibility of the patient, from mere flatulent distension of the stomach to frequent and distressing vomiting. In some of the severer cases, only the mechanical act of the vomiting is excited, and the stomach is emptied of its ordinary contents; in others, the irritation in the gall-duct excites the secreting function of the stomach, and great quantities of gastric acid are brought up by the repeated efforts of vomiting. This sympathetic disorder of the stomach, like that arising from other sources of irritation, is, as a general rule, much greater in women than in men.

A gall-stone in the common duct of course impedes the flow of the bile, so that, if the stone do not quickly pass into the bowel, the symptoms above mentioned are usually followed by jaundice. When the obstruction of the duct is complete from the first, the jaundice appears very soon—it may be, within a few hours of the first seizure. When the obstruction is partial, a week or more may elapse before the occurrence of jaundice.

The severity of the symptoms, and the time they last, are of course very variable, depending on the number, and the form, and the size, of the stones that are passing, and on the previous state of the ducts. In some cases, the symptoms cease after an hour or two, or a still shorter time, and in most instances, *suddenly*, as the stone escapes into the duodenum, the obstruction of the duct is not complete or does not last long enough for the production of jaundice, and the disorder may be taken for mere hepatic colic. In other cases, where the stone is larger, or the passage less free, or where many stones pass in succession, the paroxysms of pain and spasm may continue to recur, with intervals of comparative ease—and jaundice, with varying degrees of intensity, may persist—for many weeks.

The passage of gall-stones does not produce, at first, either tenderness of the side or fever. On the contrary, the pain is generally somewhat eased by firm pressure; and, during the severe paroxysms of pain, the skin is cold and the pulse slow or weak. If, however, the stone be long in passing, some degree of fever is set up, the epigastrium becomes tender, and the tongue foul. These symptoms are probably owing to inflammation of the ducts, caused by the mechanical irritation of the stone. Besides tenderness at the epigastrium, there is general soreness of the belly, from the repeated efforts of vomiting, and from the spasmodic action of the muscles during the paroxysms of pain.

When the stone is long in passing, the sensibility of the nerves about the gall-ducts is heightened, and, in addition to the functional disorder of the stomach before described, the patient now and then has hiccough, or a peculiar catch in the region of the gall-duct on drawing breath, and sometimes feels as if there were a knot there in the constricting cord. The liver grows larger from retention of the bile within it; there is often a manifest fulness of the right hypochondrium from distension of the gall-bladder; sometimes a throbbing is felt there; and the thin edge of the liver may be traced much below its natural limits.

Another common symptom in severe and protracted cases is a shivering fit which recurs generally at irregular intervals, but sometimes almost with the regularity of ague. The rigors probably depend on *distension* of the bladder or ducts. Rigors of the same kind not unfrequently occur from distension of the urinary bladder in consequence of stricture, or from the introduction of a catheter, and now and then from distension of the large intestine by feces.

The passage of a gall-stone through the ducts, though productive of alarming symptoms, is attended with little immediate danger to life. It can only prove fatal when the stone gets long fastened in the common duct, but, as before remarked, the common duct is larger and straighter than the cystic duct, so that a stone which has passed through the cystic duct, generally passes through the common duct as well. The stone, after having caused the most agonizing pain (continued, perhaps, with short intervals of comparative ease, for several days, or, it may be, for several weeks), and great exhaustion, and juandice, passes into the intestine, and the alarming symptoms at once cease. It does, however, now and then happen, that a person dies from the pain and vomiting, and the great depression of the heart's action, that are caused by the passage of a gall-stone through the common duct. An instance of this is recorded by Abercrombie (*Diseases of the Stomach*, &c., 2d edit., p. 389); and several other instances of the same kind have been published.

Instances are also recorded where a gall-stone in the common duct has proved speedily fatal, by causing bursting of the gall-bladder, or of the duct behind, in consequence of their great and rapid distension. But such events are extremely rare. When a gall-stone in the common duct proves fatal, it is generally by causing permanent closure of the duct, and lasting jaundice. A fatal issue, in any way, is, however, of comparatively rare occurrence. In the great majority of instances the stone passes into the intestine, and the chief danger is over.

If the time of its passing has been short, the patient is then well, or suffers merely from the exhaustion consequent on the severe pain and the repeated efforts of vomiting, and from the irritation and obstruction which the stone may afterwards occasion in its passage through the bowel. But if the stone have been long in passing, and have produced jaundice, the patient, after it escapes into the duodenum, has the tenderness and the fever consequent on the injury done to the ducts, and the additional disorder caused by long pent-up and irritating bile flowing suddenly into the intestine.

Gall-stones in their passage through the intestine frequently produce slight colic and tenesmus, but seldom other evils unless they are very large. When this is the case they may obstruct the bowel and cause constipation, or even fatal ileus. Many instances of this kind are recorded;[1] but in most of them, I believe, the gall-stone was too large to pass through the gall-duct, and had escaped *by ulceration*, from the gall-bladder or the common duct, into the intestine.

A *small* gall-stone, like any other small hard body, may, in its passage through the intestine, get lodged in the vermiform appendix, and may cause ulceration or sloughing, and perforation of the appendix; and, as a consequence of this, a circumscribed abscess in the cavity of the peritoneum, or general peritonitis that proves rapidly fatal—according as the contents of the intestine ooze into the cavity of the peritoneum or are poured into it at once. Several instances of this kind have been recorded, and one has fallen under my own notice. Such an event is, however, very rare, and in general the passage of a gall-stone through the intestine causes no other inconvenience than a little colic and tenesmus.

The symptoms hitherto mentioned result merely from the mechanical effects of the stones in the gall-bladder, or in their passage through the gall-ducts and the bowel. But persons who have gall-stones have frequently other ailments which result from the faulty assimilation that led to the gall-stones, and perhaps in part from the irritation of the stones, even when they do not cause the severer symptoms that mark their passage. These ailments are usually of a very vague and uncertain charac-

[1] A case of this kind has been published by Abercrombie (2d ed., p. 133), and one by Cruveilhier (liv. xii., pl. 4, p. 3); and two others referred to in an elaborate paper on gall-stones, by M. Fauconneau Dufresne, published in the first volume of the *Revue Médicale*, for 1841 (p. 194).

ter. In one person they are principally nervous, and consist in hypochondriasis, or depression of spirits, or other nervous disorder; in another, they are chiefly disorders of digestion that are complained of; in a third, the urine is unhealthy, and frequently deposits lithic gravel, and the chief complaint is of irritation of the kidneys or bladder. Persons of middle age, or older, who have urinary calculus, have not unfrequently gall-stones as well. Numerous examples of this were collected by Morgagni, who inferred from them that gall-stones and urinary calculus are often caused by the same conditions; and that the presence of a urinary calculus in a person who has reached middle age, should strengthen any suspicions of the existence of gall-stones which other symptoms may awaken. (Epist. xxxvii., art. 43.)

Many of the various ailments that are found associated with gall-stones are, no doubt, mainly owing to the faulty assimilation in which these originate; but it would seem that in some cases they are attributable in great part to the mere irritation kept up by the gall-stones themselves.

The mechanical irritation of the stones, even when contained in the bladder, sometimes greatly disturbs the stomach, causing not only vomiting, but also an abundant and unseasonable secretion of gastric acid; and the irritation is now and then reflected upon the kidneys. I have been informed by a person who has several times passed small angular gall-stones that the illness attending their passage always began with pain in the loins and the passing of a large quantity of urine. It seemed that the irritation of the stone in some part of its course through the ducts—probably in the cystic duct—was, in this instance, reflected upon the kidneys so as to excite an abundant secretion of urine. Disease or irritation of other parts seems occasionally to excite through the same nervous agency the action of the kidneys.

A person who has once suffered from the passing of a gall-stone is very liable to suffer in the same way again. Where there are many gall-stones in the bladder, a few only, or even a single one, may pass at a time; or after all that were in the bladder have come away, others may form in their place. Now and then, a person, after having suffered from the passing of gall-stones at irregular intervals for years, has freedom from such suffering for the rest of his life. This may happen from the cystic duct becoming blocked

25

up by a stone—an event which allows no others to form, or, at any rate, to pass; or it may happen from all the stones in the bladder being at length discharged, and no others forming in their place. It has been already remarked, that when there are many gall-stones in a bladder, they have usually the same characters, and appear to have been formed at the same time. The immediate cause of their formation is probably the deposit of some of the principles of the bile in solid form, in consequence of some passing fault of the bile, or of unusual retention, which may not again occur.

From the account that has been given of the symptoms produced by gall-stones, it will appear that, before any have passed, while they are still lodged in the bladder, or when one has become impacted in the cystic duct, it is impossible to detect them. They then give rise to no symptoms, or merely to some pain or uneasiness in the region of the gall-bladder, with certain obscure derangements of health, which may equally result from ulceration of the gall-bladder, from organic disease of the liver itself, from disorder of the stomach or of the large intestine, and from various other causes. No constant or peculiar constitutional symptoms, indicative of gall-stones, have been yet noticed, and our knowledge of the circumstances under which gall-stones occur is too meagre to give meaning to symptoms otherwise vague.

When gall stones are passing, the symptoms are more significant, but even then may not be so peculiar as to give assurance of the fact, unless the person have had former attacks of the same kind, and have ascertained that they resulted from gall-stones. Sometimes, indeed, the passing of gall-stones causes but a few severe paroxysms of pain, or a few sharp twinges, which, unless it be known that the person has passed gall-stones before, may be attributed to various other conditions.

Now and then, similar attacks of pain in the region of the liver, more severe in paroxysms and unattended by fever, are brought on in highly sensitive persons by what seem to be very trivial causes of disturbance. They are of the kind we are in the habit of calling *nervous*—that is, they owe their chief severity to the peculiar state of the nervous system, and are most common in unmarried or hysterical women. In such persons they may generally be distinguished from the paroxysms of pain produced by the passing of gall-stones by the circumstances under which they occur, and by the general condition of the patient. They have been preceded by hysterical pain, or spasm, in other parts of the body; or the paroxysms are brought on by emotion, or fatigue; and, as in other painful hysterical disorders, there is exquisite and widely-diffused tenderness.

In persons of feeble digestion, a solid mass of undigested food, which cannot readily pass through the pyloric orifice of the stomach, may cause pain and spasm, and great depression of the heart's action; and may thus excite the suspicion that gall-stones are passing. If the disorder continue a day or two, as sometimes happens, the secretion of bile may be checked so as to produce slight jaundice, and the train of symptoms may be still more like that which results from gall-stones. Such attacks, moreover, like those produced by gall-stones, are very liable to recur. Several cases have been referred to me, in which a disorder of this kind, brought on by some indiscretion in diet, has been wrongly attributed to gall-stones.

Where, without there having been any particular indiscretion in diet, the illness begins suddenly with pain starting from the region of the gall-bladder, accompanied by a sense of spasm and *by a feeling of constriction round the lower part of the chest;* where the pain recurs in excruciating paroxysms, attended with vomiting, but at first without tenderness of the side and without fever, and where these symptoms are followed, at the end of a day or two, by jaundice: where, moreover, the patient is of sedentary habits, and of middle age, or older—the condition of life and the age in which gall-stones are common—there can be but little doubt that the illness is owing to the passage of gall-stones. The presumption that such is the case is still stronger if similar attacks have occurred before, and if in these the violent symptoms have ceased, as they began, suddenly. Such a succession of events is proof of an intermitting stoppage of the common gall-duct, and almost proof of the passage of gall-stones, or, at least, of the passage of gritty and irritating bile. It may, indeed, be caused, as we have seen above (p. 292), by a wart-like body growing from the mucous membrane of the common duct, but such disease is very rare in comparison with gall-stones.

The symptom which, more than any other, is significant of mechanical stoppage of the common gall-duct, is the feeling of constriction round the lower part of the chest, which varies in definiteness according to the degree of obstruction and the nervous susceptibility of the patient. When the obstruction is incomplete, a sense of tightness only is usually felt, which, as the obstruction increases, sometimes goes on to a distinct sense of constriction, as if a cord were tied tightly round the waist. Extension of the pain to the back about the angle of the right scapula is another circumstance that affords strong presumption that the disorder originates in irritation of the gall-ducts. It frequently happens, however, that the symptoms are of more doubtful character. The stoppage of the duct may not be sufficiently complete or may not last long enough for the production of jaundice: or the stone pass into the bowel by ulceration, or even through the ducts, without any very severe paroxysms of pain: and in a first attack the evidence furnished by the mere repetition of similar attacks is of course wanting. On all these accounts it often happens that we can only *guess* that gall-stones are passing.

In all cases where the illness is suspected to result from gall-stones, the matters discharged from the bowels should be examined, with the view to discover the stones. It is always satisfactory to *see* the stones; and we may besides draw important inferences from their size and form. If only one stone is discovered, and this is of considerable size, and round, or oval, we may infer that there are no others in the bladder, and that if the patient change his mode of life he may not suffer in the same way again. If the stone be of considerable size, but, instead of being round or oval, have smooth or polished faces, we may be sure that there were others, but probably not many, in the bladder with it, and which perhaps are still there. If the stone be small and angular, with polished faces, or even if many such stones are found, the probability is still greater that others are yet left in the bladder which will pass out, and the patient may expect at uncertain intervals a recurrence of similar attacks. It often happens, however, that when search is made no gall-stones are found, even when the train of symptoms has been precisely such as the passage of gall-stones occasions. The failure to find the offending bodies is no doubt owing in many cases to the incompleteness of the search ; but in some cases it is attributable to the fact, that severe paroxysms of pain and spasm are sometimes caused by a mere gritty state of the bile, or by what may be more properly called biliary gravel than gall stones—and that in the discharges from the bowels the particles that have caused so much irritation are difficult to detect. Dr. Prout recommended that, when the passage of gall-stones is suspected, directions should be given to mix the feces with water, on the surface of which, he says, the stones, if present, will be found floating. But this certainly will not always be the case. Most gall-stones, when fresh from the bladder, are heavier than water. They become, indeed, lighter than water by drying, and will then float in water until they have imbibed a certain quantity of it, when they sink slowly to the bottom. Dr. Watson has also recommended the adoption of this method of finding the stones, but he adds—"I never but once succeeded in thus catching a concretion in the evacuations of a patient, whose symptoms had led me to search for it." (*Lectures on the Practice of Physic*, vol. ii. p. 527.)

In the *treatment* of gall-stones three distinct objects have been proposed: 1st. To calm the pain and spasm while the stone is passing; 2d. To dissolve any stones that may remain in the bladder; 3d. To prevent fresh stones from forming.

While a gall-stone is passing nothing calms pain and spasm, and prevents, therefore, the exhaustion it occasions, so much as opium. This should be given in large doses, and is generally best given in a pill; for, from the irritability of the stomach, liquids are usually almost immediately rejected. Occasionally opium may be given with advantage in effervescing draughts, which allay the irritability of the stomach, and for a time enable the patient to retain the opium. In some cases much relief is obtained from sulphuric ether or chloric ether, in conjunction with opium. But, as was stated by Dr. Prout, more immediate relief is often afforded by large draughts of hot water, containing bicarbonate of soda in solution (in the proportion of from one to two drachms of the bicarbonate to a pint of water), than by any other means yet recommended. "The alkali counteracts the distressing symptoms produced by the acidity of the stomach; while the hot water acts like a fomentation to the seat of the pain. The first portions of water are commonly rejected almost immediately; but others may be repeatedly taken; and after some time it will be usually found that the pain will become less, and the water be retained. Another advantage of this plan of treatment is, that the water abates the severity of the retching, which is usually most severe and dangerous where there is nothing present on which the stomach can react. This plan does not supersede the use of opium, which may be given in any way deemed most desirable; and in some instances a few drops of laudanum may be advantageously conjoined with the alkaline solution, after it has been once or twice rejected." (Third ed., p. 263.)

The *hot* bath, fomentations with hot water, alone or with opium or decoction of poppies, or other appliances of like effect, but more especially the hot bath, should be had recourse to at the same time, and will often much alleviate the patient's sufferings. If these means fail, trial may be made of very cold applications—as a bladder of pounded ice—which have been much recommended by several writers, and, it would appear, have often been productive of benefit.

These means not only mitigate the pain and spasm, but in so doing doubtless promote the escape of the stone, and thus lessen the danger of ulceration or permanent obstruction of the duct.

It seems to have been formerly a common practice to give emetics or strong purgatives, to quicken the passage of the stone; but this practice has been justly reprobated, on the ground that it increases the pain before the ducts are sufficiently dilated to allow the stone to pass. A certain time is requisite for the necessary dilatation of the ducts; and when the stone is in the common duct it is sufficiently urged forward by the constant and gradually increasing pressure of the accumulated bile behind.

When the symptoms lead to the inference that the stone has passed into the duodenum, purgatives and copious injections of warm water should be given to hasten its discharge from the bowel, and with it the discharge of the accumulated and irritating bile.

If any tenderness and fever should come on during the passage of the stone, leeches should be applied at once to the tender part. These symptoms show that inflammation of the ducts has been set up, which may produce ill effects of various kinds. We have considered in a former chapter the nature of these effects, and the great importance of the early employment of local remedies—leeches and blisters—when the symptoms lead to the inference that inflammation either of the gall-bladder or of the gall-duct exists. In the present instance, the tenderness and the fever, from the peculiar symptoms that precede them, are unusually significant of inflammation of the ducts, and of inflammation excited by a local cause, and, therefore, to be chiefly relieved by local remedies.

The second object proposed in the treatment of gall-stones, is to endeavor by medicines to dissolve any stones that may yet remain in the bladder. Various medicines have at different times had the credit of doing this. The alkaline carbonates were long held in repute as solvents of gall-stones, and a plausible reason of their having such virtues has been assigned in the great solubility of the cholesterates of potash and soda. Soda is a natural constituent of bile. It is probable, therefore, that salts of soda, given as medicine, may be in part excreted in the bile, and may tend to form a soluble compound of cholesterine.

But the medicine that has been most celebrated as a solvent for gall-stones is a combination of sulphuric ether and turpentine. This was at one time much relied on in France, where it was brought into great vogue by Durande, a physician of Dijon, who published the details of many cases for the sake of establishing its efficacy. Durande's remedy, which consisted of a mixture of three parts of ether with two of essence of turpentine, became in consequence very famous. It has never been much employed in this country, and latterly has lost much of the credit it at one time had in France.

It is clear that it must be extremely difficult to obtain satisfactory evidence in favor of such virtue for any medicine. Before gall-stones have passed we can never be sure of their existence; and after a person has once passed gall-stones, he may go on for years, or even for the rest of his life, without passing others. All the stones in the bladder may have come away at once, and no others may form; or those which remain in the bladder may be too large to pass out; or one may have permanently blocked up the cystic duct: or, if the person continue to pass gall-stones, he may suffer much less in the subsequent attacks than at first, on account of the dilatation of the ducts which was then effected, or the smaller size of the stones. When, therefore, a person who has once passed gall-stones, passes no more for the future, or if he have other attacks, suffers less in them than in the first, we must be very cautious in assuming that this happy circumstance is the effect of our remedies.

Medicines whose efficacy is so difficult to establish, however real their efficacy may be, almost inevitably fall after a time into comparative disrepute. This has happened for taraxacum, and for most other medicines that have been supposed to increase the quantity and to alter the qualities of the bile. Few practitioners have the same faith in the reputed virtues of *cholagogues* and alteratives of the bile, as they have in medicines which increase the quantity or alter the qualities of the urine, because, although analogy leads us to conclude that some medicines have such virtues, there is not equal proof that the virtues actually belong to the particular medicines to which they have been ascribed. The natural tendency, therefore, seems to be, to estimate too low the value of such medicines, and perhaps of late the notion has been too much discarded, that gall-stones once formed in the bladder may be again dissolved. Combinations of ether and turpentine, if they do not dissolve gall-stones, seem occasionally to have done good—probably by relieving the pain and spasm which the irritation of gall-stones occasions.

The third object of treatment is, when gall-stones have been formed and passed, to prevent others from forming in future. For this, chief reliance must be placed on free exposure to the fresh air, on exercise, and on proper diet. The chemical composition of gall-stones and the facts well established by observation, that they are most common in persons of sedentary habits, and that they very rarely occur at the time of life when respiration is most active, tend alike to show that free exposure to the air must have great influence in preventing their formation. The patient should therefore be much in the open air, and sleep in an airy bedroom; he should rise early, and take plenty of exercise; should abstain as much as possible from fat or gross meats and heavy malt liquors; and, with the view of preventing undue concentration of the bile in the gall-bladder, should take diluents rather freely, and not make the intervals between meals too long. The bowels should be duly regulated, if need be, by the habitual use of rhubarb, or rhubarb and aloes; or by mild saline purgatives, as the Pülna water; and the action of the skin should be kept up by an occasional warm bath.

In addition to these means, we may endeavor to render the bile more healthy by some of those medicines which are supposed to alter its quality. In some persons who suffer from gall-stones and other disorders that arise from an unhealthy state of the bile, no medicine does such signal good as mercury, in small doses, continued for some time. It seems to increase the quantity of the bile, and at the same time to render it more healthy, and certainly often improves in a striking manner the general health. The best preparation of mercury for this purpose is the blue pill. It may be given most safely, and with best chance of benefit, to persons of full habit who have lived freely, and in whom there is no reason to suspect organic disease.

Where the patient is thin, or has lived badly, or where there is reason to fear organic disease of the liver, or of some other organ, it is safer and wiser to abstain from mercury, and to be content with taraxacum, or muriate of ammonia, or the alkaline carbonates, or other mild medicines that are supposed to alter the qualities of the bile. Where the secretion of bile has been long disordered, and the health is much broken, great benefit sometimes results from a mild course of the natural alkaline or saline waters. The alkaline waters of Vichy and Ems, and the waters of Carlsbad, on the Continent; and in this country, the saline waters of Cheltenham and Leamington, and the sulphurous waters of Harrowgate, are those whose efficacy in such cases is best established. The waters of Vichy, in particular, are very highly thought of by French physicians, and probably with sufficient reason.

CHAPTER IV.

DISEASES WHICH RESULT FROM SOME GROWTH FOREIGN TO THE NATURAL STRUCTURE.

SECT. I.—*Cancer of the liver—Origin of cancerous tumors of the liver—their growth, dissemination, and effects—Encysted, knotty tubera of the liver.*

HAVING considered the inflammatory diseases of the liver, and the diseases which result from impaired nutrition of its tissues, and from faulty secretion, there remain for us to consider those which consist in some growth foreign to the natural structure.

The most important member of this class is *Cancer*, which is more frequent in the liver than in any other organ. Indeed, no serious organic disease of the substance of the liver is, in this country—at least among people who have never drunk hard—so frequent as cancer.

In some instances, the liver is the only organ infected with cancer, or is the organ in which the cancer originates; but far oftener the formation of cancerous tumors in it is consequent on cancer of some other part, especially the stomach and the breast.

In the *Anatomie Pathologique* of Cruveilhier, the *Clinique Médicale* of Andral, and the little work by Dr. Farre on the *Morbid Anatomy of the Liver*, twenty-nine cases are recorded in which cancerous tumors were found in the liver. In three only of these cases was the disease confined to the liver. (*Cruv.*, liv. xii. pl. 2, p. 8; *Clin. Méd.*, iv. p. 445; *Farre*, Case 2.) In another case (*Cruv.*, liv. xxxvii. pl. 4, p. 3), the lungs and the liver were the only organs in which cancerous tumors were noticed; in another (*Clin. Méd.*, iv. 433) the liver and the gastro-hepatic omentum. In all these cases it is, perhaps, fair to conclude that the disease originated in the liver.

In the remaining twenty-four cases, other parts of the body were affected with cancer, as well as the liver. In thirteen of them there was cancer of the stomach; in five, cancer of the breast. Some particulars of these cases will be presently mentioned, which leave little doubt that in most of them, if not in all, the disease was propagated to the liver from the stomach and the breast respectively.

Many circumstances conspire to render the liver, more frequently than any other organ, the seat of both disseminated abscesses and disseminated cancer.

One of these is the great vascularity of the liver, and the slowness with which the blood, already retarded by passing through a system of capillary vessels, traverses the dense plexus of vessels that goes to form its lobular substance. But a circumstance much more influential, is that the liver is the organ through which the blood, returning from the intestinal canal, first passes. When the stomach or intestines are ulcerated, the blood that flows to the liver from these parts is liable to be contaminated by pus and other noxious matters, which cause inflammation that rapidly leads to abscess. When the stomach is the seat of cancer, the portal blood is liable to be contaminated by cancer-germs, which, being stopped in their passage through the liver, are there developed into cancerous tumors. In such cases, the abscesses and the secondary cancerous tumors are usually found only in the liver, which seems to detain all the pus-globules and cancer-germs that are brought to it by the portal blood. It rarely happens that any of these seeds of mischief pass through to cause abscesses or cancerous tumors in the lungs and other organs.

It is seldom that a *single* cancerous growth is found in the liver. There are usually scattered through its substance a great number, often hundreds, of round tumors, some of them so small as to be distinguished with difficulty, others of the size of a bean, of a walnut, or of an orange. Sometimes, indeed, cancerous tumors in the liver grow still larger, especially when there are but few of them; for, as Cruveilhier has justly remarked, their size is usually inversely as their number.

When they are numerous, it is generally plain, from their difference of size and texture, that they are of different ages: so that in the same liver they are often seen in various stages of growth.

The first token of the deposit of cancerous matter, discoverable by the naked eye, is a change of color, which is limited to two or three contiguous lobules, or even to a single lobule. The tainted lobules, instead of being of their natural tint, are whitish or black, according to the variety of cancer, and their consistence is altered, but they remain unchanged in size and form; thus showing that the disease originates in the lobules, and not in the areolar tissue in the small portal canals.

Not unfrequently, in a small cancerous tumor, throughout, and near the circumference in large tumors, when they are cut across, a mottled appearance is seen, like that of the lobular structure of the liver, and clearly resulting from this structure having been involved in the cancerous growth.

A cancerous tumor in the liver grows larger by infiltration of the cancerous matter into the contiguous liver-substance, which becomes gradually converted into cancer. In this way, a great portion of the proper liver-substance may be entirely replaced by the new structure. I have more than once known the left lobe of the liver undergo this transformation in its entire thickness, so that, as in a case related further on, when a vertical slice was made a little to the left of the suspensory ligament, the cut surface, from front to back, exhibited nothing but white cancer. The cancerous tumor grows, also, by addition to its own proper mass, and may thus come to project above the surface of the liver, and in the substance of the liver may, to a certain extent, push aside and compress adjacent tissues.

One effect of the pressure, not unfrequently observed when the cancerous tumors are thickly studded, is partial biliary congestion. Portions of the hepatic substance between the tumors are of a dark green, or an olive color, in consequence of compression of the small gall-ducts. The cancer may afterwards invade these portions, and the corresponding parts of the cancerous growth will be deeply colored with bile. I have more than once found parts, near the circumference, of large cancerous tumors, and small cancerous tumors throughout, tinged of a deep green, evidently from the cancer having invaded portions of the hepatic substance already gorged with bile.

The hepatic substance immediately surrounding a cancerous tumor not unfrequently, however, exhibits a change which cannot, perhaps, be attributed to pressure. It is pale and fatty, while other portions are not so. As before remarked, such a partial deposit of fat round a cancerous tumor is not peculiar to the liver, but is often found also in cancer of the omentum and of other parts.

Those cancerous tumors which originate near the surface of the liver, in growing project above it, so as to render it knotty or uneven. When the projecting tumors are large, the centre of the projecting portion is often somewhat depressed or cupped; an effect, it would seem, of strangulation of the central part of the tumor. The tumor is more freely supplied with blood, and grows faster, round the edge. This cupped form is not peculiar to cancerous tumors of the liver, but is sometimes observed also, though much less frequently, in cancerous tumors of the lung, when these are large and project above the general surface of the pleura.

Cancerous tumors in the liver, as in other parts, differ much in firmness, vascularity, and color, in different cases. Sometimes the tumors are white and fibrous, or, as it is termed, *scirrhous;* but far more frequently, especially when numerous, they are soft, or *medullary.* Instances are now and then met with, in which, in the same liver, some tumors are hard, and others soft.

Soft cancer presents the same varieties in the liver as in other organs. Most commonly the cancerous mass contains but few vessels, and is pulpy and whitish, or of a grayish-white—presenting that striking resemblance to brain rather softened, which led Laennec to apply to it the term *encephaloid.* In other cases, the tumors are extremely vascular, presenting the appearance known as *fungus hematodes.* In others, again, they are *melanotic.* Indeed, every variety of cancer, excepting, perhaps, *gelatiniform,* or *colloid* cancer, has been met with in this organ.

The color of melanotic tumors of the liver varies, according to the quantity of pigment-granules they contain. In the same liver tumors may sometimes be found of every shade from light brown to black.

Melanosis, whatever be its primary seat, becomes disseminated sooner, and more widely, than any other variety of cancer. I am not aware that melanotic tumors have ever been found in the liver without being found, at the same time, in other organs; and when they exist in the liver, they are usually in very great number. Sometimes, indeed, the whole liver is thickly studded with small black grains, giving to a section of it an appearance compared by Cruveilhier to granite, or black mica. This appearance is represented in Plate 4, which was made from a preparation in the Museum of King's College. (Prep. 324.)

Large cancerous tumors, whether hard or soft, white or melanotic, are usually slightly lobulated, from there having been greater impediment to their growth in some directions than in others; and they are united to the substance of the liver in which they are imbedded only by areolar tissue and vessels. It happens, however, now and then, though very seldom, that tumors of medullary cancer are surrounded by a well-defined cyst. The cyst, as was observed by Laennec, is a smooth membrane, about half a line in thickness, of fibrous texture, and silvery white color, imperfectly transparent, and easily separable from the mass it incloses.

Encysted cancerous tumors are always very soft and fluctuating, having much the feel of an abscess. When cut across and macerated, the pulpy matter is washed out, and a beautiful filamentous mass is left. We are ignorant of the circumstances which determine the formation of the cyst. Melanotic tumors, as well as common encephaloid tumors, are sometimes encysted; and some tumors in a liver may be encysted, while others are not. (*Cruv.*, liv. xxiii. pl. 5, p. 5.) It may be, that the cyst is owing to the development of cancerous matter from the inner surface of a gall-duct. The cyst is very like that of the knotty tumors containing a cheese-like matter, which are sometimes found in the liver, and which (as will be seen towards the end of this chapter) appear to originate in inflammation of a small gall-duct.

It now and then happens that cancer is found in the gall-bladder, as well as in the substance of the liver. Sometimes the cancer of the gall-bladder is distinct from the neighboring cancerous masses; in other cases it results from a cancerous tumor in the substance of the liver involving the gall-bladder in its growth.

Not unfrequently, too, cancerous matter may be found in the veins of the liver, and, as happens for the gall-bladder, this may grow from their inner surface, and be distinct from the neighboring cancerous masses, or it may result from a cancerous tumor involving, and penetrating, as it grows, the coats of the vein from without.

When a liver contains numerous masses of cancer, it is generally much enlarged, extending far below the false ribs, and sometimes even to the brim of the pelvis. Its increased size is in most cases owing entirely to the presence of the cancerous tumors; and, indeed, when these are removed, the hepatic substance is found to be diminished in volume. As before remarked, portions of the lobular substance are involved in the tumors; and other portions, especially between contiguous cancerous masses, are sometimes found pale and atrophied, and even converted into fibrous tissue, probably from their supply of blood being stopped by the pressure of the cancerous masses, or by cancerous matter within the veins, or by adhesive inflammation of the inner surface of the veins, which is very common in the neighborhood of cancer in some other parts.

From the tumors thus invading the lobular substance of the liver in their growth, and from their causing atrophy of other portions, the organ may contain numerous masses of cancer, and yet be smaller than in health.

But this happens very seldom. In almost all cases, the tumors more than compensate in bulk for any destruction or wasting of the lobular substance which they occasion; and sometimes the bulk of the organ, without the tumors, is much increased from the presence of an unusual quantity of fatty matter, or other products of secretion, in the lobular substance.

Even when the cancerous masses have grown rapidly, there are seldom any marks of inflammation in the hepatic tissue around them. The tumors owe their development, not to any process of inflammation, but to their own independent vitality; and the hepatic tissue in which they are lodged generally presents no other changes of structure than those produced by pressure and defective nutrition.

But although cancerous growths do not cause inflammation of the surrounding hepatic tissue, they now and then, when superficial, cause inflammation of the peritoneum above them. But even this happens seldom. The liver is often found much enlarged from cancerous tumors, and much deformed by some of these tumors projecting above its surface, without any traces of inflammation of its capsule. When inflammation occurs, it is probably caused by rupture of the peritoneal coat and escape of cancerous matter.

The character of the peritoneal inflammation which is excited by cancer has been already noticed (p. 147). It is always *adhesive*, and is generally very partial, causing the effusion of only a very small quantity of lymph. The usual traces of it found after death are, opacity and apparent thickening of the peritoneum above the projecting tumors, or very delicate, thread-like bands, uniting these tumors to the opposite surface of the diaphragm or abdominal walls. Sometimes, however, the inflammation is more extensive, and it may involve the entire surface of the liver, and even that of the peritoneum.

But it is a property of cancer to invade and destroy all structures within its immediate reach; and in consequence of this, if a cancerous mass be on the convex surface of the liver, it may eat through the diaphragm, and cause adhesive inflammation of the pleura. (*Cruv.*, liv. xxxvii. pl. iv. p. 4.)

Cancer of the liver may perhaps, also, like cancer of other parts, cause adhesive inflammation of contiguous veins. Inflammation of the adjacent veins is very common in cancer of the uterus, and it is in such cases that the inflammation of veins which is produced by cancer has been most studied. The uterine, and often one or both of the iliac veins, are found blocked up with fibrin. Lower down in the veins, proceeding against the course of the circulation, there may be small collections of pus, bounded above and below by fibrin; and sometimes the veins of the leg for a great length are found filled with pus. I met with an instance of this, in the spring of 1843, in a poor woman who died under my care in King's College Hospital.

She had cancer of the neck of the uterus, which had eaten into the bladder in front, and into the rectum behind, so that, for many weeks before her death, both the urine and the feces were continually passing through the vagina. She had constant severe pain in the lower part of the belly, and occasional pain in the region of the liver. Two or three weeks before her death she began to complain of severe pain in both legs, which became very much swelled.

The intestines in the lower part of the abdomen were found matted together, while those in the upper part were free and presented no traces of inflammation. On separating the adherent coils, two pouches of the peritoneum filled with pus were opened.

The lumbar glands were cancerous, and the liver was studded with medullary tumors, of various sizes, of which many of those that were superficial were united to the opposite surface of the diaphragm, or abdominal walls, by thread-like bands of false membrane. In the lower lobe of the left lung was a small whitish mass, which was inferred to be cancer. No cancerous tumors were discovered in other parts of the body.

The internal iliac vein on each side was blocked up with fibrin, while the femoral and popliteal veins, and the veins of the legs as far as they were traced, were filled with pus. The left knee-joint contained a large quantity of pus, but there was none in any other joint, nor were there any abscesses in other parts of the body. The fibrin that plugged the upper portion of the vein prevented the pus from contaminating the circulating blood.

Cruveilhier has distinctly remarked that, while it is very common, in cancer of the uterus, for small isolated collections of pus to form in the veins of the pelvis or of the legs, it very seldom happens that abscesses form in other parts of the body, or that the patient presents the general symptoms of contamination of the blood by pus. The pus is prevented from mixing with the circulating blood by adhesive inflammation of the upper portion of the vein. It would seem that adhesive inflammation is first set up in this portion, and that afterwards, suppurative inflammation is excited in the portion below. This sometimes happens in inflammation of veins from other causes; and it would almost seem that adhesive inflammation of the trunk of a vein may of itself lead to suppurative inflammation of the branches through which the flow of blood is thus prevented.

In cancer of the liver, I have more than once found some veins of this organ blocked up with what I took for coagulated fibrin, but have never found any filled with pus. Inflammation of the contiguous veins is most common in cancer of the uterus and cancer of the breast, in consequence of the great frequency of *ulceration* in cancer of those parts. The ulceration produced by cancer, like that from other causes, is adequate, of itself, to cause inflammation of adjacent veins.

It not unfrequently happens that, with cancer of the liver, a collection of serous fluid is found in the cavity of the peritoneum, even when this membrane presents no trace of inflammation. The serum is probably effused in consequence of obstruction to the passage of blood through part of the liver from some of the veins being blocked up by cancerous matter, or by fibrin, or from their being simply compressed by the cancerous tumors.[1] The quantity of fluid in the peritoneum in such cases is usually small, and is very seldom sufficient to cause that *distension* of the belly which is observed in cirrhosis, where the passage of blood through every part of the liver is impeded.

A similar effect is frequently produced by cancerous masses in

[1] In a preparation in the Museum of King's College (No. 288), large branches of the hepatic vein between contiguous masses of cancer are seen to be flattened.

the *lung*. Serous fluid collects in the cavity of the pleura without any inflammation of the serous membrane, or, at any rate, without inflammation that leaves other permanent traces.

But there may be impediment to the flow of blood and partial œdema in the cancerous matter itself. The centre of a large cancerous tumor in the liver has not unfrequently a gelatinous appearance, and when this part is punctured, and the tumor pressed, a transparent, *serous* fluid escapes, very unlike the opaque, white fluid of cancer. This œdema is very common in the projecting tumors whose surface is cup-shaped.

Another occasional event in the soft and vascular varieties of cancer of the liver is hemorrhage into the cancerous mass. This sometimes takes place to such an extent as to cause a rapid increase in the size of the liver, and almost to produce the alarming symptoms of copious internal hemorrhage. Now and then, indeed, the capsule of the liver is ruptured, and the blood escapes in large quantity into the sac of the peritoneum. When only a small quantity of blood is effused in the substance of the tumors, the serum and the coloring matter may be absorbed, and small masses of fibrin be left.

But the most remarkable property of cancer—a property which often influences the condition of the patient more than any damage the disease does to the part in which it first appears—is its power of dissemination. This varies much in degree, according to the variety of cancer and the part of the body in which it originates.

The laws which regulate the dissemination of cancer have not been fully made out, but there is clear proof that the dissemination may take place in two ways: 1st. By *inoculation*, or by the mere contact of a sound part with a part affected with cancer, without any direct vascular connection between them; 2d. By cancerous matter conveyed by lymphatics and veins to other parts of the body.

In the belly, where the relative motion between the surfaces is great, we have now and then distinct evidence of inoculation, in finding cancer communicated from one surface to another by mere contact without adhesion. In a woman who lately died in King's College Hospital, of cancer of the liver, there were small cancerous tubercles on the under surface of the diaphragm corresponding to a projecting cancerous tumor of the liver, although there were no unnatural adhesions between the liver and the diaphragm, and no cancerous tubercles on other parts of the reflected peritoneum. In another woman who died of cancer, which involved all the organs in the pelvis, and led to secondary cancerous tubercles of the peritoneum covering the intestines, the under edge of the liver, which had touched the tainted parts, had its surface studded with cancerous tubercles, while the substance of the liver, and the upper part of its surface, which was shielded by the ribs, were free from them. It was impossible to doubt that the edge of the liver had been infected by contact with the cancerous mass below.

In 1847, I met with another striking proof of the dissemination of cancer in this way in a woman who died in King's College Hospital of a cancerous cystic tumor of the ovary. The reflected layer of the peritoneum and the coils of intestine in contact with the tumor were studded with cancerous tubercles. There were only a few scattered tubercles on the coils of intestine above the umbilicus, which were not in contact with the tumor; but the surface of the liver was adherent to the diaphragm, and between them there was a continuous layer of cancerous tubercles. There were no cancerous tumors in the substance of the liver or in the lung, and there could be no doubt that the cancerous tubercles on the *surface* of the liver originated from germs which were transferred to that part from the original tumor in the lower part of the belly.

Cruveilhier mentions a case in which he found cancer of the left extremity of the pancreas with cancer of the upper part of the left kidney. (Liv. xii. pl. 2, p. 5.)

It is chiefly in this way—namely, by inoculation—that *gelatiniform* cancer of the stomach or intestines becomes extended to other organs in the cavity of the belly. In this variety of cancer the cancer-cells are too large to be readily transmitted by the veins so as to infect distant parts. It would seem, indeed, that cells of gelatiniform cancer, when detached from the outer surface of the stomach, may, like the fibrin which is effused in inflammation, become adherent to any part of the serous membrane with which they are accidentally brought in contact, and may be nourished from the vessels of that part.

But the widest dissemination of cancer is effected by the transfer of cancerous matter to distant parts of the body through the lymphatics and veins. The dissemination effected in this way usually takes place in the direction of the current of blood, or lymph. This is well shown by contrasting the organs that become infected from cancer of the breast, a part from which the blood is returned immediately to the vena cava, with the organs that become infected from cancer of the stomach, a part from which blood is returned to the portal vein. To take merely the cases recorded by the writers before referred to—Cruveilhier, Andral, and Farre. In the *Anatomie Pathologique* of Cruveilhier, there are, as before remarked, five cases (liv. xxiii. pl. 5, p. 1; id., p. 2; id., p. 3; id., p. 4; liv. xxxi. pl. 2, p. 3) in which cancerous tumors of the liver were consequent on cancer of the breast. In all these cases, with the exception of one (liv. xxiii. pl. 5, p. 1), in which the state of other organs is not mentioned, the lungs were infected as well as the liver. The cancer-cells had to pass through the lungs, before they could arrive at the liver.

But although cancer of the breast seldom causes cancer of the liver, without also causing cancer of the lungs, it not unfrequently gives rise to cancerous tumors in the lungs, without giving rise to any in the liver. In the *Anat. Path.* of Cruveilhier, three cases of this kind are recorded. (Liv. xxvii. pl. 3, p. 1; id., p. 5; liv. xxxi. pl. 2, p. 2.) Cruveilhier asks how it happens, that in some cases of cancer of the breast secondary cancerous tumors form chiefly in the lungs; while in other cases they form chiefly in the liver? The circumstance may be accounted for from the variable size of cancer-cells, which, in some cases, can pass readily, in others only with difficulty, through the capillary vessels of the lungs.

When cancer originates in the *stomach* secondary cancerous tumors form in the liver before they form in the lungs; undoubtedly from the blood infected with the cancerous matter having to pass through the liver first. Indeed, it very seldom happens that the lungs become affected at all. As before remarked, all the cancerous matter brought in the portal blood is usually detained in the substance of the liver, as are the globules of pus in purulent phlebitis, instead of passing through to contaminate other organs. In the works already referred to there are thirteen cases in which cancerous tumors in the liver seemed to be secondary to cancer of the stomach. In nine of these cases the liver was the only organ, besides the stomach, in which cancerous tumors were found. In the remaining four cases there was cancerous disease of some part of the mesentery, or of the glands about the aorta, as well as of the liver. It is a striking fact, that in not one was any cancer remarked in the lungs.

Cruveilhier relates seven other cases of cancer of the stomach. In four of these the disease was confined to the stomach; in the remaining three, all of them of gelatiniform cancer, there were likewise cancerous tubercles in the mesentery, but in no other organ.

When cancer originating in the kidney becomes disseminated, the lungs are infected more frequently than the liver. It might have been imagined that the same law would hold for the uterus which, like the kidney, returns its blood immediately to the vena cava; but it sometimes happens, as in a case before related, that in consequence of cancer of the uterus, cancerous tumors form in the liver, without any forming in the lungs. This results from the primary cancer extending to the rectum, and involving the hæmorrhoidal veins, which return their blood to the vena portæ.

All these instances are sufficient to establish the fact that cancer often becomes disseminated by means of cancerous matter which is conveyed onwards in the venous current. We have additional proof of it, in the points of resemblance, before noticed, between secondary cancerous tumors of the lungs and liver and the scattered abscesses which form in these organs in consequence of suppurative phlebitis.

It would seem, indeed, that cancer may even be propagated by inoculation, or by injection of cancerous matter into veins from one animal to another.

Professor Langenbeck injected into the veins of a dog some pulp taken from a cancer which had just been removed from a living body. At the end of some weeks the dog began to waste rapidly. It was then killed, and several cancerous tumors were found in its lungs.

Another instance to the same effect, taken from a German periodical, is related in the *Provincial Medical Journal* for September 23, 1843, in the following words: "Some cells were collected from a black liquid in the orbit of a mare affected with melanosis, and were inoculated into the conjunctiva and lachrymal gland of an old horse. These merely caused a black spot on the conjunctiva, which extended very slowly; but about the sixteenth week after inoculation, melanosis of the lachrymal gland was very decided; it had invaded the whole organ, and pushed the globe of the eye forward. Some of the melanotic matter, taken from the same mare, was injected into the veins of the neck of a dog, who died suddenly whilst hunting, three weeks after the operation. There was found in the left lung a melanotic tumor, which was ruptured, and which contained a brown, coffee-colored fluid, abounding in cells."

So many instances have occurred of cancer of the penis in men whose wives had cancer of the womb, that many physicians have been led to believe that the disease in these instances was propagated by contagion.

But the most obvious, if not the most common mode in which cancer becomes disseminated from the part in which it first appears, is by transmission of the cancerous matter through the lymphatics. It is through these vessels that cancer is so constantly propagated from the breast to the glands in the axilla. The small cancerous tubercles that are sometimes found surrounding a cancer of the breast of long standing are also, as was beautifully shown by Sir Astley Cooper, seated in the lymphatics.

Cancer of the stomach may, as we have seen, give rise to disseminated cancer of the liver, or to cancerous tubercles in the mesentery. In some instances of the latter kind the presence of the tubercles in the mesentery may be best explained by supposing cancer-cells to have been detached from the outer surface of the stomach, and to have been transferred, mechanically, to other parts of the serous membrane; but in other instances, the secondary tumors are clearly under the peritoneum, and in the mesenteric glands, and the germs of the disease must have been transmitted by lymphatics and lacteals.

When cancer is disseminated *from* the liver, it is usually through the lymphatics, and not through the veins. The lymphatic glands along the common gall-duct and in the belly, to which the lymphatics of the liver run, and some of the lymphatic glands in the mediastinum, usually become affected before cancerous tumors form in the lung.

In the *lymphatics* cancer is propagated, not in the natural direction of the current of lymph only; it is sometimes propagated backwards, as when, in cancer of the breast, cancerous tubercles are found under the skin, not in the direction of the axilla merely, but surrounding the breast. This propagation of the disease backwards through the lymphatics probably depends chiefly on the onward course of the lymph being impeded. Cruveilhier has remarked that cancer of the breast leads less frequently to cancer of internal organs when the disease is thus disseminated outwardly.

It may be readily conceived that obstruction in the course of the lymphatics leading to the axilla, or in the axillary glands, or that adhesive inflammation of the veins, by blocking up the usual channels for the transmission of the cancerous matter, may favor the dissemination of this matter in the opposite direction, and thus lead to the formation of cancerous tubercles in the neighborhood of the primary disease.

Admitting all these means for the propagation of cancer, there are still cases occasionally met with, which they do not enable us to explain satisfactorily, and which strongly favor the inference, that the cancerous tumors found in different parts of the body are not offsets from one primary cancer, but are the result of a peculiar disposition to the disease. There are, perhaps, few cases in which such a supposition is more needed than in cases of primary cancer of the liver. In these cases, as when cancerous tumors form in the liver in consequence of cancer of the stomach, the infection does not often pass much beyond the liver, but there are almost always a great number of cancerous tumors in the liver itself. We have at present no evidence that these are, in all cases, derived from a single parent tumor, but it seems probable that more careful observation will hereafter prove them to be so. It is clear, at least, that dissemination may take place within the liver in various ways; through the lymphatics, and through the veins; and, as before explained, in a twofold direction in both.

Cancerous tumors may form in the liver, *as a consequence of cancer of some other part*, at any period of life. They are in that case dependent on the primary cancer, and of course are most frequently found in conjunction with cancer of particular parts at the periods of life when those parts are most liable to the varieties of cancer which become readily disseminated. For the *breast*, this is, perhaps, the period comprised between the ages of thirty and fifty. Under the age of thirty, cancer of the breast, of any kind, is very rare; and beyond the age of fifty, the disease is frequently *scirrhous*, of slow growth, containing but few vessels, and, in virtue of these conditions, less apt to become disseminated than other varieties of cancer.

Cancer of the *stomach* does not occur so early in life as cancer of the breast. It is very rare in persons under the age of forty. Twenty cases of cancer of the stomach, recorded in the works of Cruveilhier, Andral, and Farre, have been already referred to. In eighteen of these the age of the patient is noted, and in all of them it was above forty, with the exception of one, in which it was thirty-eight. In eight of the cases, or nearly one-half, the patient was sixty or upwards.

Dissemination from cancer of the stomach is not much influenced by age, but it seems to be much favored by the occurrence of ulceration. In the great majority of the cases just referred to, in which cancerous tumors were found in the liver, the cancer of the stomach was ulcerated. This may, however, be partly explained from the circumstance, that the soft varieties of cancer, which are most readily disseminated, are also the most prone to ulcerate.

Cancer of the *uterus* follows nearly the same laws, with respect to age, as cancer of the breast; and cancer of the *colon* and *rectum* the same as cancer of the stomach. But cancer of the uterus, and of the large intestine, becomes disseminated much less frequently than cancer of the stomach or breast.

The parts above specified are by far the most frequent seats of primary cancer; and since this disease occurs in them only in the middle and advanced periods of life, disseminated cancer of the liver is also most frequent at those periods. But cancerous tumors may form in the liver at any age, as a consequence of cancer of some other part. Dr. Farre has related the case of an infant, three months old, in which there was fungoid cancer of the left kidney, with fungoid tumors in the liver and lungs; another case in a boy, two years and a half old, in which numerous cancerous tumors of the liver, and a single cancerous tumor of the lung, were consequent on fungoid cancer of the testicle; and a third case in a boy of the same age, in which there was a melanotic tumor in the pelvis, with cancer of the lumbar glands and cancerous tumors in the liver and lungs. Indeed, secondary cancerous tumors form much more frequently in the liver in children affected with cancer than in grown-up persons, because children are subject only to the soft and very vascular varieties of cancer, which, by reason of their softness and vascularity, are the varieties which become soonest and most widely disseminated.

But, although cancerous tumors may form in the liver, in consequence of cancer of a distant part, at any period of life, the disease seldom, if ever, originates in the liver until the age of 35. In the five cases before alluded to, in which cancerous tumors seemed to have formed primarily in the liver, one of the patients was 37 years of age, two were 39, and two were 45. The disease often occurs in persons much more advanced in life, and now and then in extreme old age. The period from 35 to 55, in which functional disorder of the liver is most common, appears to be that in which cancer most frequently originates in this organ.

Nothing more than this is known of the conditions that dispose to primary cancer of the liver. We have no evidence that it is more frequent in hot climates than in our own; or in persons who drink spirits to excess than in those who abstain from them. It has been found, with more perhaps than the average frequency, in conjunction with gout and gall-stones; so that it is probable that high living and indolent habits, which favor the production of these latter diseases, may also dispose the liver to become the primary seat of cancer. It seems, to judge by my own experience, to be more common in the middle classes than among the poor.

In speculating on the cause of cancer, the question at once arises—Is the germ of the disease a true parasite, introduced from without; or is it generated within the body, and of the materials of the body, under the influence of certain agencies?

The strongest argument in favor of the first supposition, is, that cancer originates in various organs, and has, in all of them, independent vitality and powers of growth. This is shown in the continued increase of the primary tumor, without any process allied to inflammation, whatever be the age of the patient; and still more strikingly by the fact, which seems fully established, that the mere lodgment of one or more germs from the original tumor in a *distant part*, is sufficient of itself, and independently of constitutional predisposition, to communicate the disease to that part. In cases in which the disease is propagated from one animal to another, by inoculation, or by injection of the cancerous matter into veins, it may, indeed, be considered *parasitic*, in the strictest sense of that word.

But although cancer is capable of being thus directly implanted from one individual to another, it occurs in almost all cases in circumstances in which it is difficult to believe that any such inoculation or infection has taken place; and not unfrequently it appears to originate in some direct injury, or in prolonged irritation of the part.

Thus cancer of the breast is frequently ascribed to a blow, and instances are now and then met with in which it is difficult to avoid the conclusion, that it really had this origin. Cruveilhier relates a case in which cancer of the breast in a man, which is a very rare disease, was consequent on a sabre-cut received there.

Cancer of the lip is much more common in persons addicted to smoking, than in others; and probably originates in the irritation of the pipe, or tobacco-juice. It is hardly ever met with in woman; and almost invariably occurs in the lower lip.

Cancer of the penis is found in undue proportion in men with congenital phimosis—an effect, probably, of irritation by long retained and acrid secretions.

Cancer of the anus or rectum is said to be especially frequent in persons who have had syphilitic vegetations or piles. (*Cruv.*, liv. xxv. pl. 3, p. 2.)

These instances go to bear out the old doctrine, that a disease, which is not primarily malignant, may become so—a doctrine which is in some degree at variance with the notion, that the germs of cancer are always introduced from without.

Another instance to the same purport, more convincing than any of those yet adduced, is the cancer of chimney-sweeps, which appears to originate in prolonged irritation of soot.[1]

Perhaps the facts that cancer does not occur in the mamma, or in the uterus, before puberty; and that it originates in the liver chiefly in the middle period of life—give further support to the doctrine, that the disease results from depraved nutrition of one of the normal constituents of the part.

[1] An interesting case in which cancer of the hand was produced by the handling of soot, in a gardener, who had long been in the habit of spreading it over his beds as manure, is related by Mr. Travers, and is cited by my brother, Dr. William Budd, in a paper published in the *Lancet*, in 1843, in which the origin and propagation of cancer are fully considered, and from which some of the instances adduced in the text have been borrowed.

The structure of cancer affords additional reasons for rejecting the notion, that the germs of the disease are always introduced from without. The essential elements of a cancer, as of other tissues, are nucleated cells and fibres. These cells multiply by throwing off the germs of fresh cells from their outer surface; and sometimes also, as in colloid cancer, from their inner surface.

All these circumstances give powerful sanction to the opinion, that cancer originates in depraved nutrition of the original nucleated cells of the part in which it first appears. We are ignorant of the conditions which lead to this depraved nutrition, except in the comparatively few cases in which the disease can be traced to some direct injury, or to some palpable cause of irritation.

Cancer seems to depend less on the general state of nutrition, and more on accidental conditions affecting the particular part, than some other diseases—for instance, consumption, and scrofula—which likewise result from faulty nutrition. It is not hereditary in the same degree, and it very seldom originates, as the last-named diseases do, at the same time, or nearly at the same time, in fellow-organs, on the two sides of the body. It occurs also in persons who are plethoric and seemingly robust.

Symptoms.—Cancer of the liver comes on without marked constitutional disturbance, and its early symptoms are very obscure. When the disease originates in the liver, the patient usually complains, first, of uneasiness and of a sense of fulness and weight in the right hypochondrium, and of failing strength, attended very commonly with impaired appetite, flatulence, and other disorders of digestion.

After these ailments have lasted some time, the medical attendant, or perhaps the patient himself, discovers that the liver is enlarged. The liver is felt extending across the epigastrium, or below the false ribs, sometimes reaching as low as the umbilicus, or lower, and not unfrequently an unevenness of its surface, caused by the cancerous tumors projecting above it, or even a palpable tumor, can be distinguished through the walls of the belly. The patient now, or even before this, suffers more or less pain in the region of the liver, and the functions of the organ are often hindered. In one case the flow of bile through the large ducts is stopped and there is jaundice; in another, without this, the passage of the blood through the liver is impeded, and there is slight ascites: sometimes, both these events occur in succession.

In addition to these local symptoms, there often exists some of the *sympathetic* disorders—vomiting, a short dry cough, rigidity of the abdominal muscles, pain in the right shoulder—which have already been noticed as frequently occurring in abscess of the liver.

As the disease progresses, the patient falls away more and more in flesh and strength, and generally becomes very anemic; the spirits are depressed; and pains are felt in the back and loins, caused most probably by cancerous contamination of the abdominal glands to which the lymphatics of the liver run. The functions of the stomach are variously performed. In some cases the appetite is good, at times almost ravenous, and digestion is easy; in other cases the appetite is much impaired, and there is frequent vomiting or retching, with other disorders of digestion. When the tumors grow rapidly, some degree of fever is set up: the pulse is habitually rather frequent; the skin of the hands is often hot; the tongue is red and furred; and the urine is high-colored, and throws down a lateritious sediment, which is not unfrequently pinkish.

In advanced stages of the disease there is often, as in cancer of other parts, profuse sweating; the patient is much wasted and very anemic, has aphthæ of the mouth, colliquative diarrhœa, and other tokens of defective nutrition, and at length dies of exhaustion.

Such is the usual course of primary cancer of the liver, but the remark which was made in a former chapter on abscess of the liver, applies equally here—namely, that the local symptoms, on which we rely most in forming our diagnosis, are far from being uniform, or constantly present. The degree of enlargement of the liver, and of pain or tenderness, and the presence or absence of jaundice and of ascites, depend mainly on the number, and size, and situation, of the tumors, on their rate of growth, and on the inflammation which they happen to excite in their neighborhood—circumstances which vary in every separate case.

Enlargement of the liver, which is the most constant, and by far the most significant, of these local symptoms, in most cases varies in degree with the number and size of the cancerous tumors. If the tumors be few in number, and small, there may be no enlargement of the organ that can be discovered while the patient is alive. But this very seldom happens. Almost always the liver is perceptibly enlarged, and in some cases it attains a prodigious size. A case is related by Dr. Farre, in which the liver, which was thickly studded with cancerous tumors, was more than *fifteen pounds* in weight. The enlargement of the liver is constantly progressive, and in the soft and vascular varieties of cancer is so rapid, that, week after week, a further increase in the size of the organ may be noticed.

An important circumstance that may serve in some degree to distinguish enlargement of the liver caused by the presence of cancerous or other tumors within it from the fatty or scrofulous enlargement and the enlargement that takes place in cirrhosis, is, that the lower edge of the liver is not uniformly thick and blunt, as in the latter diseases, in which the enlargement is owing to a change that affects every part of the organ alike.

The degree of *pain* and *tenderness* depends, perhaps, chiefly on the situation of the cancerous masses and on their rate of growth, and varies very much in different cases. In some cases, even when the liver is much enlarged, and deformed by cancerous tumors projecting above it, there is very little distinct pain, and pressure may be made on the liver, or the tumors themselves may be freely handled, without exciting complaint. In other cases, with much less amount of disease, the pain and tenderness are great.

The pain has not any particular or constant character that might serve to distinguish it as belonging to cancer. In some cases it is lancinating; in others, not.

When the liver extends far below the false ribs, it may occasionally be remarked that the tenderness is greater at some points than at others. It is greatest at those points where tumors project and where circumscribed inflammation has been excited in the serous membrane above them.

The presence or absence of *jaundice* depends, not so much on the number and size of the tumors and on their rate of growth, as on their being so situated as to prevent the flow of bile into the intestine. The liver may be tripled in volume, and a considerable part of its proper substance be converted into cancer, without jaundice; and, on the other hand, there may be deep jaundice, without appreciable enlargement of the organ, and when the amount of disease is small.

Jaundice is a frequent symptom in cancer of the liver; occurring probably, sooner or later, in the majority of cases. When it has once come on, it continues till the death of the patient. It results, in most cases, from some of the gall-ducts being compressed by the cancerous tumors; but it may also result from the ducts being closed by the growth of cancerous matter within them.

Ascites occurs much less frequently than jaundice. Its presence or absence, like that of the latter condition, seems to depend more on the situation of the tumors than on their number and size. Circumstances have already been mentioned which render it probable that the ascites results from obstruction to the flow of blood through branches of the portal or of the hepatic vein, either from the pressure of neighboring cancerous tumors, or from the presence of cancerous matter, or of fibrinous coagula in the vein itself. The immediate cause of the ascites is clearly different from that of the jaundice. Ascites may exist without jaundice; and jaundice without ascites.

The quantity of fluid effused is generally small. As before remarked, it happens but seldom that the belly is *distended* by fluid, as it is in the advanced stages of cirrhosis.

The ascites may come on without pain. In some cases, indeed, its occurrence relieves the pain which previously existed, by preventing the tender surface of the liver from rubbing so much against the walls of the belly.

When ascites has occurred, it is generally permanent—a circumstance which tends further to show that it results from some mechanical impediment to the passage of the blood.

Now and then, however, the ascites, after having existed for a time, disappears, to recur again at a future period.

The degree of *constitutional disturbance* excited by cancer of the liver, when other organs are sound, depends chiefly on the rapidity with which the cancerous tumors grow and multiply. When the tumors are of slow growth, and multiply slowly, they may, from their situation, produce local, or special symptoms—pain, or jaundice, or ascites—but they cause little fever, or other disturbance of the system at large than what results from these several conditions.

When, on the contrary, they multiply and grow rapidly, there is usually an irritative fever, the pulse is habitually more frequent than natural, and the patient wastes rapidly, and becomes rapidly anemic. When the disease has existed a few months, the pallor is often very striking, if there be no jaundice to conceal it. The impoverishment of the blood results partly from derangement of the functions of the liver and stomach, but more especially from the rapid growth of albuminous tumors, which must be formed ultimately from the albuminous constituents of the blood.

The following case, and I have seen several like it, is an instance of extreme anemia brought on by the rapid growth of cancerous tumors, without much pain or other suffering:—

John Clewer, a carpenter, forty years of age, was admitted into King's College Hospital on the 17th of May, 1855. He came of a healthy stock—his father and mother were both living—his habits had always been temperate, he had never had severe troubles, and his health had been constantly good until his present illness, which commenced soon after Christmas with indigestion and occasional vomiting. Up to Christmas he was very strong and healthy, capable, as he assured us, of as much work as any man in his trade. The vomiting recurred for a time about once in two or three days, and he began to fall away in flesh and strength. About two months before his admission to the hospital, he discovered a globular tumor in the epigastric region. This went on increasing in size for about a month, and then, as he judged, ceased to enlarge further. It was at the beginning hard to the feel and painless, and so it continued. A week before his admission to the hospital his feet and ankles began to swell.

On the 17th of May, when he entered the hospital, he was much emaciated, and *strikingly pallid.*

The liver was found to be much enlarged, its edges reaching below the umbilicus. In the epigastric region there was a large and apparently somewhat globular tumor, evidently projecting from the surface of the liver, and so situated that a vertical line from the ensiform cartilage to the umbilicus would pass through its centre. The tumor felt hard, and could be freely pressed and examined without causing pain. In the right side of the belly, the edge of the liver could be felt not thickened. There was a conspicuous network of enlarged veins over the chest, especially over the left side of the chest, the enlargement of the veins seeming to begin at the epigastric tumor.

There was not the slightest tint of jaundice, but there seemed to be some liquid in the peritoneal sac, and the feet and ankles were œdematous.

He had pain or uneasiness in the stomach, when the stomach was distended, and pain round the waist, with a sense of constriction when he lay on his right side. Otherwise he was free from pain. His pulse was high—generally about 100 a minute—but he slept well. His tongue was clean, and he had desire for food, but refrained from eating much, from fear of exciting pain in the stomach. The urine was 1015, acid, and free from albumen.

He was put on milk diet, and ordered small doses of hydrocyanic acid and morphia.

From this time his appetite was very variable. On some days he had desire for animal food; on others he could eat little of anything. The tongue remained clean, the bowels were regular, and the sleep was generally good. The pulse gradually mounted from 100 to 120; he complained very little of pain, but grew daily weaker, and died on the 25th.

On examination of the body, the liver was found to be greatly enlarged, and to weigh 9 lbs. 4 oz. The left lobe was almost entirely converted into cancer. When it was cut through by a vertical slice a little to the left of the suspensory ligament, nothing was seen in the cut surface, in the entire thickness of the liver at that part, but white cancer. The cancer diminished in amount in moving to the right, and the extreme right of the right lobe (about one-fifth of the original entire liver) was but little tainted—contained only a few small cancerous tubercles. The gall-bladder and larger gall-ducts were free from disease and unobstructed—a circumstance which explains the absence of jaundice. Many of the deep mesenteric glands—gastric and lumbar—were enlarged and cancerous. The coats of the stomach along the lesser curvature were somewhat thickened, and obviously infected with cancer. A series of enlarged cancerous glands were found in the posterior mediastinum, reaching as high up as the upper extremity of the sternum. The lower lobes of both lungs were thickly sprinkled with small bodies looking like tubercles, and many of the lymphatics of the lung were distended and of an opaque white, so that they were plainly seen by the naked eye under the pleura. Under the microscope the small masses in the lung and the matter distending the lymph-ducts presented the appearance of cancer. No other disease worthy of note was found in the body.

In this case the patient died after an illness of only five months; and at the time of death the cancerous tumors in the liver and elsewhere, consisting for the most part of solid albuminous matter, must have weighed at least five pounds. Now the blood does not contain more than one-fifth of its weight in albuminous substances, so that in the growth of these tumors there must have been expended, on a very moderate calculation, twenty pounds of blood. No wonder the patient became rapidly blanched. It is worthy of remark, that there was not the slightest tint of jaundice, although the cancer was so extensive that not more, it was estimated, than one-fifth of the original liver-substance remained. The absence of jaundice is attributable to the circumstance, that the large gall-ducts were free from disease and unobstructed.

Instances have been before related of equal or even greater destruction of the liver-substance from cirrhosis without any decided jaundice, and they strongly favor the opinion that the coloring matters of the bile are formed, for the most part, not in the blood, but in the tissues of the liver itself.

The case is still further interesting from the evidence it affords in favor of the opinion I have before advanced, that extension of the disease from the liver takes place, not through the bloodvessels, but through the lymphatics. There was a series of enlarged cancerous glands in the posterior mediastinum, the lymph-vessels under the pleura were rendered white and conspicuous by cancerous matter within them, and small cancerous tubercles were scattered through the lower lobes of the lungs. It was impossible in this instance to resist the conviction that the lymph-ducts conveyed the cancerous matter to the lungs.

In some instances cancer of the liver, without setting up any inflammatory process, causes great pain, and, as has been already remarked, the character of the illness may be further diversified by the occurrence of jaundice.

We are ignorant of the conditions which dispose to primary cancer of the liver, or which immediately give rise to it, so that in the diagnosis of this disease we are little helped by knowing the previous habits of the patient, or the circumstances in which he has lately been placed. We know only that the disease does not occur before the age of thirty-five. In persons above this age it can only be discovered by the intrinsic import of the symptoms. But in the early stages of the disease, and while the liver is still shielded by the ribs, the symptoms are vague, and such only as are common to various derangements of this organ. They may justly excite our fears; but they cannot give us assurance that the liver is the seat of cancer.

The most significant symptom is enlargement of the liver. When this comes on in the middle period of life, attended with gradual wasting and such serious disorder of health as may justify the suspicion of cancer, and especially when the enlargement is progressive, and when other conditions that may equally give rise to it are wanting—when there is no obstacle to the circulation in the chest, when the patient is not consumptive and has no chronic disease of the bones, when his habits have not been such as to lead to the suspicion of cirrhosis, and when, from the absence of jaundice, the enlargement of the liver cannot be ascribed to stoppage of the common gall-duct—it affords, of itself, strong presumption that the disease is cancer. The presumption is much strengthened if, on a careful examination of the liver, any tumors are discovered in it, and if the lower edge of the liver is felt to be not thickened, as it is in the fatty and in the scrofulous enlargement and in the enlargement that results from cirrhosis. When, with the conditions mentioned above, the liver is of very great size and its surface can be felt to be nodulous or uneven, there is no longer much room for doubt.

Another symptom, which is of very frequent occurrence, and which may help to distinguish this disease from some others in which the liver is likewise enlarged, is pain and tenderness of the liver itself, and pain, more widely diffused, in the back and loins, resulting, perhaps, from cancerous contamination of the glands to which the lymphatics of the liver run.

A small, permanent collection of fluid in the cavity of the peritoneum, when there is no reason to believe it to be the result of cirrhosis, is another significant token of the presence of cancerous tumors in the liver. A large quantity of fluid in the peritoneum is less significant of itself, and it may even increase the difficulty of diagnosis, by preventing our feeling the large and nodulous liver.

A circumstance to be especially attended to when cancer of the liver is suspected is the time the disease has lasted and the general condition of the patient with reference to it. Cancer of the liver generally grows and multiplies rapidly, and generally causes, therefore, rapid wasting and anemia, when no other exhausting influences exist. Sometimes, as we have seen, the growth of the cancer is so rapid, and so much blood is taken to feed it, that, after an illness of no more than five or six months, the patient dies greatly emaciated, and almost as much blanched as if death had been caused by an issue of blood. In other cases, the progress of the disease is slower, and life may be protracted to a year and a half or two years, but the cancer always gradually reduces the strength and impoverishes the blood, and the patient dies at length wasted and anemic. If, therefore, a disease of the liver has existed a year or two, or if it has existed several months without causing much wasting and anemia, the presumption is strong that the disease is not cancer.

Cases as difficult of diagnosis as any are those in which the cancerous growth stops the common gall-duct and causes persisting jaundice before the liver has become much enlarged or any tumors can be detected in it, and before the patient is much wasted. In such cases the subsequent enlargement of the liver may be ascribed to accumulation of bile in it from closure of the duct and the subsequent wasting to the jaundice—and for some time it may be impossible to say that the jaundice and enlargement of the liver do not result from stoppage of the common duct by a gall-stone or by inflammatory thickening, or through simple enlargement of a contiguous lymphatic gland. When, however, the common duct is stopped by a cancerous tumor, other tumors soon form in the liver itself, the patient wastes more rapidly and the enlargement of the liver is more continuous than in the other diseases just referred to, and after a time, on a careful manipulation of the liver, some tumor or small projecting nodule can often be discovered in it.

When cancer of the liver is consequent on cancer of some other part, its detection is much easier, because, from our knowledge of the frequent dissemination of cancer, symptoms, which are in other circumstances trivial, then acquire great significance. In a woman who has ulcerated cancer of the breast, with the general symptoms of the cancerous cachexy; or in one who has cancer of the uterus, which has eaten into the intestine; or in a person who has presented for some time the symptoms of cancer of the stomach—pain and tenderness in the region of the liver, or a slight increase in its volume, with jaundice, or slight ascites, or even one of these symptoms, is sufficient evidence that cancerous tumors have formed in this organ. The same symptoms, occurring soon after an injury to the head, or after amputation of the leg or arm, together with the constitutional symptoms of suppurative phlebitis, would scarcely leave a doubt that abscesses were forming in the liver. The diagnosis is formed, not so much from the intrinsic value of the symptoms, as from the significance which these derive from the circumstances under which they occur.

The *treatment* of malignant disease of the liver should be simply palliative. Practitioners have, indeed, hoped to destroy cancerous tumors by some powerful alterative, or, if not to destroy them, at least to retard their growth. Various powerful medicines—alkalies, mercury, arsenic, iodine—have been tried in turn with this view, and all—it is almost needless to remark—have signally failed. They have aggravated suffering and hastened death, by adding their own noxious effects to those of the malady; but there is no evidence that they have ever in the slightest degree retarded the growth or prevented the multiplication of the tumors. We can, indeed, hardly expect ever to effect this by medicines of any kind—seeing that cancer is not destroyed by any injury short of entire removal, and that it never loses its vitality by any change in the patient's constitution. The objects of rational treatment are, then, to mitigate the pain and any inflammation that may be caused by the cancerous tumors; to procure sleep; to remedy, as far as is possible, the various disorders of digestion; and in these and other ways to retard the emaciation and exhaustion that attend the disease.

For the relief of the pain, which is often quite independent of inflammation, and to procure sleep, no means are available but narcotics, which are very useful for this end, more especially in advanced stages of the disease. The most efficient of these remedies are the extracts of belladonna and conium, and the different preparations of morphia.

Any inflammation of the peritoneum that may be excited by cancer of the liver will be best relieved by the application of a few leeches, or a blister to the side. The diminution of tenderness from these means is often great, and before the strength of the patient is much reduced there are no countervailing evils which should deter us from their use. When the patient has become somewhat low in condition, we should, of course, be chary in taking away blood; and but little benefit can be expected from other active measures. Any good to be obtained from blisters, or other modes of counter-irritation, will seldom compensate for the torture and the weakness they occasion. In the advanced stages of the disease blisters are never advisable, since in the cachectic condition produced by cancer, and, indeed, in persons much reduced by any organic disease, they often cause severe pain and give rise to irritable ulcers of the skin.

The strength of the patient should be supported by a light, nourishing diet; and we should carefully abstain from mercury, iodine, strong purgatives, and all other powerful and lowering medicines. The wisdom of the practitioner is best shown in his abstaining from all fruitless interference.

In no cases, perhaps, has the specific influence which has been long attributed to mercury in the treatment of liver diseases done so much harm as in cases in which this organ has been the seat of cancer. In its early stages the disease is often set down vaguely as enlargement or obstruction of the liver, and mercury is given in consequence. In this country, indeed, a few years ago, the patient was fortunate if he escaped salivation, even after the tubera could be plainly felt, or when the existence of cancer elsewhere should have left no doubt as to the nature of the disease of the liver. In eight out of ten cases which have been recorded by Dr. Farre, the patient was mercurialized. In some of these cases mercury was given, or its use was continued, after the tumors in the liver were felt. In three of the cases in which it was given the patients were young children.

In cases such as these it is happy for the patient if the physician sees the true scope of his power, and is especially careful to do no harm where, confessedly, he can do but little good. Dr. Farre makes some judicious remarks on the error that was committed in the cases which he has recorded, in making ineffectual efforts to cure, where the treatment should have been simply palliative. As he well observes, "the perfection of medicine consists, not in vain attempts to do more than nature permits, but in promptly and effectually applying its healing powers to those diseases which are curable, and in soothing those which are incurable."

Encysted Knotty Tumors of the Liver.

In connection with cancerous tumors of the liver, it will not be altogether out of place to describe tumors which are now and then met with in this organ, and which, although essentially different from cancerous tumors, resemble them somewhat in appearance, and have been generally confounded with them. The tumors I allude to are the encysted tumors, containing a cheese-like matter, which have been cursorily noticed in a former chapter (p. 200). From their nodulous form in most of the specimens which have fallen under my notice, I have ventured to call them "knotty tumors of the liver."

The first instance of this disease that I met with occurred in a man who had been a hard drinker, and who died under my care in the Seamen's Hospital, in 1838, at the age of 32. The liver presented marks of extensive adhesive inflammation. It was enlarged, its surface was uneven, its edges were rounded, and its convex surface was united to the diaphragm by tufts of old false membrane. It contained several solid tumors, the largest of them about the size of a walnut, which were composed of a uniform firm, yellowish-white substance. The disease struck me at the time as being different from cancer, but no close examination of the tumors was made. There was no similar disease in any other part of the body.

In the spring of 1844 I had an opportunity of closely examining some tumors of the same kind in a liver which was sent to me by Mr. Busk, and which was taken from a man who died in the Seamen's Hospital of fever. The liver was of moderate size, and adhered to the diaphragm in patches. It contained about a dozen firm, white, fibrous-looking tumors, from the size of a large pea to that of a walnut. Most of these tumors were imbedded in the liver, but two or three of them reached its surface, and the liver *was adherent to the diaphragm at those spots*. One of the tumors projected above the surface, and the hepatic tissue around the others seemed to be compressed. The larger of the tumors were very nodulous, and all of them, large and small, were surrounded by a thin, but well-defined cyst. They appeared to be all situated in portal canals, and were composed of a compact substance, of a dead white color, to the eye not unlike firm white cheese. This substance was tough, like the coagulated fibrin of inflammatory blood, and adhered firmly to the cysts.[1] Some of the tumors had at their centres a small cavity (about the size of a partridge-shot), filled with a greenish matter, which had the appearance of inspissated bile.

The cheese-like substance of which the tumors were composed exhibited, under the microscope, a mass of irregular granules (which was not much altered by acetic acid), with some free oil-globules, and with here and there a plate of cholesterine. No fluid could be pressed out of it, and it presented no trace of organization, no fibres or cells. A slice of it digested for twenty-four hours in cold muriatic acid, gave a violet solution, showing that it was allied in composition to albumen or fibrin.

The greenish matter which was found at the centres of some of the tumors presented, under the microscope, a great number of oil-globules, plates of cholesterine, and shapeless masses of an orange-yellow, of various sizes, mixed with irregular, transparent, color-

[1] One of these tumors is preserved in the museum of King's College. (Prep. 327.)

less granules. On a drop of nitric acid being added to the specimen under the microscope, the orange yellow masses immediately became of a rich marine blue, but remained perfectly distinct. After the glass on which the specimen was placed had been heated, these objects were indistinct, but round purplish globular masses were here and there seen.

The tumors seemed to be of long standing. There was no similar disease in any other part of the body, nor were there any marks of scrofula, and the person did not appear to be of scrofulous habit.

The hepatic substance was in an early stage of cirrhosis; and the hepatic cells were unusually small, and contained but little oil.

The bile in the gall-bladder was reported, by Mr. Clapp, who examined the body, to be of natural appearance.

A short time before this examination was made, I received from Dr. Inman, of Liverpool, some notes of a case in which tubera were found in the liver, which, from Dr. Inman's description, I inferred to be of the same kind as those which have just been described. At my request, Dr. Inman sent me one of the tumors, and my inference proved to be correct. The case is further interesting as illustrating the tendency, noticed in a former chapter, which gangrene of an external part has to produce gangrene of internal organs, and I shall therefore relate it at length in Dr. Inman's words:—

(Jan. 31, 1844.)

Maria Sprounds, aged thirty-one, a market woman, of loose habits, but not intemperate in drink, was admitted into the Lock, with deep sloughing of the vulva and perineum, which extended backwards over the whole sacrum. The day before her death, when I first saw her, the parts were black, and emitted a most disgusting smell. Her breathing was hurried, the inspirations being forty-four a minute, and she had cough, with expectoration of a thin serous fluid, not unlike apricot-juice. The odor of gangrene from the vulva was so strong that it was very difficult to say whether the breath was fetid or not. The pulse was 120, and small. She lay on her right side, and did not complain of any pain.

The following particulars I learned from her sister: She was always healthy till eighteen months ago, when she began to suffer pain in the region of the liver, which has continued, more or less severe, ever since. Six months ago she had a venereal complaint, which soon got well. She was not compelled to leave her habitual employment until three weeks before her death. She then complained of pain and swelling of the pudenda, the venereal origin of which she stoutly denied to her death. At first there was simply swelling of the labia externa, which soon became black; the skin then broke, and the whole of the vulva began to slough; the gangrene spread rapidly over the sacrum, but not laterally towards the nates. In this condition she was taken to the Lock, where she died a week after. The nymphæ, the clitoris, and the vagina, were all included in the slough.

The body was examined eighteen hours after death.

In the right pleural cavity there was a large quantity of opaque serous fluid, and both the costal and the pulmonary pleuræ were coated by a recently-formed false membrane. The lung was adherent to the side at a spot corresponding to a cavern, which existed immediately beneath the pulmonary pleura in the middle lobe. On the left side of the chest there was likewise a turbid serous fluid in the pleural cavity, and both the costal and the pulmonary pleuræ were covered with false membrane, but the inflammation had not been so intense as on the right side.

The right lung was carnified in great extent, and on its middle lobe being cut into, a gangrenous cavern was found, lined by a thin false membrane, and containing a diffluent substance, of repulsive smell, which, when subjected to a stream of water, left a rough, irregular mesh of partly mortified pulmonary substance. In the vicinity of this cavity, there were three others, which were smaller, but like it in other respects. There was also a small collection of *pus* in this lung.

The left lung contained a great many small cavities, lined by a delicate cyst, and containing a thick yellowish matter, like concrete pus or softened fibrin, which was insoluble in water, but was easily washed away. These existed in all parts of the lung, but seemed to be most numerous near its surface and edges. This lung also was carnified in great extent. No tubercles existed in either lung. There was some fluid in the pericardium, but the heart was healthy.

The *liver*, which was of natural size, contained three yellowish-white bodies, which projected a little above its surface, and were attached to the walls of the belly by bands of false membrane, about three inches in length. The smallest of these tumors was about the size of a Spanish nut, and was situated at the acute margin of the left lobe. The largest of them was situated at the junction of the right and left lobes, and appeared to be made up of several smaller ones, each of them contained in a cyst. They do not appear to have had any influence on the hepatic substance, as that part of it which is in immediate contact with them does not seem to be denser than natural.

The stomach, the intestines, the kidneys, the uterus, the mesentery, and the peritoneum lining the pelvis, were all healthy. The internal iliac veins were healthy, and contained no pus.

A portion of the liver containing one of the tumors, which was sent me by Dr. Inman, is now in the museum of King's College (Prep. 326). This tumor, which is as large as a moderate sized potato (see Plate 3, Fig. 2), is widest at the surface of the liver, and projects slightly above it. It is round, but has an irregular surface, not unlike that of a mulberry calculus. The knotty projections are not distinct tumors, as Dr. Inman supposed, but mere excrescences. They are all included in a common cyst, which, although very thin, is readily distinguished from its being more transparent than the substance it contains.

The tumor was evidently formed in a portal canal. A portal vein of considerable size can be traced into its capsule, round which it winds for some distance. The substance of the tumor is precisely of the same character as that of the tumors in the liver which was sent me by Mr. Busk. It is of a dead white, or rather faint yellowish-white, firm, smooth when cut, and apparently homogeneous, not unlike firm white cheese. As happened in the tumors before described, it adhered firmly to the inner surface of the cyst. Under the microscope, it exhibits a granular matter, and some small free oil-globules, but no plates of cholesterine. The granular matter is rendered a little more transparent, but not much more so, by the addition of a drop of acetic acid. The substance of the tumor contains less oil than that of the tumors of the same kind which I had before examined. A particle picked out from the centre of the tumor showed small orange-colored masses, which seemed to be composed of the coloring matters of bile. The substance of the tumor exhibits no trace of organization—no fibres or cells. A small slice of it, weighing 4.6 grains, which was dried by my friend, Dr. Miller, at 200° F., left an ash amounting to 0.15 grain.

In May, 1846, I met with several tumors of the same kind in a girl eighteen years of age, who was brought into King's College Hospital with dropsy from granular disease of the kidney, and died twenty-four-hours after her admission. On inquiry, I learnt that she was a prostitute, that she had drunk hard of spirits, and that she had long been an out-patient of the hospital on account of secondary syphilis. The tumors that reached the surface of the liver were all covered by false membrane.

In the museum of King's College (Prep. 328), there is another preparation, showing a portion of liver which contains three tumors, evidently of the same kind as those just described. No history of the case is given. The tumors are about the size of hazel-nuts, and reach the surface of the liver, which, at those spots, is covered by a false membrane. The material composing them is more friable than in the former cases, and exhibits under the microscope irregular granules, with here and there an orange-yellow mass, apparently consisting of biliary matter, a few plates of cholesterine, and some round solid globules, which refract light strongly, and some of which exhibit faint rays proceeding from the centre. These globules were most of them dissolved when a drop of ether was put on the glass under the microscope, and were probably composed of margarin.

A fresh section was made of two of these tumors, and a small mass of concrete biliary matter was found in the centre of each, exactly as in the tumors which were sent to me by Mr. Busk.

In this specimen there is a good deal of green biliary matter in the hepatic substance, and at a spot near the tumors a small biliary concretion.

From the examination of these tumors, it would seem that they are analogous to the glairy cysts described in a former chapter, and that they result from dilatation of portions of the hepatic ducts by matter secreted by their mucous membrane. This explains their being encysted, and also another circumstance, which I noticed when examining them—namely, that the cyst is not thicker in the large tumors than in the small. It explains, too, the presence of biliary matter in the centres of all these tumors. The circumstance that, in all the specimens, an old false membrane covered the tumors which reached the surface, but not other portions of the liver, showed that an inflammatory process attended their formation.

It would appear, therefore, that the disease commences as inflammation of the mucous membrane of the hepatic ducts—that, in consequence of this, a duct becomes closed at some particular point, and the portion behind distended into an irregular pouch by the matter subsequently secreted. This origin explains the absence of any trace of organization in these tubera. The matter which is poured out on the free surface of an inflamed mucous membrane is not susceptible of organization; but, if it be pent up in a closed cavity and do not contain much pus, it forms at length a cheese-like mass, as in these tubera.

The cheese-like matter of a scrofulous gland originates in the same way—from inflammation of the mucous membrane of the gland.

Encysted cheese-like masses of the same kind are occasionally found in the lung; and they may also form in the kidney.

Small tumors containing a cheese-like matter are now and then found under the skin, especially on the inside of the upper arm, and probably originate in circumscribed inflammation of the lymphatic vessels.

Tubera of this kind can only form in mucous tubes which are small, and which—as the lymphatics, the hepatic gall-ducts, and the small bronchial tubes—have, in fulfilling their natural office, but a feeble current through them.

Abercrombie, in his work on the Stomach and Intestines, has given a short chapter on tumors of the kind under consideration, and has classed them with glairy cysts of the liver. The chapter is headed, "Tubera of the liver without other disease of its structure." He says, "These tubera present externally a surface elevated into irregular knobs of a yellowish or ash color, and perhaps from two or three inches in diameter. Internally they exhibit a variety of texture—in some cases fibrous, in others tuberculous or cheesy, and frequently there are cysts containing a viscid fluid. It appears that they produce marked symptoms only when they are numerous, or accompanied by enlargement of the liver, or disease of its general structure; but that when the structure is otherwise healthy, they may exist without any symptoms calculated to give a suspicion of their presence. Of this I shall only give the following example." (*Diseases of the Stomach*, 2d edit. p. 367.)

The example given by Abercrombie is the case of a gentleman, aged 80, who had enjoyed uninterrupted good health until a few weeks before his death, when he became one day suddenly incoherent. This disorder of intellect was removed by purgatives, and he had not shown any other symptom of disease, when one morning he was found dead in his bed. "No morbid appearance could be discovered to account for his sudden death, except that all the cavities of the heart, the aorta, and the vena cava were completely empty of blood. On the convex surface of the liver there was a tumor about three inches in diameter, elevated into numerous irregular knobs; on cutting into it a cavity was exposed capable of holding about ℥viij, and full of an opaque ash-colored fluid, which could be drawn out into strings. The liver in other respects was perfectly healthy."

For a more particular account of these tubera, Abercrombie refers to the work on the Morbid Anatomy of the Liver, by Dr. Farre, in which, however, only *cancerous* tumors of the liver are described.

SECT. II.—*Hydatid Tumors of the Liver.*

HYDATID tumors, like cancerous tumors, are more common in the liver than in any other organ.

They consist of a sac, of peculiar character, which is closely lined by a thin membranous bladder, or cyst, and filled with a liquid, which is usually colorless and limpid as the purest water. In some cases, on a superficial examination, nothing more than this appears; but generally, in hydatid tumors in man, there are found floating in the liquid a variable number (sometimes many hundreds) of globular bladders or cysts, similar to that which lines the sac, but of various sizes, from that of a small pea to that of a walnut. To these bladders, Laennec gave the name *Acephalocyst*—from ἀκέφαλη κύστις—a bladder without a head.

The *sac*, which seems to be formed of condensed hepatic tissue and the remains of obliterated vessels, has just the same character whether it contain merely the cyst which lines it, or many floating acephalocysts besides. Its thickness varies with the size and age of the tumor, and perhaps also with the degree of resistance which it has experienced in its growth. In small and recently formed tumors it is very thin; but in large tumors of long standing it has sometimes a thickness of four or five lines. It is then white and tough, very much like cartilage, and is easily separable into many layers. The surrounding hepatic substance adheres to it closely, and when this is scraped away, the sac is left hanging on the side towards the transverse fissure, by fibrous threads (the remains of obliterated vessels), which are lost in its coats. The inner surface of the sac is generally rough and fretted, and often presents, here and there, yellowish spots, which to the naked eye are very like the yellow spots so frequently found on the inner surface of arteries.

The membranous bladder, or *acephalocyst*, by which the sac is in all cases closely lined, is not adherent, and may be readily drawn out by the forceps. Its coats, which are friable, and of the firmness of hardened white of egg, are *very finely* laminated. The layers are, indeed, far too fine to be seen by the naked eye, or even by low powers of the microscope.

Nothing varies more than the fertility, if so it may be termed, of acephalocysts. Sometimes, and such is almost always the case in the hydatid tumors of the lower animals, the cyst which lines the sac contains no floating hydatids ; in other cases, even of long standing, it contains only a few—perhaps eight or ten ; while, now and then, it is literally crammed with them, and these, again, may, it is said, contain another generation.

When the floating acephalocysts have plenty of room, they are all globes or spheroids; but when closely packed, they assume various other forms, in consequence of their mutual pressure.

The floating hydatids have externally a uniform smooth surface, and, like the primary acephalocyst, are very finely laminated. Their membrane is elastic, and, when punctured, contracts so as to spirt out the fluid it contains. It breaks down readily under the finger, like coagulated white of egg. The inner layers are softer than the outer, and, after death, sometimes separate in flakes, rendering the fluid turbid.

The membrane of acephalocysts is composed of a substance which is closely allied to albumen. In some of the acephalocysts which are preserved in the museum of King's College, numerous crystals or amorphous masses are seen under the microscope, which are soluble in acetic acid, and which seem to be composed of phosphate of lime.

The liquid of acephalocysts has a specific gravity from about 1.008 to 1.013, is neutral or slightly alkaline, as tested by litmus or turmeric paper, and has a salt taste. It contains common salt in large quantity ; extractive or animal matter, in an undefined form, in much smaller proportion ; and a trace of other saline matter—probably all the salts of the blood which are not associated with its albumen. It contains no albumen, or only a faint trace of it, and no phosphates. It shows nothing under the microscope, but when a drop of it is slowly evaporated on a plate of glass, beautiful, colorless, microscopic crystals of chloride of sodium are left.

The question for a long time engaged the attention of pathologists—What is the nature of hydatid tumors, and how do they originate? The first step towards the solution of this question was the discovery that acephalocysts are the dwelling-place of those microscopic animalcules to which Rudolphi gave the name *echinococcus*, from the cylinder of hooks which surrounds the head. It has long been known that echinococci occasionally exist in countless numbers in acephalocysts, but such cases were at one time considered *exceptional*, and the echinococci were regarded as parasites of the hydatids. An extended and more careful examination has led, however, to the conclusion, that these animalcules exist in all acephalocysts. A French physician, M. Livois, in an essay on the Echinococcus, published in 1843,[1] states that among more than 800 hydatids, from man and other animals, he did not meet with a single one without them.

The echinococci can in general be readily found even in hydatids that have been long kept in spirits. Soon after M. Livois' work appeared, I opened seven preparations of hydatids that had been many years kept in spirit in the museum of King's College, and obtained the assistance of Mr. Busk in examining them. In five of these we had no difficulty in finding echinococci, or some of their remains, in the acephalocysts. In one of these preparations, in which the acephalocysts were a good deal decayed, only the hooks of echinococci were seen, which, like the teeth and bones of larger animals, remain when the other tissues are destroyed. In two of the preparations, no echinococci were found, but their absence could be explained from the state of the acephalocysts. One of these preparations contained several hydatids, which had been *expectorated*, and were all broken; the other contained an immense solitary acephalocyst, which was turned inside out. There can be little doubt that in these two instances all the echinococci escaped on the rupture or inversion of the cysts, or that they were afterwards washed away. I examined, besides, great numbers of hydatid tumors in the livers of sheep, and only failed to discover echinococci in one or two instances.

When an acephalocyst quite fresh is opened, its inner surface may often be seen to be covered with particles of an opaque white, which are just visible to the naked eye, and which look like very diminutive fish spawn. These particles are often not adherent to the cyst, and may be readily detached by a slight shake of the fluid.

[1] Recherches sur les Echinocoques, chez l'Homme et chez les Animaux. Paris, 1843.

Sometimes they escape in great numbers in the fluid which spirts out when the cyst is punctured. Under the microscope they are found to be echinococci.

Fig. 14.

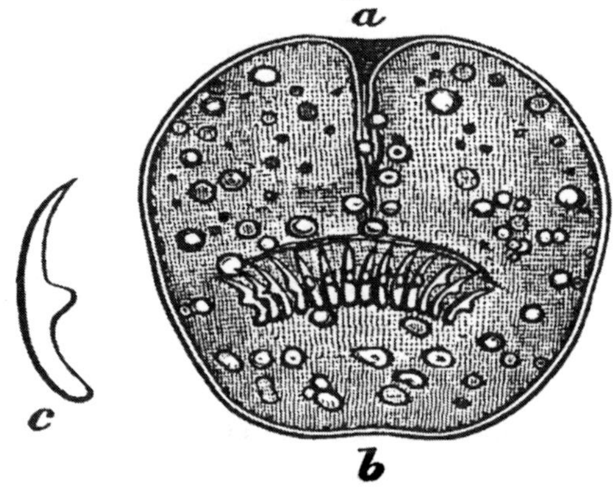

The echinococcus is a transparent, colorless creature, somewhat egg-shaped, and presenting, under the microscope, a distinct double outline, as represented in Fig. 14. The anterior end (*a*) has a depression or cleft, from which there is an evident canal or mouth, leading to a circlet of from twenty to thirty hooks within the body, and nearer the posterior end than the anterior. (*c*) represents, more highly magnified, one of the hooks or teeth, which are like those of the cysticercus. The posterior end (*b*) has also a slight depression, which has now and then a fibrous pedicle attached to it.

The creature is studded with globular corpuscles, which, from their refracting light strongly, have, under the microscope, a strong dark outline and a bright centre. They seem to be in the membrane of which the body is composed, or rather between the outer membrane and an interior solid body, and are at different depths from the object-glass, so that, while some are clear under the microscope, others are indistinct. Corpuscles of the same kind are found in all the cystic entozoa; and, according to Mr. Huxley, they are in the young and normal adult animals composed of an albuminous substance, but they frequently become calcareous from a deposit of carbonate of lime.

Commencing decomposition causes the circlet of hooks to protrude, and the creature has then the form represented in Fig. 15, or one much more elongated. The living animal seems to have the power of protruding its head, but fresh specimens have almost invariably the circlet of hooks within the body. When the head is protruded, four round disks (suckers) may be seen just below the circlet of hooks.

Fig. 15.

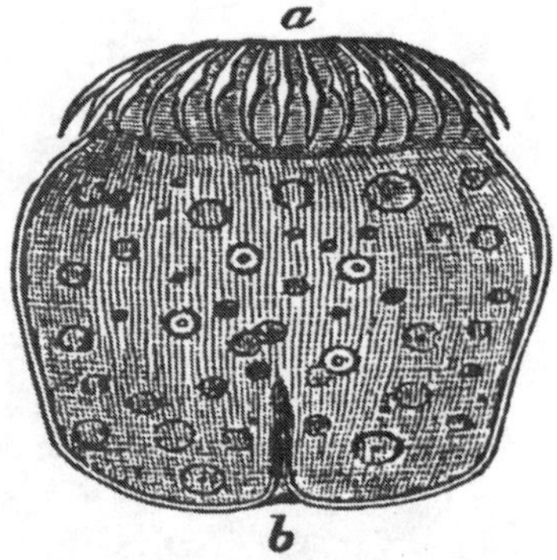

With echinococci, as above described, there are generally seen a few other bodies, which are about half their size, and which have not the same regular oval form. Their outline is single instead of double, and they present a confused mass of small granules, without any of the distinct globules which are seen in the larger ones. The body, instead of being colorless and transparent, is yellowish and opaque. The circlet of hooks is visible, but it is indistinct. These have been supposed to be echinococci not yet fully developed, but, according to Mr. Huxley, they are the creatures in a withered state.

In some hydatids, the echinococci are not seen as white grains on the inside of the cyst, and are hardly discoverable by the naked eye, but they are readily seen when a portion of the innermost layer of the cyst is looked at through the microscope.

Echinococci are not only solitary, and scattered over the inner surface of the cyst, but may sometimes be seen in small globular masses, which are inclosed in a very thin membrane, and connected with the inner surface of the hydatid cyst by a short, indistinct, fibrous pedicle, as shown in (*b*), Figure 16; in which *a* represents a portion of the hydatid cyst. *c*, in the same figure, represents one of these globular bodies, partially broken down, and shows that each individual animalcule has a distinct pedicle.

Fig. 17 represents a portion of one of the masses more highly magnified, and shows more distinctly the mutual connection of the echinococci. The animalcules in each mass are of the two kinds (*d*, *e*,) described above.[1]

[1] For the drawings given above I am indebted to the kindness of Mr. Busk, with whom I examined, some years ago, great numbers of these creatures.

The structure and mode of development of acephalocysts and echinococci, and the mutual relation of these constituents of an hydatid tumor, have been carefully studied by C. Th. Siebold, a

Fig. 16.

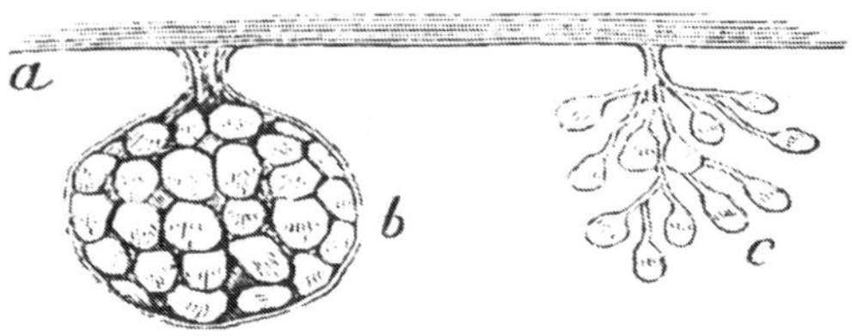

Fig. 17.

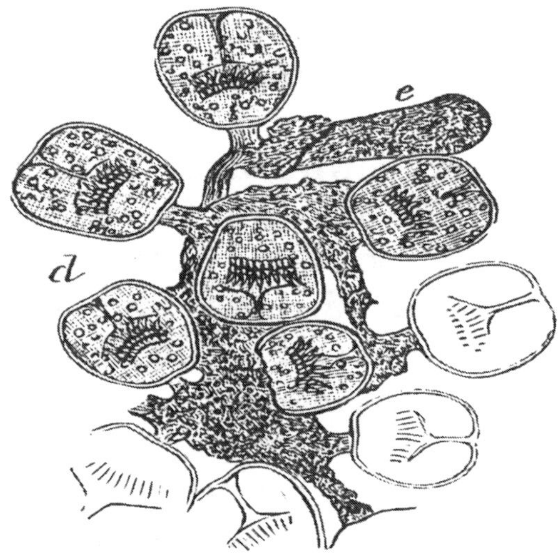

professor in the University of Munich, and by Mr. Huxley in this country. Mr. Huxley states[1] that the outer and laminated portion of the acephalocyst, to which the elasticity of the cyst is due, has no organic connection with the innermost layer, and may, with great care, be separated from it. He regards the innermost layer, which he terms the *endocyst*, as the proper body-wall of the animal, and the only active living part of the whole wall of the cyst; and considers the outer laminated portion to be a structureless cyst, formed by a process of exudation about the living organized membrane. This endocyst or innermost layer of the hydatid, which is very thin and delicate, contains echinococci in various stages of development, and exhibits, like the bladders of other cyst-worms, clear, strongly refracting corpuscles.

In the first stage of development of the scattered and solitary echinococci "elongated elevations of the endocyst are seen. Within these the circlet of hooks and then the corpuscles make their appearance; the elevation becomes a papilla, and the papilla, gradually constricting itself at the base, becomes the oval echinococcus attached by a narrow pedicle. In this state the slightest touch is sufficient

[1] Proceedings of the Zoological Society of London, for Dec. 14, 1852.

to separate the pedicle from the endocyst, and then the echinococcus is set free."

The secondary cysts are formed by groups of echinococci, which are developed, not only from the inner, but also from the outer surface of the endocyst, which thus becomes raised, with the echinococci attached to it, so as to project into the general cavity. The neck of attachment of the secondary cyst gradually narrows, and at last the secondary cyst, whose original size depends on the number of echinococci developed under the endocyst at one spot, falls into the general cavity. (*Huxley.*) The secondary cysts, when thus detached and floating in the parent cyst, grow larger, and sometimes attain the size of a small orange, but in the smallest secondary cysts the individual echinococci are as fully developed as in the large ones.

Hydatid tumors are, in this country, very common in sheep, and are occasionally found in oxen and in other herbivorous mammalia.[1] In every animal the echinococci are exactly alike, but the hydatid tumors of sheep differ in many respects from those of man. They are not regularly globular, as those of man are, and never contain more than a single acephalocyst, but, as if to make up for this, there are generally a great number of tumors in the same animal. In sheep, as in man, hydatid tumors are most common in the liver, which is sometimes found studded with them when there are none in any other organ. Often, however, the lungs are studded with them as well as the liver, and now and then there are great numbers in the peritoneum. In other herbivorous animals, hydatid tumors generally contain only a single acephalocyst; but tumors containing secondary, floating acephalocysts, have been found in the monkey, the pig, and the zebra.

The circumstance that the head of the echinococcus, when protruded, the head of the *cysticercus*, and the head of the *cœnurus cerebralis*—the many-headed bladder-worm found in the brain of staggering sheep—resemble each other, and are all like the head of the common tape-worm (Tænia solium), led some naturalists in the last century to regard these cyst-worms as modified tape-worms. Goeze, writing in 1782, describes the echinococcus-vesicles as the

[1] In the livers of sheep which are infested with hydatids, many minute pearly spots may sometimes be seen, which are too small to be recognized by the naked eye as hydatid tumors, but which, on being crushed, are found to contain echinococci as large and as perfect as those in the large hydatids.

"small social granular bladder tape-worm," and considered it an intermediate form between the cysticercus, which he termed the great globular bladder tape-worm, and the cœnurus;[1] and these surmises have been lately confirmed by direct experiment. A German naturalist, Kuchenmeister, conceived the idea of making dogs eat fresh and living cysticerci, and on making the experiment found that in the intestines of the dogs the bladder-worms were converted into tape-worms. An account of these experiments was published in 1851, and in the following year an extensive series of experiments of the same kind was made by Siebold, which confirmed and gave greater precision to the general result announced by Kuchenmeister.

Siebold found that the Cysticercus *pisiformis*, which is common in the liver and mesentery of the hare and rabbit, the Cysticercus *tenuicollis*, common in the mesentery of sheep and oxen, the Cysticercus *cellulosi*, often found in great numbers in pork, and the Cœnurus cerebralis, are all developed in the intestines of the dog into long tape-worms—the *tœnia serrata* of the dog, which he considers to be identical with the tænia solium of man.[2] He consequently considers that these various forms of cyst-worm are not distinct species, as they have been hitherto considered, but the embryos and degenerated offspring (scolex) of the same species of tape-worm.

The echinococcus (E. veterinorum) became developed in the intestine of dogs into a very diminutive tape-worm having only three joints, and which, from its small size, had escaped former observation. This tape-worm he proposes to call Tænia *echinococcus*.

By killing dogs at different intervals after they had swallowed the cyst-worms, Siebold was enabled to trace the progressive development of the worms. It appears that the bladder of the cyst-worm is dissolved by the gastric juice in the stomach of the dog, but that the head is uninjured by it and passes, still living, into the intestine, where it fastens on some point of the mucous membrane; and that, subsequently, while the head retains its original size, the

[1] See Mr. Huxley's paper, above referred to.

[2] Siebold expresses his conviction that three other varieties of tape-worm—the *Tœnia marginata* of the wolf, the *Tœnia crassipes* of the fox, and the *Tœnia intermedia* of the polecat and marten—are mere varieties of the same worm; which acquires, he believes, one form or another, according to the kind of animal in the intestine of which its development takes place.

neck lengthens and becomes marked by transverse lines, dividing it into segments—which segments, by their further growth, form the joints of the tape-worm. The different germs swallowed at the same time were found to be developed with very different degrees of rapidity. In one of Siebold's experiments a dog was made to swallow part of the large bladder of the cœnurus, and was killed thirty-eight days afterwards, when there were found in its small intestine seventy-one Tænias in different stages of development. The smallest of these were only from one and a half to two lines in length, and were but just beginning to exhibit joints: the longest were from sixteen to twenty-six inches long, and their hindmost joints contained perfectly developed eggs, and were beginning to drop off.

Since the publication of these researches on the production of tape-worms from the various forms of cyst-worm, the converse experiment has been performed, and cyst-worms have been produced from the eggs of the tape-worm. In a paper published in the *Annales des Sciences Naturelles* (tom. iv. 1855), giving an account of Siebold's researches, two experiments of this kind are referred to. In one of these experiments, made by M. Haubner, a professor in the Veterinary College at Dresden, joints of the tape-worm of the dog containing fully developed eggs were, on the 7th of January, given to many lambs with their food, and on the 20th of January all these lambs had the staggers (turnsick), while other lambs in the same fold remained in good health. The staggering lambs were killed after different intervals, and in their brains and elsewhere cyst-worms were found in different stages of development.

In the second experiment, performed by Professor Leuckart, of Giessen, mice were made to eat ripe joints of the *Tænia crassicollis* of the cat, and the result was the development of *Cysticercus fasciolaris* in the livers of the mice.

These experiments seem to be conclusive as to the mode of production of the various forms of tape and cyst-worm, and it has been inferred from them that the Tænia solium—the common tape-worm of man—is most commonly a transformation of the Cysticercus cellulosa in the so-called "measly" pork, and that the cysticercus and cœnurus of cattle is most commonly attributable to a tape-worm in the shepherd's dog; but it does not appear to be yet ascertained what animal is the usual dwelling-place of the diminutive tape-worm (Tænia echinococcus) that gives birth to hydatid tumors.

In the hydatid tumor of the human liver the sac that contains the acephalocysts, as before remarked, increases in thickness with the size and age of the tumor, but it often undergoes other change. The most common of these arises from the deposit of calcareous matter (phosphate of lime, with a little carbonate,) in its coats, so as to form ossific plates, like those so often found on the inner surface of arteries. This deposit of calcareous matter in its coats, and its ready division into laminæ, establish a striking distinction between the sac of an hydatid tumor in the liver and the cyst of an hepatic abscess. However old or large an abscess be, its cyst is always composed of dense fibrous tissue, not divisible into laminæ, and never containing calcareous matter in the form of deposit. The sac of an hydatid tumor, on the contrary, is readily divisible into distinct laminæ, and, when large and of long standing, almost always contains some ossific plates and calcareous matter in detached grains in its coats. Sometimes, this calcareous matter is in such quantity, that the entire sac is converted into an osseous cyst. In the museum of King's College (Prep. 332), there is a liver containing three large hydatid cysts, whose walls have all undergone this change.

It is probable that earthy matter is most apt to be deposited in the coats of hydatid cysts in aged persons. Some time ago one of the students at King's College brought me a liver containing an ossified hydatid tumor, which was taken from an old woman who died in one of the London workhouses, and whose body was given for dissection. In the *Edinburgh Medical and Surgical Journal*, for October, 1835 (p. 286), the case of a lady is related, who died at the age of seventy-three. Two hydatid tumors, whose sacs were almost completely osseous, and which contained a thick gelatinous matter and numerous hydatids, were found in the liver. It appeared probable, from the symptoms, that the tumors had existed from the eighth year of her age.

It has been remarked by Cruveilhier that, when ossific plates are thus formed by the deposit of earthy matter, the inner surface of the sac has a striking resemblance to that of a true aneurism, (an aneurism without rupture of the coats of the artery), empty of clots. The walls of the hydatid sac, like the walls of an aneurism, may ulcerate from distension; or may become irregularly dilated by the accumulating matter within, so as to form additional pouches springing from the primary sac. Not unfrequently the process of ulceration causes an opening from the sac into the gall-bladder, or into one of the gall-ducts.

These changes seem to be the natural consequences of the peculiar organization of the sac. They occur in hydatid tumors of the spleen as well as in those of the liver. But in some cases other changes are met with, which are produced by *inflammation* set up within the sac or in the tissue around it. In what may be called the healthy state of an hydatid tumor, and in almost all recent tumors of this kind, there are no marks of inflammation about the sac, and the hepatic tissue immediately surrounding it has its natural texture, or exhibits only such changes from the natural texture as are produced by *pressure*. But, after a time, adhesive inflammation is often set up around the sac, and coagulable lymph is poured out, which glues the sac, where it projects above the surface of the liver, to the parts—the diaphragm, the walls of the belly, the intestine—with which it happens to be in contact. Old hydatid tumors of the liver, which project above its surface, are frequently found thus united by means of false membrane to contiguous parts.

Another frequent and more serious change results from suppurative inflammation of the inner surface of the sac, converting it into an abscess. Andral, Cruveilhier, and most writers who have published a series of cases of hydatids of the liver, have given instances in which this had occurred. A great number of others are scattered through our medical journals, and three instances of the kind have fallen under my own notice. In such cases, the hydatid sac contains pus, and fragments of hydatids. When the patient dies soon after the occurrence of suppuration, some hydatids are occasionally found entire, *and containing a perfectly limpid fluid*, although the fluid in which they float is purulent. The floating acephalocysts, indeed, are not nourished by bloodvessels, and are incapable of forming pus; which is in all cases furnished by the walls of the sac. When the patient lives long after suppuration has occurred in the sac, it is sometimes difficult to discover and identify the fragments of hydatids, but even then the nature of the tumor may be at once told from the character of the sac, which differs essentially from the cysts of an ordinary hepatic abscess in not adhering so firmly to the hepatic tissue around it, in being readily divisible into layers, and frequently in containing plates or palpable grains of calcareous matter in its coats.

Cruveilhier has made the important remark that, while the fluid in hydatid cysts, in what may be termed their healthy state, is perfectly limpid and colorless, that contained in hydatid tumors of the liver which have suppurated, is almost always more or less tinged with bile. He believes that the entrance of bile into the sac, from ulceration of a branch of the hepatic duct imbedded in its walls, is the most common cause of the suppurative inflammation which converts it into an abscess. I have no doubt of the correctness of this opinion. The greenish color of the contents of the sac can only be ascribed to the presence of bile, for no such color has been noticed in hydatid tumors in other parts of the body; and the presence of bile (which, when applied to serous membranes, excites the most intense inflammation), is a sufficient cause for the suppuration of the inner surface of the sac. This circumstance explains how it happens that hydatid tumors suppurate so much more frequently in the liver than in any other organ. Suppurative inflammation of the sac may, however, be also excited by other agencies. In the spring of 1850, a woman who was long under my care in King's College Hospital, died with an enormous hydatid tumor in the liver, full of floating hydatids and of a puriform liquid, which was perfectly untinged by bile. Andral has related a case of the same kind (*Clin. Med.*, iv. p. 485), in which suppuration of the sac occurred without obvious cause, and where, after death, the pus was found to be *white* and creamy. He has also related another case (*Clin. Med.*, ii. p. 408), in which pus was found in an hydatid sac in the lung, while the floating acephalocysts contained fluid as transparent as rock water. Cruveilhier states[1] that he has found pus and fragments of hydatids in an hydatid tumor of the spleen.[2]

Inflammation, whether adhesive or suppurative, seldom occurs either around or within the sac of an hydatid tumor until the

[1] Dict. de Méd. et Chirurgie Pratiques. Art. "Acephalocyste," p. 244.

[2] The explanation of some of these cases is, perhaps, that a part of the sac imbedded in the organ became perforated from ulceration; that some of the fluid which the tumor originally contained escaped into the surrounding areolar tissue, and excited suppurative inflammation; and that some of the pus there formed got into the sac, and set up suppurative inflammation of its inner surface.

tumor has attained a certain age. It rarely happens that any traces of it are found in hydatid tumors in sheep, whose allotted duration of life, in their domestic state, is short.

Occasionally, an hydatid tumor in the liver is found filled with matter of the appearance of glazier's putty, or plaster, with fragments of dead hydatids. This matter, which may accumulate either between the sac and the acephalocyst which lines it, or within this acephalocyst, is composed chiefly of phosphate of lime and of animal matter allied to albumen. It contains also a small quantity of carbonate of lime, and, in some cases, if not in all, a small quantity of cholesterine. Three cases of this kind have fallen under my own observation, and many others have been collected by Cruveilhier, who rightly considers the secretion of a thick matter from the inner surface of the sac to be one mode of cure of an hydatid tumor. A tumor containing such matter generally looks as if it had been at some former time much larger. In some instances, no objects are to be found in it which can be recognized as fragments of hydatids, and the nature of the tumor can only be inferred from the peculiar characters of the sac.

Similar changes occasionally take place in the contents of hydatid tumors in other organs. A case is related by Cruveilhier (*Anat. Path.*, liv. 35, pl. 1), in which an hydatid sac in the spleen contained a matter like plaster or cheese, while another hydatid sac in the liver contained pus.

Cruveilhier supposes that the secretion of this peculiar matter in hydatid tumors is consequent on the death of the hydatids, but it seems not improbable that it may be the primary change, and that the death of the hydatids may result from it.

There is still another source of danger from hydatid tumors in the liver. They are apt to burst, either from blows or accidental pressure or from ulceration, and to discharge their contents into the peritoneal sac. From the nature of the fluid in healthy hydatid cysts, it might be imagined that their bursting into this cavity would excite no inflammation, and would be attended with little danger. But experience has proved the contrary. The fluid in hydatid cysts, although limpid and colorless as the purest water, is a violent irritant to the peritoneum, always exciting the most intense inflammation of it. Cruveilhier imagined that the inflammation might result from some of the hydatids escaping from the sac and irritating, *mechanically*, the surface of the serous membrane; but the same thing happens from the bursting of a solitary hydatid cyst. The bursting of an hydatid cyst, whether it contain floating hydatids or not, and when the liquid only of the cyst escapes into the cavity of the peritoneum, excites intense inflammation of that membrane, and may destroy life as soon as the bursting of the gall-bladder or of an hepatic abscess. Cruveilhier, in the paper already referred to (*Dict. de Méd. et Chir. Pratiques*, art. "Acephalocyste"), has collected from various sources four cases (*Obs.* 6, 7, 8, 9), in which the patients died very rapidly, with the symptoms of peritonitis from perforation of the bowel, in consequence of the accidental rupture of an hydatid cyst in the liver; and two cases of the same kind are related by Mr. Cæsar Hawkins, in the eighteenth volume of the *Medico-Chirurgical Transactions* (p. 124 and p. 126). In three of these six cases (Cruv., *Obs.* 6, 8, 9), the sac contained many hydatids; in the other three, the acephalocyst was solitary, and nothing but the fluid it contained and echinococci could have escaped into the cavity of the peritoneum. From these cases, and from others of the same kind, it would seem that the bursting of an hydatid tumor into the sac of the peritoneum causes death as surely, and just as speedily, as the bursting of an abscess, or as perforation of the stomach or bowel.

Ulceration and perforation of the sac may also take place at a part which is embedded in the liver. When this happens, the liquid of the hydatid tumor becomes extravasated into the surrounding hepatic tissue, and causes suppurative inflammation, and, finally, disorganization of it.

A case has been related in a former chapter (page 103), in which the liquid of an hydatid cyst seemed to be absorbed, in consequence of an injury done to the cyst, and then to cause small *scattered* abscesses in the substance of the liver. The process of suppuration in this case evidently commenced within the lobules, and most probably resulted from an attempt made by the secreting cells to eliminate the noxious matter.

When an hydatid tumor of the liver is about to open through the abdominal parietes, it sometimes causes extensive suppurative inflammation and sloughing of the cellular tissue under the skin and between the abdominal muscles—in consequence, no doubt, of the infiltration of the hydatid liquor. A case in which this occurred and proved fatal, fell, in 1855, under the observation of Mr. Fergusson and myself.

These, and other instances which might readily be cited, are sufficient to show that the liquid of an hydatid cyst—though perfectly clear and colorless, and seemingly simple in composition—is a violent irritant to many tissues.

A very important point in the history of hydatid tumors of the liver, is that very often more than one such tumor is found in the same person. Sometimes the liver itself contains two hydatid tumors; and now and then, but rarely, three or more.

But sometimes, with a single hydatid tumor in the liver, an hydatid tumor is found in the lower lobe of one of the lungs or in the lower lobe of each lung. An instance of this kind is cited by Mr. Hawkins in his paper in the eighteenth volume of the *Medico-Chirurgical Transactions.* There was a solitary hydatid in the liver, and one in the lower part of each lung. Another instance is cited by Cruveilhier (*Op. cit.*, p. 245), in which there was a multiple hydatid in the liver, and a solitary hydatid of enormous size in the lower lobe of each lung. Another instance is recorded by Andral (*Clin. Méd.*, ii. p. 408), in which, with a solitary hydatid in the liver, there was a solitary hydatid in the lower lobe of the left lung.

I am indebted to Dr. Watts, of Manchester, for details of a case that fell under his care, in which, with a solitary hydatid in the liver, there was a solitary hydatid in the lower lobe of the left lung.

The patient, a factory-man, forty-seven years of age, had good health till the beginning of the year 1842, when he became dyspeptic, complaining of pain in the stomach, and in the back, below the right shoulder-blade. In the month of April of that year, he was treated by Dr. Williams for inflammation of the left lung. He recovered from this, but the pain in the stomach and in the back continued, and he was not able to resume his work in the factory. On the 12th of April, 1843, he was taken extremely ill, with increase of pain at the stomach, together with acid eructations and with great weakness. This was followed by difficulty of breathing, and at length by symptoms of gangrene of the lung, and he died at the end of a fortnight.

On examination of the body, the liver appeared to be very large, owing to an hydatid tumor, as large as a child's head, which was imbedded in its substance, and which contained a solitary acephalocyst. The cyst was green from the imbibition of bile, and contained a green and turbid fluid.

In the middle of the lower lobe of the left lung was another hydatid tumor, of the size of a large fist, which, like that in the liver, contained a solitary acephalocyst. The lower lobe of each lung, but especially of the left, was solid, but easily broken down between the fingers, giving escape to a thick opaque matter, which had a most disgusting smell of gangrene.

The cysts were presented by Dr. Watts to the museum of King's College.

Hydatid tumors in the lung differ from those in the liver, only in the sac being thinner. In all the instances which I have found recorded, they have been in the lower lobes of the lungs. Owing, perhaps, to the thinness of the sac and to the compressibility of the lung, they sometimes attain an enormous size, almost filling the chest, and causing death by suffocation.

Hydatid tumors sometimes exist in the lower lobes of the lung, when there are no such tumors in the liver or in any other organ. A case of this kind fell under my observation in King's College Hospital, in the summer of 1851; two such cases have been recorded by Andral (*Clin. Méd.*, ii. 407 and 410); and several others have been collected by Cruveilhier.

In a remarkable case recorded by Andral, while an hydatid tumor existed in the liver, both lungs were filled with hydatids, but these, instead of being contained in a single sac in each lung, were all lodged in pouches formed by dilatation of portions of the pulmonary veins.

A man, fifty-five years of age, had all the symptoms of organic disease of the heart, and died in a state of asphyxia.

Both lungs were filled with a great number of hydatids. Andral first thought that these were in the substance of the lung, but on careful dissection he discovered that they were all lodged *in the pulmonary veins.* He traced these veins from the heart to the lung, and, on reaching their almost capillary divisions, he found that many of them presented a great number of pouches which were formed by dilatation of a portion of the vessel, and which were filled with hydatids. Beyond each of these dilated portions, the vein regained its former calibre, and a little further on became dilated again. The largest pouches were of the size of a walnut, the smallest scarcely as large as a pea. The hydatids which they contained had all the characters of acephalocysts. Many of them exhibited small spots of a dead white in their coats; others a great number of miliary granulations on their inner surface (which were doubtless echinococci).

In the middle of the liver was an hydatid sac, with cartilaginous walls, capable of holding a large orange, and containing eight or ten acephalocysts. (*Clin. Méd.*, ii. p. 412.)

It is probable that in this case hydatid germs from the liver got into the hepatic vein, and being carried to the capillary branches of the pulmonary veins, were there developed and multiplied.

An hydatid tumor of the liver is still more frequently associated with one in the spleen. An instance of this kind has been already cited from Cruveilhier. In his article on acephalocysts, which has been so often referred to, Cruveilhier has given another instance (*Obs.* 2) in which there were two hydatid tumors in the liver (not said to be multiple), and two in the spleen. Andral has given an instance in which with a tumor containing floating hydatids in the liver, there was a similar tumor in the spleen—and numerous other cases of the same kind are on record.

An hydatid sac in the spleen undergoes the same changes from distension, and from the deposit of calcareous matter as an hydatid sac in the liver, from which it differs only in the greater thinness of its coats; the consequence, perhaps, of the less degree of resistance which it experiences in its growth. It is less liable to suppurate than an hydatid sac in the liver, from not being exposed to the entrance of bile.

It is an important circumstance that an hydatid tumor of the spleen, though often associated with one of the liver, is hardly ever found alone. Another circumstance which serves to throw light on the origin of such tumors, and which, like the former, was noticed by Cruveilhier, is that an hydatid tumor is rarely found in the *substance* of the spleen. It is almost always on the posterior surface of the organ (apparently formed in the gastro-splenic omentum), and the spleen is moulded upon it.

Sometimes, with an hydatid tumor of the liver, there is a similar tumor in some part of the mesentery. Cruveilhier (*Op. cit.*, p. 216) has given the details of a case, recorded by M. Monod, in which there was a tumor of fifteen years' standing, containing numerous hydatids, in the liver; another sac of the same kind, partially imbedded in the spleen; a third, in the transverse meso-colon.

Occasionally, with an hydatid tumor of the liver, thousands of hydatid tumors are found in the belly, under the peritoneum, and between the folds of the mesentery. Cruveilhier (liv. xix. pl. 1 and 2) has published drawings taken from a case of this kind.

In the midst of the liver was a large sac containing an acephalocyst, which had collapsed, and which when filled out was three or four times larger than it at first appeared. The coats of the sac were very thick, and a gall-duct opened into it. The sac, on three-fourths of its surface, was invested by the liver; on the remaining fourth, it was confounded with the walls of a cyst of the mesentery. There were three other hydatid tumors, not altered, along the right edge of the liver, and partly sunk into it. The spleen presented some superficial hydatid cysts. Between the liver and the spleen, and below these organs, there was a large globular mass pointed below, and reaching into the pelvis This mass, when cut into, presented a number of hydatid sacs of different dimensions, communicating with each other by circular openings of various sizes. The sacs had all a fibrous structure, and contained, some a single hydatid, others two or three, or as many as seven or eight.

Another case very similar to this is related by Cruveilhier. In that case—

The liver was very large, filling all the right hypochondrium, the epigastrium, and the left hypochondrium; and the omentum was sprinkled with cysts, which extended into the pelvis. The liver contained four cysts, the largest of the size of an infant's head. An hydatid cyst in the lesser omentum compressed the spleen. The gastro-hepatic omentum and the great omentum contained, imbedded in them, more than fifty hydatid cysts, from the size of a walnut to that of two fists, and forming a kind of chaplet, which extended from the concave surface of the liver into the pelvis. The cavity of the pelvis was filled by a large cyst, situated between the rectum and the bladder, and adhering to the right vesicula seminalis, at the expense of which it seemed to be formed. (*Op. cit.*, art. "Acephalocyste," p. 226.)

A case of the same kind fell under my charge in King's College Hospital in the autumn of 1842.

Case.—George Berbick was admitted into King's College Hospital on the 31st of August, 1842. He was 28 years of age, a porter, of temperate habits, and had always resided in London. He had good health till about ten years before, when his belly began to enlarge, without his suffering any particular inconvenience from it, except that ever since he had been "troubled with bile." Five years ago he had a severe illness, which seems to have been typhus fever, lasting seven or eight weeks, during part of which he was in Charing-Cross Hospital. He recovered perfectly from this illness, but the belly continued to increase in size till three years ago, since which time, he states, it has ceased to grow larger. For the last seven years has been subject to "spasms," which of late have been less frequent than formerly. Six weeks ago was seized with sore throat and erysipelas of the head, which lasted a fortnight. Since that time has been losing flesh, and has vomited almost everything he has taken.

At the time of his admission to the hospital he was much emaciated, and his intellect was weak, so that he did not always answer questions pertinently. He vomited everything he swallowed, and had some diarrhœa. His urine and feces were passed in bed. His appetite was bad; his tongue covered with a dark coat; his pulse, 84, very weak. The belly was much enlarged, and the lower part of the chest was greatly expanded. A great number of hard tumors, about the size of oranges, were felt through the walls of the belly, but there was no fluctuation. The duluess on percussion over the liver extended considerably below the false ribs. Below this, in a line extending nearly across the belly, just above the umbilicus, was the clear sound of intestine. Over the rest of the belly percussion produced a sound, not naturally clear and not altogether dull, giving the idea of a solid layer beneath the abdominal muscles, and resting on the intestines. The chest was dull on percussion on the right side as high as the mamma, and on the left side nearly as high. The heart beat above the left mamma.

He was ordered five grains of sesquicarbonate of ammonia, and five drops of tincture of opium, every four hours; and f℥iij of wine daily.

He gradually sank, and died on the 3d of September.

The body was examined twenty-four hours after death, and the following notes of the appearances presented were entered in my case-book, by my friend and former pupil, Dr. George Johnson.

On opening the abdomen, a number of globular tumors were seen connected with the omentum. These proved to be hydatid tumors. Some of them contained a single acephalocyst, filled with a clear fluid; others contained several hydatids, from two to fifty or more; and some of them were quite solid from containing a great number of hydatids from which the fluid had escaped, and which were closely packed in their investing cyst, like a number of dried raisins.[1] The omentum was removed with these hydatid tumors connected with it, and the intestines beneath were found to be quite sound. The colon passed across where the line of resonance was observed during life. Some tumors of the same kind were connected with the liver, rendering it of enormous size. The substance of the liver was quite healthy. Some of the tumors were partly imbedded in it, and with one of these the gall-bladder communicated. The largest tumor connected with the liver contained about half a pint of fluid.

Some tumors of the same kind were also connected with the spleen; and one was connected with the summit of the urinary bladder.

All the large investing cysts were globular, as were also the contained hydatids.

In such cases, when, with an hydatid cyst in the liver, an hydatid cyst is found in the spleen, or in the omentum or between the layers of the peritoneum, there is usually no hydatid cyst in the lungs. When, with an hydatid cyst in the liver, there is an hydatid cyst in the lung, there is none in the spleen or mesentery. The disease extends from the liver forwards in the direction of the hepatic veins, or backwards in the direction of the portal veins, but not in both directions at once.

In all cases when more than one hydatid cyst exists in the same

[1] The hydatids seem to be sometimes destroyed by being packed too closely; or from the containing sac not enlarging sufficiently as they multiply.

person, we must admit—if we consider how few persons comparatively have hydatid tumors—that the different tumors originated from eggs that entered the body through the same channel at the same time, or that one tumor is the parent of others. The first supposition may seem the more natural; but the facts, that the liver is the organ in which hydatid tumors most frequently form, that there are seldom many hydatid tumors in the human liver, that when the disease extends beyond the liver it is only in one direction, and that when many tumors exist there is usually one in the liver *which exhibits marks of greater age than the rest*—all these facts favor the supposition that an hydatid tumor of the liver may be the parent of others. We have seen that by ulceration of the inner surface of an hydatid sac in the liver, the gall-ducts that adhere to its walls may become perforated and bile may flow into the sac, or, conversely, the contents of the sac may escape into the gall-ducts. It is probable that other vessels embedded in the wall of the sac may be opened by ulceration in the same way, and that thus, by the escape of germs into a branch of the hepatic or of the portal vein, or into one of the lymphatics, an hydatid tumor in the liver may lead to secondary tumors in the lungs, or between the folds of the mesentery, or in the liver itself. The supposition is still further supported by the fact, that when many hydatid tumors exist, the more advanced tumor in the liver usually presents ulceration or other marks of disease on the inner surface of the sac.

In sheep and cattle, as in man, hydatid tumors are most common in the liver, which is sometimes found studded with them when there are none in any other organ. Often, however, the lungs are studded with them as well as the liver; and now and then, as in man, there are great numbers in the peritoneum. In these animals, as in man, it seems to be a general rule, that when, with hydatid tumors in the liver, there are hydatids in the lung, there are none in the mesentery; when there are tumors in the mesentery, there are none in the lung. M. Livois states that in ten sheep that he examined, eight had hydatids in the liver and in the lungs; the remaining two in the liver and in the spleen; four oxen and two cows had them only in the liver and lungs.

It has been just stated that an hydatid tumor of the liver is associated only with hydatid tumors in the lung, or in the spleen or mesentery. There is, however, a remarkable case published by Mr. Hill, of Dumfries (2d vol. of *Medical Commentaries*, p. 303), in which an hydatid tumor (in the liver?), in a little girl, burst and discharged its contents through the walls of the belly. She got quite well from this; but, thirteen years afterwards, three large hydatid tumors, which seemed no deeper than the muscles, appeared on different parts of the belly. These tumors burst two outwards and one into the intestines, and the patient ultimately recovered.

In this instance, the secondary tumors seemed to be confined to the walls of the belly, and probably resulted from adhesion between them and the liver, and the consequent escape of an hydatid germ into one of the veins of the abdominal muscles. It is a striking fact that there were no hydatids in the lungs or in the mesentery, the parts in which they are most frequently found when there is an hydatid tumor in the liver.

The greatest objection to the hypothesis here advanced to account for the tumors in the spleen and mesentery, is, perhaps, the improbability that an hydatid germ should pass backwards in the branches of the portal vein, against the current of the blood. It seems more natural to suppose that if the tumors are related as cause and effect, the tumor in the liver is secondary to those of the spleen or mesentery, and not the origin of them. A strong fact against this latter hypothesis is the appearance of greater age in the tumor in the liver in such cases, and the circumstance that, while hydatid tumors in the liver alone are not uncommon, it seldom, if indeed ever, happens that hydatid tumors exist alone in the spleen or in the mesentery.

Hydatid tumors, having essentially the same character as those of the liver, have been found in man in other organs besides the liver, the lungs, the spleen, and the mesentery. They have been met with, but in comparatively few instances, in the kidney, in the brain, in the spinal canal, in the thyroid gland, in the subcutaneous areolar tissue, and, in one instane (*Livois*, p. 117), in the globe of the eye behind the crystalline lens. In almost all such instances on record, there has been only one hydatid tumor in the body.

Other evils than have yet been mentioned may result from an hydatid tumor in the liver. The tumor from its mere bulk may embarrass the breathing so as to destroy life; or the pus that may be formed within it, or the proper fluid of the cyst, which, to the peritoneum, and to the surrounding hepatic tissue, is, as we have seen, just as irritating as pus, may find its way into the veins, or excite inflammation of a vein, and so lead to suppurative inflammation in another part of the liver, or to inflammation of both lungs.

In the following case, for which I am indebted to Mr. Bowman, an hydatid tumor of the liver, besides producing other evils, led to disorganization of the surrounding hepatic tissue, to the formation of an abscess in a remote part of the liver, to suppurative inflammation of the hepatic veins, and to inflammation of the lower lobes of both lungs. The case is very long, but it is so well drawn up, and presents so many points of interest, that I have not ventured to abridge it.

CASE.—Judith Austin, a servant girl, aged twenty-five, was admitted into the hospital (Birmingham) on the 24th of February, 1837. According to her own account and that of her friends, she had enjoyed uninterrupted health up to the Christmas preceding, when, without obvious cause, she was seized with shivering and other febrile symptoms, together with pain in the region of the liver, which was followed after a few days by jaundice. Her disease was considered to be inflammation of the liver. Leeches and blisters were applied, she was bled from the arm, and her mouth was slightly touched by mercury. Under this treatment, she seemed to have recovered, and accordingly returned to her place of service, still, however, feeling an uneasiness in her side, and complaining of lassitude and weakness. She had scarcely been at her work a week when she was seized suddenly with a rigor, which was followed by heat of skin and perspiration. On the following morning, three days before her admission to the hospital, she found herself jaundiced.

When brought to the hospital, the jaundice was rather deep, and was attended with itching, particularly at night, and with occasional cramps of the limbs. The skin was rather dry and scurfy, of natural temperature. The pulse slightly accelerated. Respiration natural, without cough. Appetite bad. Slight thirst. Tongue foul. Occasional sickness. Headache. Bowels much constipated. Stools of a light brown color. Urine of a deep yellow, tinging the linen, and turning to an olive-green on the addition of muriatic acid. She complained of uneasiness in the right hypochondrium, especially on moving, or on lying on the left side. When in the last-named posture, she felt a weight dragging from the right side of the belly, and sometimes had nausea; and she always rested on the right side or back. She had likewise at times an aching pain in the right shoulder. On examination, there was found to be considerable fulness and firm swelling, extending from under the cartilages of the ribs on the right side and from the ensiform cartilage, as low down as the umbilicus. As far as could be ascertained, the swelling was of uniform surface, and unyielding. When firm pressure was made upon it, she complained of some pain. The swelling gave out an entirely flat sound on percussion. The rest of the abdomen was tympanitic. Her face was rather pale, and her appearance, independently of the jaundice, was that of a person considerably out of health. The catamenia were regular. A dose of blue pill and colocynth was given every night, which kept up a gentle action of the bowels, and the jaundice grew fainter.

On the 4th of March she complained of increased pain in the right side, and a blister was applied there in consequence. The blister rose well, but the pain was not relieved.

On the morning of the 8th she had a slight rigor, with headache, and thirst, and nausea; and an erysipelatous inflammation appeared around the vesication. (Tartar emetic was ordered, in doses of three-fourths of a grain, every second hour, until it should produce vomiting.)

On the 9th the erysipelas had extended upwards towards the axilla, and vesications had begun to appear on the surface first affected. She had less thirst, and no nausea. The tongue was covered with a yellowish fur; the pulse 88, and soft. (Small doses of tartar emetic and of liquor ammoniæ acetatis were given in camphor mixture; and a spirit lotion was applied to the side.)

On the 11th the erysipelas had passed away, and the cuticle was desquamating. The stools contained bile, and the jaundice had almost entirely disappeared; but the urine was still deeply tinged. The countenance, however, was very sensibly changed, being now thin and pale, and the strength was materially reduced. There was no abatement of the swelling in the hypochondrium, but the tenderness had subsided. (Small doses of sulphate of quinine, with spir. ether, nitrici, were ordered; and two glasses of wine were allowed daily.)

From this time the tumor grew rapidly larger, and towards the latter end of the month it again became very tender. She also suffered from frequent vomiting, and continued to do so up to the time of her death. On the 23d, and again on the 26th of March, she had a severe and prolonged rigor.

This did not immediately recur, but the hectic fever continued, with repeated vomiting, and with much pain in the right hypochondrium.

On the 5th of April the tenderness over the tumor had increased, and there was a superficial rounded prominence between the cartilages and the umbilicus. The jaundice had quite disappeared. The urine threw down a *pink* sediment.

On the 9th of April she had another rigor, which lasted two hours, followed by increased heat of skin, but only by very slight sweating. Percussion over the tumor gave an indistinct sense of fluctuation.

The tumor now became more prominent, and the sense of fluctuation more distinct. The bowels were costive and rather tympanitic; and the pain which she had before felt in the right shoulder was much aggravated.

She gradually sank, and died on the 12th.

The body was examined twenty-four hours after death.

The liver was found to be exceedingly enlarged, reaching as low down as the umbilicus and into the left hypochondrium. It was adherent by recently effused lymph to a great part of the diaphragm, to the walls of the belly, to the extreme right of the transverse colon, and to the right kidney. These recent adhesions having been separated by passing the finger between the contiguous surfaces, a portion of the convex surface of the liver, as large as the palm of the hand, was found to be so firmly united to the diaphragm, under cover of the cartilages, that it could not be detached. To the feel, the whole of the right lobe seemed to be little more than a great bag of fluid, although a considerable quantity of healthy structure remained towards the left. On a puncture being made, the nature of the disease was apparent. The contents consisted of more than three pints of a thinnish opaque liquid, which was deeply colored by bile, and contained pus in the proportion of about one-third, and in which floated a great number of hydatids of various sizes, some being as large as pullets' eggs while others were no bigger than peas. The larger ones were collapsed bags, more or less transparent, some containing within them similar collapsed cysts, others a gelatinous matter only, and others, merely a serous fluid.

The great cavity in which these were contained was lined by a dense whitish membrane, an eighth of an inch thick, crossed in various directions by prominent branching lines, which were themselves intersected almost at right angles by others, covered with an irregular coating of soft lymph, colored by pus and bile. These bands, which were all found to be impervious, were the remains of distended vessels. On the posterior part of the inner surface of the sac were the remains of a very thick cartilaginous cyst, which presented some calcareous plates, and was deeply stained by bile. There could be no doubt that this was an old cyst, in which the hydatids had been first contained. Several of the biliary ducts emptied themselves into the cavity ; but the most remarkable circumstance was, that the gall-bladder itself communicated with it, and contained, instead of bile, a number of hydatids floating in a gruel-like fluid. The opening into the gall-bladder was circular, about the size of a writing quill, and situated near the duct. The hydatids in the bladder were too large to pass through this opening, one of them being of the size of a filbert, and well distended. They were all globular cysts, and appeared more delicate than those in the large cavity. The mucous membrane of the gall-bladder was pale and healthy, even to the edges of the aperture. The cystic duct was not covered by bile, but had a free communication with the common duct. This and the hepatic ducts were healthy, and discharged themselves as usual.

On the outside of this immense cyst the hepatic structure was in very different states in different parts. In some parts it was redder than natural, and compressed ; in others, it was pale and soft ; while in one large portion it was disorganized to a great depth—of a light brown color, and fetid smell. The parenchyma was there almost destroyed, nothing remaining but cellular flocculi and the half-dissolved branches of vessels. The tissue of the organ generally was pale, and softer than it should be.

In the left lobe, close to the convex surface, which adhered to the diaphragm, there was an abscess of the size of a walnut, bounded by a thick membrane, containing nothing but pus. This abscess was contiguous to one of the hepatic veins, with which it communicated by an opening large enough to admit a writing quill. That part of the vessel which thus communicated with the abscess contained pus. The pus was confined on all sides by lymph, which, after lining the sides of the vessel, passed off from them towards the vena cava, in the shape of a long conical tube, the cavity of which was thus continuous with that of the abscess. At the other extremity, the lymph quite plugged up the vessel for some distance, but many of its branches in the left lobe contained small collections of pus circumscribed by lymph.

In slicing the organ in different directions, small spots were divided, which were of a bright green, apparently from the extravasation of a small quantity of bile from inflamed and ulcerated ducts. From some of them, a little pus, as well as bile, could be squeezed.

All the branches of the portal vein were sound.

The liver covered the stomach, but was not adherent to it. This viscus was of natural size. Its mucous membrane was pale throughout, and, towards the cardia, considerably softened; so that a gentle pressure of the nail was sufficient to tear it up.

The rest of the alimentary canal was quite sound. The contents of the intestines had the usual admixture of bile, but no hydatids were found among them. The spleen was rather large, but healthy. The kidneys and the urinary bladder were natural. The uterine organs presented marks of former pregnancy, but nothing worthy of notice. The pelvis contained about a pint of serous fluid, without flocculi.

The lungs were nowhere attached to the ribs. The lower lobe of the left lung was dense and heavy, and of a dark color, and it did not crepitate. When cut into, it was found to be gorged with bloody serum, and in many parts to be of a yellowish or gray color. In all these parts the tissue of the organ was very soft, the slightest pressure of the finger being sufficient to break it down. The mucous membrane of the bronchi was here and there more vascular than natural, and was everywhere covered by a somewhat viscid mucus. The remainder of this lung was healthy.

The right lung was in a similar condition to the left, except that its lower lobe was simply gorged with bloody serum, and much condensed. The morbid appearances were as marked in front as behind.

The pericardium contained about two ounces of clear serous fluid. The heart was of natural size and structure.

The brain was firm and healthy.

The researches of naturalists, respecting the organization and growth of acephalocysts, have much narrowed our field of inquiry as regards the production of hydatid tumors. It is now quite plain that these tumors are parasitic growths, and that the proximate cause of their formation is the introduction of one or more germs of the parasites into the body under conditions favorable to their development. In the production, therefore, of hydatid tumors, many circumstances, such as age, diet, and place of residence, may be very important, but merely as favoring, or not, the introduction of the germs of the parasites into the body, and their subsequent development.

From the cases which have been placed on record, hydatid tumors seem to be of nearly equal frequency in the two sexes. They are most common in persons from the age of twenty to that of forty, but may occur at any age from six years to fifty.

I have found no instance recorded in which such a tumor occurred under the age of five or six, or above that of fifty. Cruveilhier (*Op. cit.*, p. 216) has related the case of a man who died at the age of seventy-seven, with an hydatid tumor of the liver, which appeared fifteen years before—that is, when he was fifty-two. In all the other cases which he collected, and which are twenty in number, the tumor seems to have formed under the age of forty.

The conditions that favor the development of hydatids in sheep are well known. It has been long remarked that the disease they occasion is most rife in unusually wet seasons, and in ill-drained pastures; and that it is an *endemic* disease. If one sheep in a flock has it, all the others have it more or less. These circumstances, and the fact that they are not found in the purely carnivorous animals, would lead us to expect that hydatid tumors in man would occur chiefly among "vegetarians," and that they would prevail, as tape-worms do, in particular districts: but no evidence satisfactorily establishing these points has yet been collected. In this country, hydatid tumors seem to be more frequent among the poor than among the rich: a circumstance most probably attributable to the fact that the poor dwell in lower and worse-drained houses, and subsist on a diet which contains a much larger proportion of vegetable food; but they are occasionally met with in all conditions of life, almost always, however, in widely-scattered cases. Little is known of the relative frequency of hydatid tumors in different countries, or among different classes. They occur on the continent of Europe, as they do in England, not very unfrequently, but still in widely scattered cases. They are scarcely noticed by medical authors in India, and seem to be very rare in that country, where other diseases of the liver are so common. They are extremely rare among sailors. While I was physician to the Seamen's Hospital, I found a tumor containing many hydatids in the liver of a negro from the west coast of Africa, who died, under my care, of suppurative phlebitis, the result of bleeding practised for inflammation of the lung; but no other case of the kind is known to have been admitted there. Mr. Busk, who has held office in the hospital almost from its first establishment, tells me that he does not recollect another instance. It is possible that the diet of sailors, consisting, in great part, of salt meat, may be unfavorable to the development of this disease.

A curious circumstance respecting hydatid tumors in man is

that they have often been observed to form in parts that had received some physical injury. Of the published cases of hydatids of the liver there is a considerable proportion in which the tumor seems to have formed soon after a blow on the side, and, as was supposed, in consequence of it. Among the cases collected by Cruveilhier, there are four, and in the paper by Mr. Cæsar Hawkins, in the 18th volume of the *Medico-Chirurgical Transactions*, there are several others, in which the tumor was supposed to be the effect of some injury done to the side.

In some instances in which the disease was ascribed to a blow, the tumor contained a solitary acephalocyst; in others, many. In some, there was only one tumor; in others, more than one tumor in the liver, or a tumor in the spleen as well as in the liver.

If the disease in these cases really resulted from a blow, this circumstance affords an additional argument in favor of the doctrine, that, in cases in which there are many hydatid tumors in the same person, one of these tumors is often the parent of the rest.

Among the recorded cases in which an hydatid tumor has formed in other parts of the body, the proportion is still larger in which the disease has seemed the result of some physical injury. "Hydatids have been found in the humerus, the tibia, the iliac bones, and the diploe of the skull—generally in consequence of wounds." —See *Reports of the Ray Society on Zool. and Bot. for* 1845, p. 315.

The same thing has been observed with respect to the *cysticercus cellulosa.*

In the *Medical Gazette* for April 28, 1848, are notes of a case read to the Westminster Medical Society, by Mr. Canton, in which a small tumor containing a cysticercus cellulosa, in the lower eyelid of a child, was supposed to result from a slight blow from an umbrella. In the 18th volume of the *Dublin Medical Journal*, a case is related in which a tumor likewise containing a cysticercus cellulosa, in the lower eyelid of a child, was supposed to result from a blow against the corner of a coop; and reference is given to two other cases of the same kind.

It would seem, therefore, that a blow or other physical injury may favor the arrest and development of the germs of these parasites in the injured part.

When an hydatid tumor has formed in the liver, there is reason to believe that, if near the surface, it may attain a large size in a short time; but in a great majority of cases its growth is very slow.

When the tumor grows rapidly, or when, from any cause, inflammation is set up within it or around it, the patient has severe pain in the side and some degree of fever.

Under other circumstances—that is, when the tumor grows slowly and is not the seat of inflammation, it is unattended by pain, or gives rise to a sensation which the patient describes as one of weight, rather than of pain; and before it has attained such a size as to interfere mechanically with the functions of the liver, or of adjacent organs, it excites no constitutional disturbance, and is compatible with a good state of general health. Not unfrequently, indeed, the presence of a tumor of this kind in the substance of the liver is not suspected during life, and is unexpectedly made known by examination, *post-mortem*.[1]

As the tumor grows it pushes up the walls of the belly, and can in most cases be readily seen and felt. Even then, if it do not grow rapidly, and if no inflammation be set up within or around it, the tumor is not painful or tender, and causes little other disturbance than that which results from its bulk—a sense of fulness and weight in the region of the liver, more or less of gastric disorder, and some difficulty in breathing from the restrained action of the diaphragm.

Now and then, however, the tumor, from its situation or large size, compresses the portal vein or the vena cava, and causes ascites and dropsy of the legs; and in this way, and by impeding the breathing, is productive of great distress, and may even destroy life, especially when the circulation and breathing were previously somewhat embarrassed by other conditions. This happened in a case which fell under my observation in the summer of 1850.

The patient, a man of color from the East Indies, fifty-five years of age, who had for many years been employed in London as a mercantile clerk, and in the early part of his life had drunk rather freely, consulted me, for

[1] Sheep with numerous hydatid tumors in the liver and in the lungs are often in excellent condition. In these animals hydatid tumors have very little tendency to excite inflammation of the tissue or of the coverings of the organs in which they form. When there are many tumors in the lungs, the sheep are, of course, short-breathed, but they do not necessarily fall in condition. In this respect, hydatids present a striking contrast to flukes, which never exist in large numbers in a sheep without greatly impoverishing its blood.

the first time, on the 10th of July, 1850, on account of what was supposed to be an enormous enlargement of the liver. He stated that his illness commenced eighteen months before with pain in the right side, on account of which he was then bled largely: that ever since he had suffered more or less pain in the right side and back, and, for the last six months, pain also in the right shoulder. The liver extended low in the belly, and high up in the right side of the chest. The right lobe was unusually prominent, or bulging at its upper part, but no distinct tumor could be felt. He had, besides, slight chronic catarrh, and complained of shortness of breath, but was still able to perform the duties of his office; and had no vomiting, or jaundice, or other symptoms that could justify the suspicion of malignant disease. He came to my house occasionally for several weeks. Dropsical swelling of the belly and legs then came on, and he was confined to his house at Brixton, where I attended him, in consultation with Mr. Kelson Wright. My last visit to him was on the 25th of September. He was then suffering much from difficulty of breathing, caused by enormous distension of the belly, and did not live long after. The body was examined by Mr. Wright, who found that the apparent enlargement and thickening of the liver was caused by an hydatid tumor, bigger than a man's head, in the upper part of the right lobe, in contact with the diaphragm. The right lobe of the liver contained two other hydatid tumors: one, the size of an egg, projected from the concave surface of the liver, and was adherent to the colon; the other was smaller, and imbedded in the liver. The liver itself was slightly granular. There were no marks of recent inflammation about the tumors, and the only other disease discovered was slight thickening of the mitral valve.

The breathing and the circulation were, doubtless, in some degree affected by this state of the mitral valve, and by the slightly granular condition of the liver, and death resulted from the additional impediment to the performance of these functions by the presence of the large hydatid tumor.

This tumor could not be felt during life, but very strong presumption that the disease was an hydatid tumor was afforded by the bulging of the upper part of the liver; by the duration of the malady; by the absence of vomiting and of jaundice; and by the circumstance that, for more than eighteen months after the occurrence of the disease, there was not enough debility or constitutional disturbance caused by it to prevent the patient from following his usual occupation.

An hydatid tumor in the liver may continue a great number of years—indeed, for the allotted term of human life—without causing other ailments than those which result from its bulk; but the person is exposed to constant danger, and is every moment in risk of new sufferings, from the natural tendency of the tumor to discharge its contents by ulceration of the walls of the sac. The tumor may ulcerate through the walls of the belly, and its contents be discharged outwardly; or it may open into some part of the intestinal canal, and its contents be discharged by vomiting or by stool. In either case the sac may close up after a time, and the patient recover.

An instance in which an hydatid tumor in the liver emptied itself through the bowel was brought under my notice in November, 1845, by Dr. Theophilus Thompson. The patient, a man twenty-seven years of age, consulted Dr. Thompson in the beginning of November, 1845, when he had been ill nearly six months, with symptoms referable to the liver; and, during part of the time, with what was considered to be intermittent fever. The liver was then greatly enlarged, reaching as low as the umbilicus, and distending the lower part of the chest. A few days after this he began to pass from the bowels bodies which he compared to "gooseberry-skins," which proved to be hydatids; and the liver began rapidly to diminish in size. On the 14th of November he brought me three of the hydatids, of the size of large gooseberries, in which I readily discovered echinococci. He was then thin and sallow, but free from fever, The discharge of the hydatids was not attended with vomiting or diarrhœa, from which it may be inferred that the liquid of hydatids is not so violently irritating to the mucous membrane of the alimentary canal as it is to many other tissues. The discharge of hydatids from the bowel continued for four or five weeks. It then ceased, and the patient gradually improved in condition.

On the 10th of March, 1846, he called on me again, to report progress. He was then stouter than he ever was before, and was perfectly well, with the exception of slight pain under the right false ribs, and occasional attacks of shivering, which lasted about half an hour, and were followed by sweating. These attacks occurred at irregular periods, and especially after fatigue, and probably depended on the hydatid sac not being yet perfectly obliterated. While the shivering lasted, he had always a dull pain under the right false ribs.

The liver did not extend below the false ribs, and no tumor could be felt.

The danger from the tumor opening in either of the ways specified above is the greater the older the tumor, or rather, the firmer and less elastic the walls of the sac. If the tumor be of recent date, or the coats of the sac be very elastic, the sac may close up as its contents are discharged, and the patient may recover rapidly; but if the walls of the sac be firm and unyielding, so that its cavity cannot be closed, air or other matters will find their way into it, and suppurative inflammation of its inner surface will be set up, which may be so protracted as to exhaust the strength of the patient.

An hydatid tumor in the liver may also open into the lung, the hydatids be spit up, and the patient recover. Two instances of this have fallen under my own observation. When the tumor opens into the lung, the patient is constantly harassed by a hard, straining cough, and occasionally spits up an hydatid. The liquid of the hydatid tumor irritates the air-tubes, and sets up inflammation of the lower lobe of the lung into which it falls, and in this way causes hoarseness and constant expectoration of a bloody or puriform matter, which, in some instances is rendered still more irritating to the lung, and very disgusting to the patient, by admixture with bile. At first, before a free passage has been made through the lung, the hydatids expectorated are usually small, and they come away singly, at intervals, it may be, of many days. After a time, if the tumor be large and well stored with hydatids, larger hydatids are spit up, and now and then, after an unusually hard fit of coughing and straining, many are pumped up at once, or in quick succession. When large hydatids are spit up, they are almost always turned inside out, and are then bell-shaped or globular, with an open, circular mouth. The process by which their inversion is effected seems to be this: In passing through the narrow tubes of the lung, the hydatid, which is naturally filled with liquid, bursts at the foremost part, and the liquid it contains escapes. The hindermost part of the hydatid is then, by the pressure behind, pushed through the aperture in its fore part. The aperture is thus expanded, and at length, by the pressure from behind and by the elasticity of the membrane of which it consists, the hydatid is completely inverted. The elasticity of the membrane makes it again assume, in its inverted state, a globular form. The membrane has no tendency to tear in any particular direction, so that the aperture in the hydatid, as it grows larger, still remains circular, and the inverted hydatid has the form described above. When the hydatids burst or are inverted, the echinococci they contain escape, so that it is seldom any perfect animalcules can be found in hydatids that have been spit up.

The time during which hydatids may continue to be spit up depends on the size and contractility of the hydatid tumor, and on the number of hydatids it contains. A tumor which is of moderate size and not of long standing, may discharge its contents and close up in the course of a few weeks. When the tumor is old and very large, the walls of the sac are usually thick, and can contract but slowly; and if the tumor should be stuffed with hydatids, the patient may continue to spit them up for a long time. In 1852, in conjunction with Mr. Davey, of Keppel Street, I attended a gentleman who continued to cough up hydatids from an enormous tumor of the liver at intervals for nearly twelve months. Of the hydatids discharged in this way, more than enough to fill two quarts were collected, and some of them were as large as a small orange. The passage of the hydatids caused frequently-recurring inflammation in the lower lobe of the right lung, and the patient died at last, worn out by cough, and expectoration and fever. On examination after death, the tumor which had been discharging through the lung was much contracted, and contained portions of the mother cyst, but no secondary hydatids. Three other hydatid tumors, of smaller size, were found in the liver.

In the spring of the same year a man came under my care in the hospital who stated that he began to cough up hydatids about nine years before, and continued to do so occasionally—at first, two or three times a day, afterwards, once a week, or once in two or three weeks—for four years and a half. At the end of this time, after a hard fit of coughing, he brought up a large mass, looking like a cod's sound. After this, he coughed up no more hydatids, but had a constant discharge of pus. When he fell under my observation he seemed to have in the upper part of the liver a small sac containing pus, which he could empty at will by stooping forwards with his head down.

In all such cases where the tumor is large and of long standing, the harassing cough that is necessary to get up the hydatids, and the pain and broken rest, together with the constant expectoration of puriform matter, and the fever and other constitutional disturbance that results from the persisting inflammation of the air-tubes or lung, greatly reduce the strength, and now and then, as in the instance related above, their combined influence destroys life.

But instead of opening outwardly, or into the intestinal canal, or into the lung, an hydatid tumor may burst into the cavity of the belly and destroy the life of the patient by shock, and by inflammation of the peritoneum, in a few days or even in a few hours;[1] or, otherwise still, the ulceration of the walls of the sac may eat into the gall-bladder or into one of the gall-ducts, bile may flow into the sac and excite suppurative inflammation of its inner surface, converting it into an abscess; or the ulceration may eat through the sac, and the liquid the sac contains may escape into the surrounding tissue and excite suppurative inflammation there. This inflammation may by various ways be propagated back to the sac, and, as before, the sac be converted into an abscess.

[1] See Dict. de Méd. et Chirurg. pratiques, art. "Acephalocyste," Obs. 6, 7, 8, 9; and Medico-Chirurgical Trans., vol. xviii. pp. 124 and 126.

But there is still a chance of other mischief. A secondary hydatid tumor may form in the lung, which may grow rapidly and suffocate the patient; or secondary hydatid tumors may form in the liver, or in the mesentery. If there be many of these, or if they grow rapidly, the nutrition of the patient invariably suffers—he becomes thin and pallid and weak, and is gradually exhausted by diarrhœa, or carried off more speedily by the occurrence of pneumonia.

The *diagnosis* of an hydatid tumor, when it has attained such a size that it can be readily seen and felt, seldom presents much difficulty. We have, indeed, no knowledge that the disease occurs with especial frequency in any particular class, or that an especial liability to it is induced by particular habits of life, and are thus without the aid in diagnosis which such knowledge gives; but the fact that a large globular tumor, connected with the liver, *has grown slowly*, without much pain, without jaundice or ascites, and without fever or general constitutional disturbance, is almost evidence enough that the tumor is hydatid. A large abscess may form a tumor of the same size and shape, and might thus be taken for an hydatid tumor; but a large abscess never forms without a high degree of fever, and never exists without very serious impairment of health.

A distended gall-bladder, which is likewise smooth and globular and which may not be tender, may also be taken for an hydatid tumor; but great distension of the gall-bladder almost always results from some mechanical impediment to the flow of bile along the common duct, and is attended with deep jaundice, and the tumor formed by it may be further distinguished by its shape and position.

Another disease that may be mistaken for an hydatid tumor of the liver is an aneurism of the abdominal aorta forming a tumor behind the liver. This, like an hydatid tumor, may be globular, and may exist without much tenderness, without jaundice or ascites, without much disturbance of digestion, and without difficulty of breathing other than that which results from the size of the tumor and the impediment which it offers to the descent of the diaphragm. Circumstances that serve to mark the tumor as aneurismal are—the sudden occurrence of the first symptoms of the malady with a feeling, as of cramp, across the epigastrium, not attended by vomiting or purging, and not followed by jaundice; the existence of a distinct pulsation in the tumor, and a bellows-sound heard over the last dorsal, or the upper lumbar vertebræ; but, more than all, the great pain which the patient suffers in the situation of the tumor, and in various other parts of the body, especially the shoulders and the legs. An aneurismal tumor is generally very painful, and when situated behind the liver and involving the solar plexus of nerves, is attended not only with pain in the seat of disease, but with *sympathetic* pains in various parts of the body. These symptoms are absent in cases where an hydatid sac forms a similar tumor, so that by attention to them the two diseases may generally be distinguished.

A disease much more frequent, and more liable to be mistaken for an hydatid tumor of the liver is cancer. This, as we have seen, sometimes forms a tumor at the epigastrium, which is globular and hard, like an hydatid tumor, and may attain a large size without much pain or tenderness. In its form, as far as this can be made out, in its size, in its position, in its apparent hardness, and in the absence of pain and tenderness, it may be like an hydatid tumor; but, notwithstanding these points of resemblance, a cancerous tumor may generally be distinguished from an hydatid tumor by its more rapid growth, by the anemia and wasting it causes, and often by an unevenness of the surface of the liver in other parts, caused by the partial projection of other cancerous tumors.

Cases are, however, now and then met with, in which, from some unusual circumstances, it may be difficult, or even impossible, to pronounce that the tumor is hydatid. The tumor may project on the under surface of the liver, or on the uppermost part of the liver, where its outline cannot be traced, or may grow more rapidly than is usual with hydatid tumors and be attended with greater pain and fever; or, as we have already seen, it may be so situated as to compress the hepatic or the common duct, or the trunk of the portal vein, or even the vena cava, and may thus cause permanent jaundice, or ascites, or œdema of the legs. It is impossible to lay down general rules for the detection of the real nature of the disease in such cases. It is a safe rule not to pronounce a large tumor of the liver hydatid, unless there be satisfactory evidence that it has grown slowly.

If an hydatid tumor of the liver which has been long indolent should become painful and tender, and the patient should have shiverings with much fever and constitutional disturbance, it may be inferred that suppuration has been set up within the sac.

There are two ways in which an hydatid tumor of the liver may be cured: first, by the secretion of a thick matter, like putty or plaster, within the sac, either causing the destruction, or consequent on the destruction, of the acephalocysts; and, secondly, by the tumor opening and discharging itself through the walls of the belly, or through the lung, or into the intestinal canal.

The first mode of termination may be considered a *cure* of the disease, because, although the tumor does not completely disappear, it grows less, and ceases to create constitutional disturbance or to be the source of further danger.

The second mode of termination—the opening of the tumor and the discharge of its contents through the walls of the belly, or through the intestinal canal, or through the lung—is often followed by obliteration of the sac, disappearance of the tumor, and complete recovery; but it is not unattended with danger. As before remarked, by the admission of air, or otherwise, suppurative inflammation may be set up within the sac, the discharge of the natural contents of the sac may be followed at the end of some days by the discharge of pus, which may continue so as to exhaust the strength of the patient. The probability of a favorable result from such an opening is greater the younger the patient and the more recent the tumor—or rather, the greater the elasticity of the walls of the sac. It is the elasticity of the walls of the sac that closes the cavity as its contents escape, and prevents any subsequent mischief.

The chief danger of hydatid tumors of the liver arises from their liability to open by a process of ulceration into the cavity of the peritoneum, or into the vessels of the ducts of the liver itself. This ulceration of the sac, which occurs sooner or later in most hydatid tumors of the liver, seems to be owing to pressure from distension of the sac. We have good evidence of this distension in the forcible jet that sometimes issues when an hydatid tumor is punctured. The fluid secreted from its inner surface goes on stretching the sac and increasing the size of the tumor. From the property of equal distribution of pressure through fluids, the pressure on the walls of the sac from this cause must be the same at every point of its surface, and the process of ulceration will commence at that point which has the least power to resist it. Hydatid tumors of the lungs and of the spleen are, from the greater thinness and expansibility of the walls of the sac in those organs, less liable to rupture from ulceration than similar tumors of the liver.

The chief danger of hydatid tumors of the liver would then be obviated, if by any means we could so modify the fluid secreted from the inner surface of the sac as to destroy the acephalocysts without causing suppuration; or if we could merely arrest the growth of the tumor. It is not difficult to conceive that there may be medicines which have power to effect this. An agent like iodide of potassium, for instance, that is absorbed into the blood, and passes out of the body in almost every secretion, may find its way into the fluid in an hydatid sac, and although it does not destroy the vitality of the natural constituents of our organs, it may destroy the feebler vitality of the parasites and arrest the growth of the tumor.

There are, I believe, only two medicines—iodide of potassium and common salt—that have been supposed, after trial, to have the power of arresting the growth of hydatid tumors. Iodide of potassium is much confided in by many physicians in this country, and has been for some years very generally prescribed in this disease; but I have not been able to meet with any decisive or satisfactory evidence that it has the power of destroying the acephalocysts, or of stopping the growth of an hydatid tumor. Mr. Hawkins, in the paper before referred to, states that "a case lately occurred at St. George's Hospital, in which the tumor was much lessened, and ascites and other symptoms were got rid of for a time by the use of iodine;" but he makes the significant remark, that "the disease was ultimately fatal nearly a year after." I quite think, however, that our experience of this medicine encourages us to further trial of it in such cases. It will be seen that evidence of failure is much easier to be had than evidence of success, because, when the remedy fails, the diagnosis is after a time made certain. With the internal use of the iodide of potassium may be conjoined the local inunction of the compound iodide ointment.

The virtues of common salt in the treatment of hydatid tumors of the liver are much relied on by some Continental physicians, who have recommended a strong solution of it to be applied as a lotion, or in a poultice, over the tumor. It is worthy of remark, that common salt is the chief saline ingredient in the fluid of hydatid tumors. In many instances, indeed, the fluid from an hydatid cyst in the liver has been found to be quite devoid of albumen, and to be little more than pure water holding common salt in solution. Has the sac of an hydatid tumor any especial affinity for common salt, and does the accumulation of this, beyond a certain measure in the fluid within it, destroy the acephalocysts, or arrest their further multiplication or growth?[1]

The frequent failure of *medical* means to arrest the growth of hydatid tumors of the liver has led practitioners to consider the propriety of opening them—an operation that would naturally be suggested by the observation that the bursting of a tumor of this kind through the walls of the belly, or even into the intestines or into the lung, is frequently followed by perfect, and sometimes by speedy, recovery.

On many occasions, too, where an hydatid tumor has been opened by the surgeon in mistake for an abscess, the patient has speedily and completely recovered.

It is an important circumstance that in very few of these cases, if in any, has the fluid collected again in the sac. When a *serous* cyst—that is, a cyst whose innner surface has the character of a serous membrane, and secretes a *serous*, or *highly albuminous*, fluid—is thus emptied, the fluid almost always collects again, and obliteration of the sac is effected only by causing adhesive inflammation of its inner surface; but when an hydatid cyst is emptied, the creatures within it die, and the fluid is no longer reproduced.

In illustration of this, and in proof of the happy result of the puncture of an hydatid tumor in some instances, I cannot do better than cite two cases, published by Mr. Hawkins, in which the operation was performed by Sir B. Brodie.

CASE.—A boy, about twelve years of age, was admitted into St. George's Hospital, under the care of Dr. Chambers, in August, 1822, having a tumor of considerable size below the ribs on the right side, the ribs being raised by the tumor, which evidently fluctuated. He had not the least disturbance of the system, nor any derangement of the functions

[1] The great quantity of common salt in the liquid of hydatid tumors is not so singular a fact as it at one time seemed. It has been ascertained that mucus, the serum of pus, and the liquid of cancerous growths, contain a large quantity of chloride of sodium. From these, and other facts to the same purport, Lehmann conjectures that every deposition of *cells* is accompanied by an increase in the quantity of chloride of sodium. Cartilages, which, in their perfect state, abound in cells, contain a large proportional quantity of this salt. See Lehmann's Chemistry (Translation of the Cavendish Society), vol. i. p. 434.

of the liver, much less were there symptoms of abscess of that organ; the skin was quite movable, and free from inflammation, and slight inconvenience from the size and pressure of the tumor was alone complained of. After he had been in the hospital a short time, a flat trocar was introduced by Mr. Brodie below the ribs, in the part where fluctuation was most distinct, and a pint and a half of clear colorless water was drawn off, which did not appear to contain any albumen, as no coagulation was produced by heat. Pressure was made by a bandage after the operation, which appeared to produce complete obliteration of the cyst, for the wound healed directly. The boy had not the least fever or other bad symptom from the operation, and left the hospital perfectly cured. (*Med.-Chir. Trans.*, vol. xviii. p. 118.)

In the second case,

The patient was a young lady, twenty years of age, and the tumor, which was larger than in the former case, prevented her from taking exercise and from sleeping, except in a particular posture; and there seemed to be some slight inflammation, as she had some pain at the commencement of the disease, a year or two before, which was increased before the operation, and she suffered from a troublesome and almost incessant cough for the first two or three weeks afterwards. Three pints of the same watery fluid were evacuated, uncoagulated by heat, and with the smallest possible quantity of animal matter; the patient recovered, and six years afterwards had had no return of the complaint. (*Id.*, p. 119.)

In both these cases, the sac most probably contained a solitary acephalocyst.

If all cases which had been treated in the same way had turned out so favorably, there would be no doubt as to the propriety of performing the operation in question whenever the tumor was ascertained to be hydatid. But, unfortunately, against the successful cases must be set others in which the operation proved fatal; sometimes speedily, at other times by inducing protracted suppuration of the inner surface of the sac.[1]

The probability of such a result, however small, will naturally make practitioners extremely cautious in recommending the operation where the tumor produces no distressing symptoms; and perhaps few persons would be disposed to submit to an operation at all hazardous, for the removal of a disease which is attended with no urgent symptoms, and with which life may be continued in tolerable comfort for ten, twenty, or even thirty years. Life, even to the most healthy, is so uncertain, liable to be cut short by so

[1] See Dict. de Méd. et de Chirurg. pratiques, art. "Acephalocyste." Obs. 13, 14, 16, 19, 21.

many accidents, that in calculations of this kind our reason must approve the decision to which our fears and our instincts lead us, to purchase present security even by exposing ourselves to a greater danger, provided it be remote.

The dangers of opening hydatid tumors of the liver are the following:—

The first thing to fear is, that from the tumor not being adherent to the walls of the belly, some of the fluid in the hydatid sac may, in consequence of the operation, pass into the cavity of the peritoneum, and excite inflammation of that membrane, which may prove speedily fatal.

The danger of this happening will depend very much on the age of the tumor, or rather on the condition of the walls of the sac. If the walls of the sac be very elastic, as they usually are when the tumor is young, the fluid will be forced out, and the cavity close up, when an opening is made into it; and the probability is very slight that any of the fluid will escape into the peritoneal sac; but if—as is the case in many old hydatid tumors, and in most, if not in all, large abscesses—the walls of the sac have not contractibility adequate to close the opening made by the trocar, a different result may ensue. All the fluid may not escape by the canula, and after the canula is withdrawn, it may go on oozing into the peritoneal sac.

The danger from this cause may be greatly diminished by proper precautions. A bandage should be applied round the lower part of the body, so as to fix the liver as much as possible, and the operation should be performed by a very small, or, as Sir B. Brodie has suggested, by a flat trocar, so that the opening made into the sac may be small, or of such a shape as will admit of its being readily closed. Considering how limpid the fluid of hydatid tumors usually is, it seems probable that a fine-grooved needle, as recommended by the late Dr. Pritchard for drawing off thoracic and abdominal effusions, would, in many cases, be a still better instrument.

With a fitting instrument, and with proper precautions, the risk that any of the fluid will get into the cavity of the peritoneum must be extremely slight, especially in young persons, or for hydatid tumors recently formed; and in all such cases, should purely medical means fail, it will, I believe, eventually be found the best plan to evacuate the tumor, as soon as full assurance is obtained of its nature; I say, as soon as full assurance is obtained, for it would be a grievous, perhaps a fatal error to puncture a distended gall-bladder in mistake for an hydatid sac.

If the hydatid tumor be adherent to the walls of the belly, as old and large tumors very commonly are, the danger we are now considering, of course, no longer exists. It is, therefore, important to ascertain, before performing the operation, whether adhesions have formed, or not. This may often be done by the adoption of the method recommended in the chapter on abscess of the liver—namely, by marking with a pen the place of the lower edge of the liver on the walls of the belly while the patient is recumbent, and then making the patient shift his posture in various ways. If the liver be extensively adherent to the walls of the belly, its lower edge will always correspond to the inked line: if it be not adherent, the liver, during the acts of breathing, and during various movements of the body, will slide against the walls of the belly, and the position of its lower edge relatively to them will vary.

But even when the liver is adherent to the walls of the belly, there is another source of danger, the danger noticed above, that the operation may set up suppurative inflammation of the inner surface of the sac, which may be so protracted as to exhaust the strength of the patient.

This result is especially to be feared when the tumor is old and large, and the walls of the sac have lost much of the elasticity they originally possessed. In such a case, the danger of opening a large hydatid tumor is nearly as great as that of opening a large abscess; and in the one case, as in the other (see p. 134), the question may arise whether it is not more expedient to allow the tumor to open of itself.

It has been suggested[1] that electricity might probably arrest the growth of an hydatid tumor, and that it might be applied for this purpose, by affixing the poles of a suitable battery to fine needles, introduced into various parts of the tumor. I am not aware that the experiment has yet been tried.

[1] Medical Gazette, Oct. 9, 1846, p. 643.

CHAPTER V.

ON JAUNDICE.

THE chief diseases to which the liver is subject having now been passed in review, it will be expected that some remarks should be added on *jaundice*.

Jaundice is, indeed a mere symptom, and, as we have seen, may occur in most diseases of the liver: but it is a symptom so striking, and such an important element in any case in which it may happen, that a separate consideration of it is almost requisite.

Jaundice—a yellow color of the conjunctiva and the skin—arises from the presence of the coloring matter of bile in the blood and tissues. Yellowness of the skin, when it is well marked, is sufficiently distinctive of accumulation of the coloring matters of bile in the blood, but the skin may become *slightly yellow* from other causes. In chlorotic girls, and in persons who have lost great quantities of blood, the skin has often a pale yellow cast, which seems not to depend on the coloring matters of bile. It is analogous to the yellow tinge which surrounds a bruise-mark, or an ecchymosis, and has been ascribed to some change in the coloring matters of the blood. The sallowness produced in this way may be distinguished from the slighter shades of jaundice by the tint of the conjunctiva, and by the state of the urine. In persons whose skin is sallow from anemia, the conjunctiva has a bluish and pearly tint, and the urine is generally limpid, while in real jaundice, the conjunctiva is more decidedly yellow than the skin, and the urine is always tinged with bile. In cases, too, of diffuse inflammation of the areolar tissue, the skin has often a yellowish tint, which seems to depend on some change in the coloring matter of the blood, for it sometimes exists when there are no indications of bile in the urine.

Jaundice may be produced in two ways: 1st. By some mechanical impediment to the flow of bile into the duodenum, and the consequent absorption of the retained bile; and 2d. By defective action on the part of the secreting substance of the liver, in consequence of which the secretion, or the elimination, of bile is arrested.

The gall-bladder and the large gall-ducts are covered by lymphatics, which, in the natural state, seem to absorb chiefly the water of the bile. If bile be retained for some time in the gall-bladder, it becomes dark-colored and concentrated, from the absorption of part of its water. But the coloring matter is absorbed as well, though in less proportion. If the cystic duct be completely closed, the bile previously in the gall-bladder gradually disappears, and, after a time, its place is occupied by a colorless, or only slightly yellow, mucous fluid, secreted by the coats of the bladder. When, however, the passage of the bile through the common duct is impeded, and the gall-bladder and gall-ducts are in consequence much distended with bile, the bile passes into the lymphatics much more rapidly. This was ascertained by Dr. Saunders, more than fifty years ago, by direct experiment. He tied the hepatic duct in a dog. Two hours afterwards, the dog was strangled, and the absorbents of the liver were found to be "very much distended with a fluid of a bilious color, and their course, which was very conspicuous, could be traced with the greatest ease to the thoracic duct, the contents of which seemed only moderately bilious." (*Saunders on the Liver*, p. 90.)

Saunders also endeavored to prove by experiment that, under these circumstances, bile is likewise absorbed by the veins. "A second dog was procured, and a ligature made on the hepatic duct, as in the preceding experiment. Two hours afterwards, blood was taken from the jugular vein and set to rest, in order that it might separate into its *serum* and *crassamentum*. The liver was then drawn down a little from the diaphragm, and blood taken from one of the hepatic veins. This blood, as well as the former, was allowed to separate into two parts, and on immersing pieces of white paper into the *serum* of each, *that* taken from the hepatic veins gave the deepest tinge, the *other* produced *only* a very slight degree of discoloration."

Many other pathologists have also observed the coloring matters of bile in the lymphatics coming from the liver, in cases in which the gall-ducts have been obstructed. "Tiedemann and Gmelin, after tying the *ductus choledochus* in dogs, found the lymphatics of the liver filled with a fluid of a deep yellow color; the lymphatic glands which these lymphatics passed through were yellow; and the yellow fluid taken from the thoracic duct contained the components of the bile."[1]

These observations clearly prove the absorption of the coloring matters of bile in considerable quantity when there is an impediment to the flow of the bile into the intestine. The inference has been drawn from them that in such cases the jaundice is produced *solely* by absorption of the retained bile; but this inference is not warranted by the facts. A mechanical impediment to the passage of the bile through the gall-ducts leads to an accumulation of the secreted bile in the lobular substance of the liver, and, in so doing, lessens the secretion which is there going on, and impairs the nutrition of the cells. The result is that, with absorption of the retained bile, there is scanty and defective secretion. We have seen, indeed, that in fatal cases of jaundice from permanent closure of the common duct, the cells in the lobular substance of the liver are sometimes found after death completely broken up, so that, at the time of death, the liver must have been incapable of any longer secreting bile.

But in many cases of jaundice, perhaps in the greater number, there is no impediment to the flow of bile through the large ducts. In fatal cases, it sometimes happens that, although the passages of the bile are unobstructed, the gall-bladder and gall-ducts are found empty and unusually pale, and the liver itself is smaller than it should be, and not deeply stained with the biliary pigment, showing that no bile, or but little, was secreted. The jaundice results solely from suppressed or defective secretion.

It has long been a question whether the blood in jaundice contains perfect bile or some of its principles merely. It evidently contains the biliary pigment in the state in which it exists in the bile itself, for the addition of dilute sulphuric acid in sufficient quantity to the serum of the blood in jaundice, even in jaundice arising from suppressed secretion, changes, after a few minutes, its yellow color to the characteristic green color of acid bile. Some chemists, among them Orfila, state that they have found the resinous matter of bile in the blood in jaundice; but others have failed to detect it. Lecanu, whose investigations on the composition of

[1] Müller's Physiology. Dr. Baly's Translation, p. 276.

the blood in different diseases are among the most recent, and seem to have been conducted with much care, states that the blood in jaundice contains the coloring matter of bile, but that he has never been able to find in it any of the other ingredients.[1] This discrepancy in the results of the analysis of jaundiced blood made by different chemists may be accounted for by the fact that the peculiar biliary acids are still but imperfectly characterized, and are readily decomposed, and enter readily into new combinations; and, perhaps, in part, by the supposition that the condition of the blood may vary, according as the jaundice depends on a mechanical impediment to the passage of bile through the ducts or on suppressed or defective secretion.

A fundamental question as regards the production of jaundice, is, Where is the biliary pigment formed? Glisson supposed that bile exists ready formed in the portal blood, and is merely separated from it in the liver, as he expressed it, *peculiari colatorio*—by a kind of filtration; just as urea and some other components of the urine are now known to exist ready formed in the blood, and to be separated from it merely by the kidneys. But the most skilful chemists who have recently analyzed the portal blood have failed to detect the biliary acids in it, and have come to the conclusion that these, at least, are formed in the liver. Lehmann, who has investigated with great care the changes which the blood undergoes in its passage through the liver, states also that the peculiar coloring matters of bile cannot be detected in the portal blood, and infers that these, as well as the biliary acids, must be formed in the liver itself. The inference is to some extent supported by the fact that in cirrhosis, in cancer of the liver, and in other diseases, a great portion of the lobular substance of the liver is sometimes destroyed without the occurrence of jaundice. This fact is not, however, conclusive on the point, because great destruction of the lobular substance of the liver from chronic disease is always attended with great anemia, and the portion of liver still effective may be sufficient to produce the needful purification of the diminished quantity of blood. The strongest argument which pathology furnishes in favor of the opposite opinion—that the coloring matters of bile

[1] Similar testimony has recently been given by Scherer, who states that he has failed to discover the biliary acids in blood and urine deeply jaundiced when he has sought for it most carefully, and even with the aid of Pettenkofer's test.—See *Chemical Gazette*, vol. iii. p. 207.

exist ready formed in the blood—is drawn from those cases in which jaundice arises from suppressed or defective secretion. In fatal cases of this kind, although up to the time of death the skin and the urine were deeply stained with the biliary pigment, the gall-bladder and gall-ducts are sometimes found almost empty of bile, and the liver itself, instead of being enlarged from retention of bile, is shrunk, and instead of being deeply colored with the biliary pigment, as we might expect on the supposition that it is the source of the pigment that causes the jaundice, is not more deeply jaundiced than many other tissues. In these cases the most obvious explanation of the facts is that the biliary pigment exists in the blood, and that, in consequence of defective action of the secreting cells, it is not eliminated, as it should be, in the liver.

The natural constituents of the blood seem at first to be little affected by the retention, or the reabsorption of the principles of the bile. When jaundice has lasted some time, the globules of the blood are always in less than the proportion of health; but this probably results, not so much from the mere presence of the principles of the bile in the blood, as from diminution of these reparative changes which the blood naturally undergoes in its passage through the liver, and from the impaired digestion consequent on defective action of the liver and on the absence of bile in the intestines. Andral states that he has many times analyzed the blood of persons with jaundice, but never found the fibrin in greater proportion than in health. From this it can only be inferred that in these instances the jaundice was not the effect of extensive inflammation; but from the frequent occurrence of petechiæ on the skin and the general disposition to hemorrhage in protracted jaundice, it seems probable that in most cases of jaundice the fibrin of the blood is reduced after a time in still greater proportion than the globules.

When the coloring matter of the bile is in such quantity in the blood as to produce jaundice, it is eliminated in most of the secretions. It passes off most abundantly in the urine, to which, when the urine is collected in considerable quantity in a deep vessel, and is otherwise healthy, it gives a dark, almost black color, with somewhat of a greenish tint—not unlike that of a strong infusion of senna. The urine in a shallow white vessel appears of a brilliant yellow. The presence of the coloring matter of bile is readily detected in urine by the yellow color which it gives to a piece of white linen dipped in it, or by the urine—which appears yellow in a shallow white vessel or in a test tube—becoming of a dark green, and afterwards purple, on the addition of a sufficient quantity of sulphuric acid. The coloring matter of bile may be detected in this way in the urine even before the skin becomes yellow, and in some cases the readiness with which it passes off in the urine seems to prevent the occurrence of jaundice—the skin retaining its natural color, while the tint of the urine attests the presence of bile. It is astonishing, however, how deeply the urine may be tinged with bile, and yet the jaundice persist. This is attributable to the intense color of acid bile, and to the circumstance that a small quantity of it, like a small quantity of blood, makes a great show when mixed with water.

The coloring matter of the bile is eliminated by the kidneys, at least in part, as in the liver itself, through the agency of the secreting cells. If the urine be examined under the microscope, cells from the convoluted tubules of the kidney may often be seen deeply colored with bile.

Under certain circumstances it is eliminated by the salivary glands. In a woman who was under my care in King's College Hospital, in the autumn of 1855, with jaundice from closure of the common duct by a gall-stone, salivation was caused by mercury, and the saliva was deeply colored with bile.

The coloring matter of bile passes off also by the skin, and if the patient perspire much, his linen is stained yellow. This has been repeatedly noticed; but the most striking instance of it I have read of, is recorded by Dr. Cheyne, of Dublin. In his account of a case of jaundice, he says: "The indisposition was so slight, that the individual in question had no intention of sending for a physician, till she discovered that the bilious tinge of her skin was imparted to her linen. To satisfy my doubts, she repeatedly wiped her face with a cambric handkerchief, which thereby acquired a saffron color."[1]

The tears (and the fluid of serous cavities) have likewise been found tinged with the coloring matter of bile; and more than one physician has remarked it, or something like it, in the milk. Dr. Marsh mentions, that in examining the body of a woman who died in the Lock Hospital, Dublin, of protracted disease with jaundice

[1] Dublin Hospital Reports, vol. iii. p. 269.

"the mammæ appeared full; and by moderate pressure, there were obtained from them several ounces of a yellow, tenacious fluid, having all the properties of pure bile." In a case recorded by Dr. Bright, of a woman who suckled her child within three weeks of her death: "The adipose matter was deeply stained with jaundice, as was the secretion which flowed from the lactiferous tubes, on cutting through the mammary glands."[1]

Mucus contains the coloring matter of bile much less frequently than other secretions. The mucus secreted by the stomach and intestines has never, I believe, been found tinged with it, except when bile has continued to flow into the intestines. Mucus brought up from the lungs has occasionally been remarked to be yellow or green; but it not unfrequently has this color in cases of inflammation of the lung, when there is no jaundice, and it is then certainly owing, like the green or yellow color of a bruise mark, not to the elimination of the coloring matter of bile, but to some change in the coloring matter of the blood which has exuded from the vessels.

The different tissues in the body are tinged in jaundice in very different degrees. In all cases in which the jaundice depends on closure of the common duct, the liver itself is more deeply jaundiced than any other organ or tissue. If the jaundice have lasted long, the liver has a deep olive color from the retention of bile. Where, on the contrary, the jaundice depends on suppressed secretion, the liver is not more deeply jaundiced than many other tissues. Instead of being of an olive color, it has some tint compounded of pale yellow and brown or red.

After the liver, the skin is perhaps the tissue that becomes the most deeply jaundiced. The tint of the skin in jaundice varies, in different cases, from a bright lemon color to a dark olive, according to the natural hue of the complexion, the quantity of fat, and the quantity of biliary pigment retained in the skin. In young persons, who are plump, and naturally fair, the tint of the skin is a bright yellow, the depth of which depends on the degree of jaundice; while in the wrinkled skin of thin old age, when the jaundice results from closure of the common duct and has lasted some time, the tint is olive or dark green.

[1] Guy's Hospital Reports, vol. i. p. 623.

The yellow color of the skin in jaundice remains a considerable time—especially in elderly persons—after the flow of bile into the intestine has been restored, and when the urine is no longer much tinged with it. The stain of the skin from the retention of the biliary pigment, after the hepatic obstruction is removed, is diminished in a very striking manner by warm baths. We should be careful not to be misled by it, and thus to continue active remedies when they are no longer necessary. Persons with jaundice from temporary obstruction of the gall-ducts are sometimes drugged with mercury long after the function of the liver is re-established, on account of a yellowness of skin for which warm baths, and whatever causes perspiration, are the proper remedies.

The biliary pigment seems also fixed in an especial manner in the adipose cellular tissue, as if there were some affinity between the coloring matter of bile and fatty substances. In some races, indeed, the fat is naturally of an orange color. It is so in the cows of Guernsey; and I have more than once remarked it in negroes from the west coast of Africa, who were not jaundiced.

The biliary pigment is not retained in the same special manner in other tissues. The lungs and the kidneys, though they may contain as much blood, have not the green color of the liver or skin.

The mucous membranes are the tissues that are among the least tinged in jaundice. The tongue and the inside of the lips, in jaundice, have not the yellow color of the skin; and the mucous membrane of the intestines is sometimes quite white. It has already been remarked that mucus is less frequently jaundiced than other secretions. The mucous membrane of the intestines seems, indeed, never to eliminate the coloring matters of bile.

It sometimes happens that the cornea, or the humors of the eye, become jaundiced, and all objects appear yellow. The notion seems to have formely prevailed that this is generally the case in jaundice, but it happens, on the contrary, very rarely. The error of supposing it of constant, or of frequent occurrence, doubtless originated, as Morgagni suggested, from the yellow color of the conjunctiva in jaundice.

Besides the color of the different secretions and of the skin, which characterizes jaundice, there are other symptoms, which depend on the absence or the deficiency of bile in the intestines, and on its presence in the blood, and which may therefore be considered symptoms of jaundice, without reference to the particular condition of the liver on which the jaundice depends.

Thus, from want of bile in the intestines, the bowels are apt to be confined, and the evacuations are pale, or of a drab color, and sometimes unusually offensive. These characters of the evacuations are not, however, observed in all cases, but only where the flow of bile into the intestine is completely stopped. Bile enough may flow into the intestine to give to its contents their usual characters, and yet the secretion may be inadequate to free the blood of all the coloring matters of bile, and the person may be jaundiced. Not unfrequently, in slight cases of jaundice, especially where this results from suppressed secretion, the discharges from the bowels present no striking deviations from their natural state.

In almost all cases of jaundice, the patient grows thin, and, as before remarked, the blood becomes much impoverished, the globules and the fibrin falling below their natural standard. When the jaundice results from simple closure of the common duct, the impairment of nutrition is, however, in some cases not very marked, even after the jaundice has lasted a considerable time. More than one instance has fallen under my observation in which, six or seven months after bile had ceased to flow into the intestine, the patient was able to walk three or four miles without fatigue; a more remarkable instance has been related above (p. 233), in which a poor woman became deeply jaundiced from complete and permanent closure of the common duct by a gall-stone, when four months gone in pregnancy, but nevertheless, brought forth her infant at full time, and, although she lived badly, had many privations, and lost much blood during her *confinement*, suckled it for three months afterwards, when she died, not simply from the gradual exhaustion produced by the jaundice, but from intestinal hemorrhage as well.

A general disposition to hemorrhage very commonly exists in jaundice, and is probably owing to the impoverished state of the blood; but, besides this, in jaundice that results, not from stoppage of the gall-duct, but from suppressed secretion of bile, there is an especial disposition to *hemorrhage from the stomach*, which seems owing to congestion of the stomach, caused by the arrest of secretion in the liver. In jaundice that results from simple closure of the common gall-duct, a similar disposition to hemorrhage from the stomach frequently exists after the jaundice has lasted a long time, when the secreting cells of the liver are destroyed. The arrest of secretion in the liver impedes the passage of blood through it, and leads, in this way, to congestion of all those organs which return their blood to the portal vein. It seems to lead especially to congestion of the *stomach*, perhaps by disturbing that intimate relation, electrical or other, which naturally exists between the two organs. In consequence of this, or from the greater disposition to hemorrhage from the stomach, owing to its greater vascularity and more active function, the blood oozes from the mucous membrane of the stomach more frequently than from that of any other part of the intestinal canal.

It not unfrequently happens in jaundice, especially in that which results from closure of the ducts, that some pain or uneasiness is occasionally felt in the loins, which is probably owing to irritation of the kidney, caused by the passage of the biliary pigment, or some other irritating matter, through it. We have seen that in jaundice some of the epithelial cells in the secreting tubules of the kidney are often shed, and may be found, deeply colored by bile, on microscopic examination of the urine.

Another symptom frequently observed in jaundice is a very troublesome itching of the skin. This does not occur in all cases of jaundice, and is, I believe, most frequent in the jaundice that results from closure of the ducts. When it does occur, it sometimes ceases after a short time, and may come and cease several times in a lingering case. The itching seems not to depend on the coloring matter merely of bile. It does not vary with the depth of the jaundice. In a former chapter (p. 204), a case of jaundice originating in inflammation of the gall-bladder has, indeed, been cited from Dr. Graves, in which excessive itching of the skin preceded the jaundice, and ceased as soon as the jaundice appeared.

In some cases, jaundice is attained with but little general disorder—and the patient, if he were not yellow, would not consider himself ill. But, very commonly, besides pain or tenderness in the region of the liver and disorder of digestion, there is a sense of languor and debility, the person complains of being drowsy, and the pupils are dilated. These symptoms have been ascribed to the presence of bile in the blood, which has been supposed to lower, in some way or other, the nervous energy.

Now and then, the drowsiness passes into delirium or coma, and the patient dies very speedily from disorder of the brain.

The interesting question, which has been considered in a former chapter (p. 278), at once occurs—On what does this fatal disorder of the brain depend? It is clear that it does not depend merely on an unusually large quantity of biliary pigment in the blood, because it very seldom occurs in the jaundice that arises from complete closure of the common duct, which is deeper than any other jaundice.

It occurs, as before remarked, peculiarly, indeed almost exclusively, in jaundice which results solely from suppressed secretion. Dr. Alison has endeavored to explain this, by supposing that bile retained in the blood is much more hurtful than bile reabsorbed after having been secreted. But this supposition is inadequate to explain the fact: for, where jaundice results primarily from closure of the common duct, the lobules of the liver soon become gorged with bile, and the nutrition and secreting function of the cells is in consequence impaired—so that even in such cases there is, after a time, not only obstruction to the flow of bile through the large ducts, but defective secretion of it. The inadequacy of the supposition is clearly shown by cases related above (pp. 227 and 234), in which, from long-continued closure of the common duct, the cells of the liver were at the time of death completely destroyed, so that the secretion of bile must have been completely stopped, and yet there was no appreciable disorder of the brain almost to the last days of life.

There is reason to believe that the delirium and coma, which sometimes occur in these terrible cases after the jaundice has lasted for weeks without presenting any alarming symptoms, depend, not merely on arrest of the secretion of bile, or on the presence of the principles of the bile in the blood, but on some peculiarly noxious matter which is evolved, *in consequence of decomposition*, in the lobular substance of the liver. (See p. 278.)

Jaundice, as already remarked, is rather a symptom of disease than a disease of itself, and may arise from various causes, which it is very important that we should be acquainted with; since a knowledge of the cause, or of the circumstances under which the jaundice arose in any particular case, often gives us an insight into its real nature which we could scarcely obtain from considering the symptoms merely.

The most obvious cause of jaundice, and which was, therefore, the earliest assigned—which was, indeed, at one time assigned almost to the exclusion of all others—is some obstruction in the gall-ducts, preventing the flow of bile into the intestine. This obstruction may arise in various ways.

It may be caused by a gall-stone passing out of the gall-bladder and becoming impacted in the common duct. The jaundice that occurs during the passage of gall-stones is caused in this way. It is generally of short duration, soon going off when the obstructing stone has passed into the intestine. But it now and then happens that a gall-stone becomes permanently fixed in the common duct, or leads to permanent closure of the duct by inflammation, and, of course, the resulting jaundice is permanent.

Another cause of jaundice from obstructed gall-ducts, is cancerous disease of the liver or of the pancreas. In such cases the obstruction is permanent, and the jaundice continues till the death of the patient.

Jaundice, from closure of the ducts, now and then occurs in that form of adhesive inflammation of the liver brought on by spirit-drinking, which sets in with severe inflammatory symptoms, and which leads to adhesive inflammation of the capsule of the liver, and to the effusion of much lymph in the portal canals. In such cases the jaundice generally goes off when the inflammatory symptoms subside; but sometimes the common duct becomes permanently closed or narrowed by the contraction of lymph effused on its outer surface, and the jaundice is permanent.

Jaundice from obstruction of the gall-ducts may also be caused by inflammation originating in the ducts, which, from their small size, must be readily closed by viscid mucus, or by inflammatory swelling of their lining membrane. It is probable that this is a frequent cause of jaundice; but at present jaundice so produced cannot be surely distinguished from that which results from suppressed secretion.

The flow of bile may be stopped, and jaundice be caused, by simple enlargement of one of the lymphatic glands that are contiguous to the common duct.

Jaundice occasionally arises from constipation, in which case it is probably caused by the loaded intestine pressing on the common duct, and thus impeding the flow of the bile. It soon disappears when the cause is removed.

Jaundice, brought about perhaps in the same way, occasionally occurs during pregnancy. It goes off after childbirth, and may sometimes be removed before by efficient purgatives.

Spasm of the gall-ducts has also been assigned as a cause of jaundice, and was at one time advanced to explain all cases of it in which no mechanical impediment to the flow of bile was found after death; just as spasm of the intestines was supposed to be the cause of colic, and spasm of the bronchi the cause of difficulty of breathing, in all cases in which no other ready explanation of these symptoms could be found. Spasm of the gall-ducts is, however, something more than a mere hypothesis. The common gall-duct, like the intestines, is, when empty, commonly found contracted after death, by the rigor mortis; and its contractibility, as well as that of the efferent ducts of other glands, has been further proved by direct experiment. Müller states that by irritating mechanically, or by galvanism, the *ductus choledochus* of a bird just dead, he has frequently produced a very strong contraction of it, which continued some minutes; after which the duct resumed its previous state.[1] We must, then, admit the muscularity of the gall-ducts, and the consequent possibility of their being contracted by spasm; but it is difficult to conceive the spasm to be lasting enough to cause jaundice. If jaundice be produced by mere spasm of the gall-ducts, it must surely be very slight and transient.

But, although a mechanical impediment to the flow of bile into the intestine is sometimes the cause of jaundice, it is much less frequently so than was formerly imagined. In a large proportion, perhaps in the greater number of cases in young persons, jaundice results primarily, and solely, from the secretion of bile being suppressed or defective.

The secretion of bile may be suppressed, or be rendered inadequate, by various conditions:—

1st. It may be rendered inadequate by most of the structural changes that have been described in the foregoing pages. Thus,

[1] Kölliker has lately, by means of an electro-magnetic apparatus, excited contraction in the veins of an amputated leg; and has discovered a low form of muscle, consisting of a thin layer of peculiar cells, which he designates "muscular," or "contractile fibre-cells" in the bloodvessels, and in many other contractile tissues in which no muscular fibres had been previously recognized. (See *Kölliker and Siebold's Zeitschrift*, 1849; or, Todd's *Cyclopædia of Anatomy and Physiology*, art. "Vein.")

in high degrees of congestion, however produced, when the capillary vessels of the liver are gorged and the blood flows tardily through them, the secretion and the elimination of bile are impeded, and a sallowness, which sometimes passes into jaundice, results.

Again, in suppurative inflammation of the liver, the inflamed portion ceases to perform its office, and, if this portion be large, the action of the entire liver is so deranged that jaundice results.

In adhesive inflammation of the liver brought on by spirit-drinking, when severe inflammatory symptoms exist, there is frequently jaundice; but, as before remarked, the jaundice here seems to result from the gall-ducts being closed by the pressure of the lymph effused in the areolar tissue about them. This form of inflammation seems not to involve, *primarily*, the lobular substance of the liver, so much as the areolar tissue in the portal canals and the small twigs of the portal vein. In the end, however, by obliterating branches or small twigs of the portal vein, it leads to atrophy of the secreting substance of the liver, and in this way also may cause jaundice. But the jaundice in the advanced stages of hob-nailed or granular liver, unless the hepatic or the common duct be at the same time closed or narrowed, is always very slight, —in most cases a sallowness, rather than decided jaundice.

But jaundice occurs from other changes in the secreting substance of the liver, which are not attended by the effusions characteristic of inflammation. It has been remarked by Abercrombie and by Andral, that jaundice now and then comes on in the course of pneumonia of the lower lobe of the right lung. I have witnessed this occurrence two or three times. The jaundice seems to depend on a change which the secreting substance of the liver has undergone, and which is different at least from ordinary inflammation. The substance of the liver near the diaphragm is paler and softer than it should be, and the capsule can be readily stripped off, but no pus or lymph is seen there.

2d. The secretion of the liver may be suppressed, so as to cause jaundice, by mental shock, by long-continued anxiety or grief, and, I believe, by exhausting dissipation.

The jaundice so produced is often attended by no alarming symptoms; but, now and then, after it had existed for some time without any symptoms indicative of especial danger, disorder of the brain, which proves rapidly fatal, comes on. After death in such cases, portions of the liver are sometimes found completely disorganized. It would seem that some virulent poison is generated in the liver, which deranges and then paralyzes the brain, and, after death, causes softening and disorganization of the liver itself.

It is not on the secretions of the liver only that mental emotions have such influence.

The passions of fear and anger may check the secretion of the gastric juice, and thus suspend or retard the process of digestion. The secretion of milk may be suppressed by fright; and not only may the secretion of milk be checked, but its *quality* even may be changed by anxiety or grief.[1]

3d. The secreting function of the liver may be so suspended as to cause jaundice, by various poisons in the blood.

Jaundice is sometimes produced by the salts of copper, by opium, by mercury, by the poison of serpents; and it often occurs, obviously from the poisoned state of the blood, in the course of fevers, especially the virulent fevers of tropical climates.

It not unfrequently occurs in hard-working medical students, most probably from the noxious effluvia to which they are often exposed when in a state of depression from work; and, now and then, as we have seen, it occurs, with peculiar characters, in several members of a family, or in several persons living together, in quick succession—where it can only be attributed to some peculiar poison.

Certain forms of gastric disorder, attended by an inordinate secretion of acid in the stomach, may likewise check the secretion of bile, and cause, after some days, a slight degree of jaundice.

Jaundice occurs in various other circumstances, as the result either of arrest of secretion, or of inflammation and consequent closure of the gall-ducts. I have met with several instances in which it occurred, with symptoms of much depression, in young persons affected with severe primary syphilis. In two of these instances it occurred before mercury had been taken, and before there were any of the recognized *constitutional* effects of the syphilitic poison. It seems probable, therefore, that the jaundice in such cases results from suppressed secretion, and is caused by the mental distress which severe syphilis often occasions.

[1] Instances in proof of this are cited in Todd's Cyclopædia of Anatomy and Physiology, art. "Secretion."

Dr. Graves has remarked that jaundice followed by urticaria now and then occurs during the course of arthritis. He says: "A person laboring under inflammation of the joints gets an attack of hepatitis, accompanied by jaundice, and this is followed by urticaria. I have observed this sequence of disease in eight or nine cases. The first was in a gentleman residing in Lower Mount Street, whom I attended with Dr. Cheyne. This gentleman, in consequence of exposure to cold, was attacked with arthritic inflammation and fever. After he had been ten days ill, he became suddenly jaundiced, and in a day or two afterwards a copious eruption of urticaria appeared over his body and limbs. Exactly the same train of phenomena, and in a similar order of succession, were observed in a man treated in the Meath Hospital, in 1832. A short time before this, I had been attending a medical friend in Baggot Street, who had been affected in the same way; and I mentioned to the class, as soon as I perceived the man was jaundiced, that he would most probably get urticaria. I made a similar prediction in a case which occurred recently in our wards, and it was verified by the event. Now, this is not a mere fortuitous occurrence; the various symptoms must be connected in the relation of cause and effect."—*Clinical Medicine*, p. 564.

Since, then, jaundice may arise from such various causes, and be a symptom in diseases so different, it is clear that we cannot foretell its issue in any given case, or have well-grounded confidence in our treatment, unless we can pass from the jaundice to the particular disease of the liver on which it depends, or to the particular cause by which it is produced.

In some cases there is little difficulty in doing this. We can generally, for instance, interpret the slight shade of jaundice that occurs in the granular or hob-nailed liver. We are sufficiently informed of the nature of the disease by the previous habits of the patient, and by the symptoms of impeded circulation through the liver that are almost always present in these cases when there is jaundice. Frequently, too, we can interpret the jaundice that occurs during the passage of a gall-stone, or in the course of cancer of the liver, by the presence of other symptoms indicative of those diseases.

When, again, there has been, for a considerable time, *deep* jaundice, without any bilious tinge in the matters discharged from the bowels, and without alarming head-symptoms, we may be sure that the common or the hepatic duct is closed in some way or other, and that the jaundice results from mechanical impediment to the flow of bile into the intestine.

But in many cases, with our present knowledge, it seems impossible to trace the jaundice to its source, and especially to tell whether it depends on inflammation of the gall-ducts, or on suppressed secretion of bile.

In a former chapter (p. 250), the details of several cases were given, in which jaundice from suppressed secretion proved fatal, and in which the lobular substance in some parts of the liver was found to be completely disorganized, or very much softened. These cases were placed together with the view of exhibiting the characters of this obscure disease, which is far more important than one would be led to suppose from the fatal cases merely, which are few. It is clear from the instances in which jaundice occurred in several members of a family in succession (p. 290), that jaundice of this kind does not always prove fatal; and that occasionally it is attended by no alarming symptoms. There is reason to believe that in a considerable proportion of the cases of jaundice that occur in young persons, the jaundice arises from suppressed or defective secretion.

It appears, from the cases before related, that, in mild forms of the disease, the patient's illness begins with general disorder; with languor or listlessness, vague pains in the belly, and sometimes with vomiting, but without much fever. In a day or two, jaundice comes on, but the flow of bile into the duodenum is not always *completely* stopped; the matters brought up by vomiting, or passed by stool, are still bilious. The jaundice may continue some time with no more alarming symptoms, and may then go off gradually, and the patient gradually recover. But now and then, after it has continued in this state from a few days to several weeks, delirium comes on, and the patient soon dies in a state of coma.

In more acute forms of the disease, the illness begins with symptoms more like those of remittent fever: with fever, vomiting, and thirst, and furred tongue, and headache, and restlessness. In a day or two, jaundice comes on, soon followed by drowsiness or active delirium, which, as in the former class of cases, speedily passes into coma.

Two circumstances that may serve to distinguish this variety of jaundice are: 1st, that the liver is not enlarged, generally, indeed, in the cases that prove fatal, it is found to be much smaller than natural; and, 2d, that the flow of bile into the duodenum is seldom completely stopped; the discharges from the stomach and bowels are still tinged with bile.

The treatment of jaundice must, of course, be guided chiefly by reference to the particuluar condition of the liver on which the jaundice is supposed to depend.

Where there is reason to believe, from tenderness in the region of the liver, or fulness in the right hypochondrium, and other circumstances, that the jaundice results from inflammation in the substance of the liver, or in the excreting ducts, leeches or cupping, fomentations, saline purgatives, and diet, are the remedies that should first be employed. In adhesive inflammation of the liver, and in inflammation of the gall-ducts, local bleeding always produces great relief. When the activity of the inflammation has been somewhat subdued by these means, recourse may be had to mercury, in order to promote the absorption of effused lymph, or to correct the acrid quality of the bile, which seems frequently to cause, and to keep up, inflammation of the ducts.

In other cases, where jaundice occurs without previous organic disease, and, there is reason to believe, from suppressed secretion merely—where the patient feels languid and oppressed, and has occasional vomiting, and the pupils are dilated, while there is no fulness, and not much tenderness, in the region of the liver, and the flow of bile into the intestine is not quite stopped, the propriety of bleeding, or of giving mercury, is very doubtful. From what we yet know of the pathology of such cases, these measures seem much more likely to do harm than to do good. It is safer to be content with diaphoretics and with alkaline saline purgatives, than to use, as it were, in the dark, and at hazard, our more powerful remedies.

If the patient should become very drowsy, and especially if sluggishness of the pupil and other symptoms should betoken approaching coma, strong purgatives should be given so as to cause copious discharges, and at the same time an attempt should be made to rouse the brain by blisters to the scalp and by other excitants. Cases have been before related (p. 281) in which recovery took place under these measures, even after the patient had fallen into a state of almost complete coma. The tendency of free purging to remove the coma, or lessen the stupor, when this exists, leaves little doubt that it tends also to prevent it, and suggests the propriety of the systematic and active use of saline purgatives in this variety of jaundice.

Mild saline purgatives, as the Seidlitz, Pullna, or Cheltenham waters, continued for some time, seem often of great service during the decline of jaundice, and when the time for more active measures is past.

In the jaundice that results from long-continued closure of the common duct, it is clear that mercury and all lowering remedies must generally do harm. When the closure of the duct is caused by inflammatory thickening about it, or by simple enlargement of one of the contiguous lymphatic glands, benefit may, indeed, result from a mild course of bichloride of mercury, or blue pill; but when, as is oftener the case, the closure is caused by a gall-stone, or by malignant disease, there is little more to be done than to regulate the diet; to remedy, as far as possible, the disorders of digestion; to prevent the accumulation of noxious matters in the bowels by an aloetic pill, or other warm purgative; to keep up the action of the skin by an occasional warm bath; and to take care to do nothing likely to disorder the action of the kidney, through which the bile finds its way out of the system.

Itching of the skin, which is most common in this kind of jaundice, may be somewhat relieved by the use of the flesh-brush, and by warm baths.

APPENDIX.

The liver-fluke—Its effects on sheep and other graminivorous animals. Flukes found in the gall-ducts, in the duodenum, and in branches of the portal vein, in man.

THE gall-bladder and gall-ducts of most of our graminivorous animals, and especially of the sheep, are frequently infested by two kinds of parasites—the *Distoma Hepaticum* and the *Distoma Lanceolatum*—which are often found together, and are commonly confounded under the term *liver-fluke*. They are the cause of the distemper in sheep, which is known as the *rot*, and which is so justly dreaded by the farmer.

The Distoma *hepaticum* is, in shape, very like a small sole or flounder, and, when full grown, is, in the sheep, from three-quarters of an inch to an inch and a half in length, and from one-third to half an inch wide, at the widest part. It has two suckers, hence the name, *Distoma*. One of these is at the extremity of the head (*a*), Fig. 18, and is a little turned downwards; the other (*b*), which is the larger of the two, is on the under surface of the body, at the base of the neck. The first leads to the alimentary canal, and is pierced by the mouth; the hinder one is imperforate, and is a mere organ of adhesion.[1]

Fig. 18.

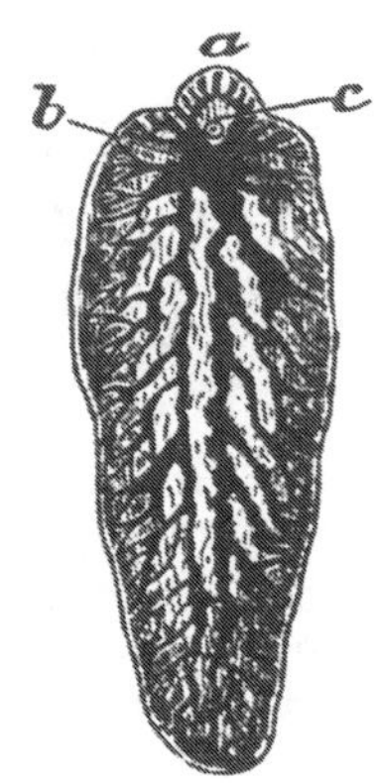

Distoma hepaticum, from a sheep. Natural size.

Between the suckers is a small depression (*c*), in which are the two genital pores.

The alimentary canal is, for a very short distance from the first sucker, a single tube, and then divides into two, which diverge a little to embrace

[1] See Owen's Lectures on the Comparative Anatomy of the Invertebrate Animals, from which the account of the anatomy of the liver-fluke in the text is chiefly taken.

the genital pores and the hinder sucker, and then run parallel to each other along the middle of the body to near the tail, where their ends are closed. These parallel tubes send off many branched tubes from their outer sides, which extend nearly to the margins of the body. The ends of all these tubes are closed or blind.

The organs of both sexes are in the same individual. The male organs are situated between the alimentary tubes. Convoluted seminal tubes, which may be recognized by their opaque white color, occupy a great extent of the middle part of the body, and terminate by two trunks in a common canal, which ends at the base of the penis. The penis, when flaccid, is spiral, and not unfrequently may be seen projecting from the anterior genital pore. The ovaria occupy the whole margin of the body for a line in breadth. They consist of minute branched tubes in which the ova are developed. The oviducts terminate in a single large canal which opens by a distinct pore, immediately behind the male bursa, after making many convolutions between this and the hinder sucker.

Fig. 19.

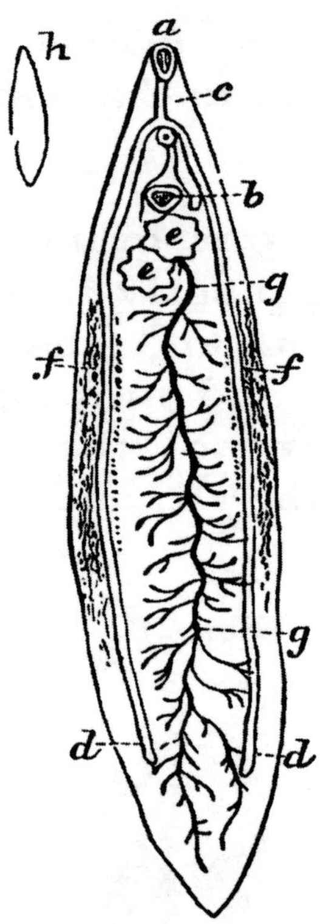

Distoma lanceolatum, magnified. *a*, *b*, the suckers; *c*, *d*, *d*, the alimentary canal; *e*, *e*, male organs; *f*, *f*, ovaria; *g*, *g*, the ramified uterine tube. *h*, outline of D. lanceolatum, of natural size. (*Owen.*)

The body is soft, almost of gelatinous consistence, and semitransparent; and of a whitish color, variegated near the margins by the yellow ova, and within by the double ramified alimentary canal, which is greenish or brown from containing the coloring matter of bile.

The Distoma *lanceolatum*, which was at one time regarded as the young of the Distoma *hepaticum*, is much smaller, being commonly about a quarter of an inch in length, very seldom half an inch. It also differs in shape from the Distoma hepaticum. The outline of the body, instead of being rounded at each end, as in the latter, has each end *lancet-shaped;* the end terminated by the head being much the narrower or more pointed of the two. The sucking cups are placed as in D. hepaticum, but are larger.

There are also differences in the internal structure of the two varieties.

In the D. lanceolatum, the alimentary canal does not ramify as in D. hepaticum. It is a single tube to the genital pore, which is here midway between the suckers, and then divides into two, which go along near the margins of the body, without sending off any branches, almost to the tail, where their ends are closed. The male organs are contained in the anterior part of the space between the alimentary tubes. The ovaria are situated at the margins of the middle third of the body, outside the alimentary tubes. The oviducts run transversely and terminate in a common uterine tube, which is very long and tortuous, occupying all the hinder part of the space between the two alimentary tubes.

In sheep, these parasites are often found in great numbers. Many hundreds may sometimes be counted in a single liver. They produce remarkable changes in the gall-ducts they inhabit, and through them in the adjacent parts of the liver. The gall-ducts infested by them become dilated, and their coats much thickened. In cutting across the liver, after the rot has lasted for some time, many branches of the hepatic ducts are seen of the size of a large quill, with thick coats having much the look of soaked leather. These ducts are stuffed with flukes, and often with a dirty greenish matter, the excrement and ova of the flukes, enveloped in mucus. The ova are egg-shaped bodies, all nearly of the same size—$\frac{1}{200}$ of an inch long, and about $\frac{1}{330}$ of an inch broad. Under the microscope, they are yellow by transmitted light, have a distinct single outline, and appear solid and filled with very fine granular matter.

At first, only the larger branches of the hepatic duct are changed in the way described. The smaller branches, which are not yet reached by the flukes, are healthy. It often happens, too, that while some of the larger ducts are so changed, others contain no flukes and are quite healthy. After a time, the infested gall-ducts are still more changed. Those near the under surface of the liver often form white tubes, the largest the size of the thumb, or larger, which project above the surface, and in some parts are visible, without dissection, quite to the edge of the liver. On the convex surface of the liver, the dilated tubes, being deeper seated, are not visible except in a spot, here and there, near the edge. The coats of these white prominent gall-ducts are much thickened, and have the look and almost the toughness of cartilage. On tracing them from trunk to branch, we sometimes find one closed, or blind, at the further end, from obliteration of the smaller branches which went to form it. These blind tubes are filled with mucus and the remains of flukes, which die when deprived of the bile on which they subsist. It now and then happens, too, that a portion of a dilated duct becomes separated from the rest, so as to form a cyst, which is filled with mucus.

Those parts of the liver in which the ducts are much dilated are more or less atrophied, from pressure and from obliteration of some of the small ducts, and are *pale* and shrunken, as compared with other parts of the same liver in which the ducts are less diseased. Occasionally, a thin false membrane is found on the convex surface of the most diseased portion of the liver, and uniting this by threads to the contiguous organs.

Later still, the inner surface of the ducts becomes incrusted with chalky matter (carbonate of lime), which, in the end, transforms them into bony tubes. Now and then there is found a small cyst filled with chalky matter and completely isolated from the tubes; the remains, perhaps, of what was at one time a mucous cyst.

The effects which these parasites have on the health of the sheep are also very striking. At first the sheep has a remarkable aptitude to grow fat, and, if the accumulation of fat only be regarded, may be prepared for the butcher perhaps weeks sooner than a sheep perfectly sound. This circumstance has even been turned to profit. Sheep nearly ready for slaughter have been purposely placed in a pasture that gives the rot, that they might fatten more quickly. But, unfortunately, while they grow fat, their muscles waste, and, from the first, they are weak and languid. They soon become anemic, and now and then slightly sallow. They are recognized by butchers as having the rot, chiefly by an unusual whiteness of the eye, which does not show the red vessels seen in the eye of a healthy sheep. The caruncle, too, at the corner of the eye, is pale, and often slightly yellow; and the skin, when the wool is parted, does not exhibit the ruddy hue of health, but is pale and sometimes sallow. There is also a tendency to œdema, which is first conspicuous in dropsical swelling of the legs just above the hocks; but before this appears the skin is looser than in a healthy sheep—it is more readily stripped off by the butcher.[1]

[1] These symptoms, from being so obvious, were early noticed. They are pointed out very distinctly in the famous Booke of Husbandrye, published more than three centuries ago (the Booke of Husbandrye, by Sir Anthony Fitzherbert, 1532), when from the general want of draining, the rot must have been more destructive in this country than now. "Take both your handes, and turn up the lid of his eye, and if it be ruddye and have red stringes in the white of the eye, then he is sound, and if the eye be white like tallowe and the stringes dark coloured, then he is rotten."

"And also take the shepe upon the wol on the side, and if the skin be of a ruddey colour and dry, then he is sound, and if it be pale-colored and watery, then he is rotten." (*Library of Useful Knowledge.* Treatise on the Sheep, p. 446.)

As the disease goes on, the fat disappears, and the animal loses flesh rapidly, and grows extremely feeble. The appetite fails and the bowels are irregular—sometimes costive, at other times much purged. The œdema increases, the skin in consequence becomes loose and flabby, and gives out a peculiar crackling sound when pressed, and the belly also gets dropsical. The wool now comes off at the slightest pull, the skin often becomes spotted with yellow or black (probably from ecchymosis), and the animal dies a mere skeleton—generally from two to six months from the commencement of the disease. The rot, however, is not inevitably fatal. Sheep frequently recover, if early removed to a healthy pasture.

It will at once be seen that the chief symptoms of the disease and its fatal issue depend, not so much on the changes of structure in the liver, striking as these are, as on an unhealthy state of the blood. The disease may prove fatal when part only of the liver is involved, and when more than enough is left for all the purposes of secretion. The sallowness of the *caruncula lachrymalis* and of the skin, occasionally noticed, is always slight, never amounting to jaundice, and depends probably more on anemia than on bile. The blood becomes impoverished in this disease just as it does from granular degeneration of the kidney, in man. The paleness of the conjunctiva and of the skin, that may be noticed even at an early period, show diminution in the proportion of globules in the blood. M. Andral has ascertained that when the disease has gone on to dropsy, the proportion of albumen is likewise much diminished, and he considers this circumstance to be a strong argument in favor of the opinion he has advanced, that the dropsy from granular kidney, and in this disease as well, is caused immediately by loss of the albumen of the blood. In sheep infested with flukes, the kidneys are pale like the other tissues, but not otherwise altered in structure; and the urine does not contain albumen. The yellow and black spots on the skin often noticed in the advanced stage of the disease, if they result from hemorrhage, as they probably do, would favor the inference that at this date, the proportion of fibrin in the blood is also diminished. The blood becomes at length so drained of all its organic constituents—globules, albumen, fibrin—that it is no longer fit to nourish the body and maintain life. The death of the animal is hastened by diarrhœa, which recurs frequently, especially towards the close of the malady, occasioned probably by irritating matters passing into the intestines from the gall-ducts.

No one, I believe, has inquired how flukes in the liver work this change in the blood. It cannot be by merely consuming the bile, unless this is much more necessary for digestion in sheep than in man; and flukes have no organs which can enable them to penetrate a sound surface, and thus to draw blood or the serum of blood, from it.[1] Do they not, by the irritation caused by their adhesion or presence, excite a serous discharge from the lining membrane of the gall-ducts, which, by its amount, greatly impoverishes the blood?

I have described thus fully the characters of this disease in sheep, not only on account of the intrinsic interest which it must have for the pathologist, but also on account of its great national importance—which alone is a sufficient reason why it should be investigated by medical men, who are the persons best qualified by previous education for such a task, and who are many of them placed in circumstances very favorable for it. Some notion of the importance of this disease may be formed from the statement made by a high authority on the diseases of cattle, that more than a million sheep and lambs die of it annually in this country.[2] In some seasons, this number, vast as it is, is much exceeded. In the winter of 1830–31, it was far more than doubled; and in some of the midland, eastern, and southern counties, where the pestilence was most rife, the existing race of sheep was almost entirely swept off.

Besides the sheep that actually die of the disease, vast numbers of those which are slaughtered are infected with it, and their flesh, we may suppose, is less wholesome and nutritious in consequence. In the spring of the present year (1844) a considerable portion of the sheep that were brought to the London market were infested with flukes. I had no difficulty in getting from the butchers any number of diseased livers to examine.

But the disease is not confined to England. It prevails in other countries of Europe, as far north as Norway, and in the most

[1] The anterior sucker, or mouth of the fluke, is a simple pore, unprovided with teeth or with a proper suctorial margin. The only real sucker is the posterior one, and this would seem to be solely for the purpose of adhesion.

[2] Library of Useful Knowledge. Treatise on the Sheep, p. 445.

southern provinces of Spain. It occasionally prevails likewise in North America; and in Van Dieman's Land and Australia it has been at times quite as destructive as in England.

Flukes in sheep have, I believe, been found nowhere but in the liver, or duodenum. They usually inhabit the gall-ducts, where, as we have seen, they produce countless numbers of ova, or spawn, most of which must pass into the intestine, and be dropped by the sheep on the pastures. It is stated that from November to April, minute oval particles, which are doubtless these same ova, may occasionally be seen in swarms in the droppings of the infected sheep. They probably, under favorable circumstances, retain their vitality for a long period. The rot is most probably propagated by the sheep swallowing the produce of the ova thus dropped on the pastures;[1] and by the young flukes passing instinctively from the duodenum into the gall-bladder and gall-ducts. (*Owen.*)

But although the disease is so far propagated by infection, other conditions, of soil and season, are necessary for its spread.

The rot is almost confined to marshy or wet grounds, and is unusually destructive after a wet summer or autumn, or during a wet winter. It does not spread in dry seasons, or during hard frosts, and never shows itself on dry sandy soils, except after long rains. Autumn and winter are the seasons in which it prevails most. Meadows which are very destructive in autumn and winter, may often be safely pastured in spring. Another circumstance of practical importance, and which also seems to be well established, is, that, season and soil alike, the disease spreads much more in lands that are over-pastured. This has been attributable, in part, to the ground being then broken by numberless footmarks, which are so many cups in which the water collects.

It is generally believed, too, that at night, or while the dew is on the grass, the infection spreads much more than by day; and it has been in consequence laid down as a precept, that when a pasture is

[1] Animals of the class *Trematoda*, to which flukes belong, afford an illustration of what has been lately termed the "alternation of generations." In their larva state, before they pass into the bodies of the animals they infest, they are minute, almost microscopic creatures, somewhat resembling tadpoles in their outward form, which move freely about in water, and have been known to naturalists under the generic name of *Cercaria*. (See *On the Alternation of Generations; or, the Propagation and Development of Animals through Alternate Generations*. By J. J. S. Steenstrup. Translated from the German, by George Busk. Printed for the Ray Society, 1845.)

suspected to be rotting, the sheep should be folded early in the evening, and not be released till the dew is partly evaporated.

In an infected pasture, a whole flock of sheep may be tainted in a very short time. Of this some very striking instances have been recorded, in a manner so circumstantial, that, considering their antecedent probability, there seems no reason to doubt their reality. The two following will perhaps suffice:—

"A farmer in the neighborhood of Wragby, in Lincolnshire, took twenty sheep to the fair, leaving six behind him in the pasture on which they had been summered. The score sent to the fair, not being sold, were driven back, and put in the same field in which the six had been left. In the course of the winter every one of them died of the rot, but the six that had been left behind all lived and did well. There could be no mistake with respect to this fact, as the sheep sent to the fair had a different mark from that of the six that were left at home. The loss of these twenty sheep can only be accounted for on the supposition that they had travelled over some common, or other rotting ground, and there became infected."

The second instance is still more conclusive:—

"A sheep, belonging to a lot of twenty, being lamed in consequence of a broken leg in getting out of Burgh fair, in Lincolnshire, the nineteen were suffered to range on a common at the end of the town until a cart could be procured to carry the maimed sheep home. The nineteen all died rotten, while the sheep with the lame leg continued perfectly free from the disease."[1]

It follows at once from these observations that the most effectual way to prevent the rot is to make the pastures dry by thorough draining. In order that the disease may spread, it seems necessary that the soil should be wet or marshy, or at least that there should be stagnant water on it. It is perhaps enough that there be stagnant ditches about a field, though the field itself be dry. Sheep, more than any other of our domestic animals, require a dry soil.

Oxen are likewise infested with flukes, but in much less degree. They are not *rotted* by them, like sheep, and will thrive on pastures destructive to sheep. I have learned from a farmer in Devonshire, that in some rich meadows on the banks of the Taw, where the beautiful North-Devon cattle are bred and thrive, sheep can never be kept for any length of time. They almost invariably die of the rot in less than twelve months from their being brought there.

[1] Lib. of Useful Knowledge. Sheep, p. 453. Quoted from Parkinson on Live Stock, vol. i. p. 421.

The meadows, though drained enough to produce rich grass, are low, and divided by ditches in which the water is almost stagnant.

Various other precepts for the prevention of the rot may be drawn from the observations that have been mentioned, but which it would be out of place to dwell on here. They are, most of them, obvious enough, and are well expressed in works on this and similar subjects,[1] and are, besides, pretty generally known and acted upon by prudent farmers. The great point to inculcate is the importance of thorough draining. More ills of man and beast than we yet suspect are probably owing to the want of it; and it is fortunate for the future generations of both in this country, that farmers are now becoming sensible of the remarkable effect of thorough draining in increasing the fertility of land, and are thus led to undertake it by the only motive that is generally efficient—the expectation of a profitable return.

When sheep are once infected, there is little hope for them unless they be speedily removed to a healthy pasture. When this is done, many may still die, for they carry with them the parasites, which, once in their appointed abode, will perhaps continue to find there all that they require for their nourishment and growth; but many of the sheep will recover.

The medicine, whose efficacy is best established in this disease, is common salt, of which as much should be given as the sheep will eat. It has been long known that sheep hardly ever become rotten in salt marshes, except in years when the disease is extraordinarily rife; and that they usually recover when placed in such pastures, if they be only slightly tainted. Of late years, many agriculturists have given strong testimony in favor of the efficacy of salt sprinkled on the animal's food, or given to it forcibly, not only in preventing the rot, but in curing it when not far advanced. (*Op. cit.*, p. 459.)

It would seem that the salt not only prevents the further multiplication of the flukes, but that it destroys those that already exist in the liver of the animal.

[1] I would especially refer the reader who is desirous of more information on this subject to the very elaborate and interesting treatise on the sheep to which I have already referred.

Condiments of various kinds seem to have similar efficacy. Gentian and ginger are those most in repute. They have been recommended to be given in powder, in conjunction with salt. It is probable that various aromatic herbs have similar virtue, and that good might result from planting in lands that give the rot some such herb, of a kind that will grow there and that sheep will eat. In high grounds, where sheep feed on dry aromatic herbs, the rot never occurs.

Other graminivorous animals are liable, like sheep, to be infested with flukes. Hares and rabbits that feed on the same pastures, are *rotted* like sheep. They become thin and pot-bellied, and lose their flax, and at length die much wasted. Oxen also are infested by them, but much less than sheep, and they do not suffer in health in the same degree. Flukes have also been found in the liver of the deer, and of the pig—and, in a few instances, in man; but not in the Mammalia that are exclusively carnivorous.

In man, liver-flukes are so rare, and when present are generally so few in number, that they must be considered a curiosity rather than a cause of disease.

Bucholz found a considerable number of flukes in the gall-bladder of a prisoner who died of putrid fever. Rudolphi, who got possession of some of them, states that they were precisely like the Distoma *lanceolatum* of the sheep. Rudolphi had many other specimens, also of Distoma lanceolatum, that had been passed by a girl after having taken a dose of *Chabert's* empyreumatic oil. He states that he could not find an authentic instance of a specimen of Distoma *hepaticum* having been found in the human liver.

Brera found some flukes in the gall-ducts of a man who died of scurvy complicated with dropsy, which were larger than those found by Bucholz, and which were considered to be of the variety D. hepaticum.

A few years ago, a single fluke was discovered by my colleague, Mr. Partridge, in the gall-bladder of a person who died in the Middlesex Hospital. Mr. Partridge was present at the examination of the body, and was struck with the appearance of the gall-bladder, which, instead of being stained by bile, as is usual, was perfectly white. He took the gall-bladder away, to make of it a preparation to show the natural structure, and, on laying it open, discovered the fluke. He presented the fluke to Professor Owen, who considered it to differ in no respect from the Distoma hepaticum of the sheep. The gall-bladder and cystic duct, which were perfectly healthy, are preserved in the museum of King's College.

In the winter of 1843, fourteen flukes were found by Mr. Busk in the *duodenum* of a Lascar, who died in the Seamen's Hospital. There were none in the gall-bladder or gall-ducts. These flukes were much thicker and larger than those of the sheep, being from an inch and a half to near three inches in length. They resembled the Distoma hepaticum in shape, but were like the Distoma lanceolatum in structure; the double alimentary canal, as in the latter variety, being not branched, and the entire space between it towards the latter part of the body being occupied by a branched uterine tube. Two of these flukes, which were given me by Mr. Busk, are in the museum of King's College (Prep. 346), and from one of them, which is injected with size and vermilion, the annexed wood-cut (Fig. 20) was made.

Fig. 20.

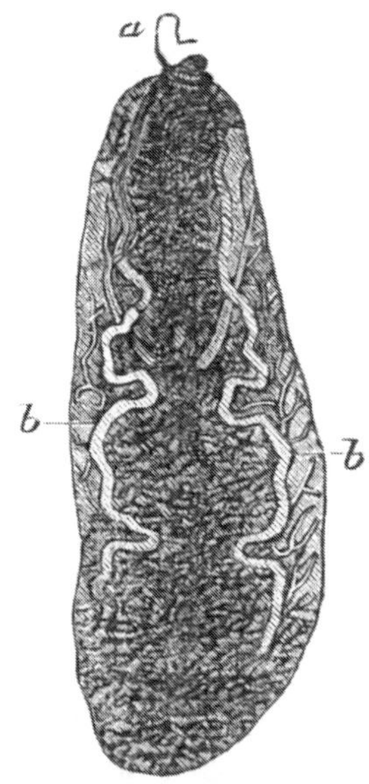

Fluke, from the duodenum of a man, (natural size,) injected. *a*, ligature round the neck; *b*, alimentary tube.

Some flukes were also found by Brera in the human duodenum; where they doubtless subsist, as in the liver, on the bile.

Rudolphi mentions, merely to deny the assertion, that some authors, to whom he gives no reference, have stated that flukes occasionally inhabit also the branches of the portal vein. An observation, however, made some years ago by M. Duval, a physician at Rennes, confirms these statements. In the beginning of April, 1830, M. Duval, while engaged on the veins, in a course of anatomy, had, to illustrate his lectures, the body of a man, about forty-nine years of age, who died in an hospital at Rennes. While demonstrating the portal vein, at lecture, M. Duval discovered that there was a foreign body in its trunk, and, on carefully laying the vein open, he found that this was a Distoma hepaticum, of large dimensions, in the midst of a little fluid blood. Subsequently, in tracing the hepatic divisions of the vein, he found four or five others

32

of the same kind. There were none in the mesenteric branches that go to form the trunk of the portal vein. The branches of the vein that contained the flukes presented no erosion, nor any marks of inflammation, and had quite their natural appearance. The liver elsewhere was sound, and, excepting the flukes, nothing particular was remarked in the body. The man was brought into the medical wards of the hospital on the 24th of March, and died on the 28th. No particulars of his case are given. The flukes are preserved in the museum at Rennes. In 1842, when they had been twelve years in spirit, they were found to be from eleven to fourteen lines in length, and from four to five lines wide.

From M. Duval's account, which is very detailed, there seems to be little doubt that these parasites were really specimens of Distoma hepaticum. M. Duval states that he found them to accord with plates of the D. hepaticum in the *Encyclopédie*; and that he subsequently showed them to M. Dujardin, a high authority, he says, in such matters, who pronounced them to be really of this species.[1]

In this instance, the flukes obtained, immediately from the portal blood, the means of subsistence, which they generally draw from the bile. It is remarkable, considering the great changes that are produced by flukes in the texture of the gall-ducts in sheep, that there were here no marks of disease in the coats of the veins which the flukes infested. Is it (as the symptoms of the disease which they occasion in sheep render probable) that flukes require for their support some of the principles of the blood as well as bile, and that in the gall-ducts they obtain these principles by causing a drain of serum from their coats? It is remarkable, too, that their excrement and spawn should not have set up disease in the substance of the liver, and thus have led to appreciable changes of texture. But perhaps the greatest puzzle is: how did the flukes get into the vein? We are led to infer that they grew up there, from there having been no erosion of the coats of the veins, nor any other marks of disease in them. Besides, there were no flukes in the gall-ducts, nor any signs of flukes having been there at some former time. But supposing that the flukes grew in the vein, how did their eggs, or larvæ, which are so much larger than blood-globules, get there?

[1] Gazette Médicale de Paris, 3 Decembre, 1842.

The supposition that the Distoma cause, in some way or other, a serous discharge from the gall-ducts they inhabit, accounts for their producing less effect on larger cattle than on sheep, hares, and rabbits. A loss of albumen that would exhaust these small animals would have little effect on an ox.

THE END.